Liver Biopsy Evaluation

Liver Biopsy Evaluation

Histologic Diagnosis and Clinical Correlations

Gary C. Kanel, MD

Professor of Clinical Pathology
University of Southern California
Associate Pathologist
Rancho Los Amigos National Rehabilitation Center
University of Southern California Liver Unit Laboratories
Downey, California

Jacob Korula, MD

Professor of Clinical Medicine
Division of Gastroenterology and Liver Diseases
University of Southern California
Los Angeles, California

W.B. SAUNDERS COMPANY

A Harcourt Health Sciences Company

Philadelphia London Toronto Montreal Sydney Tokyo

W.B. SAUNDERS COMPANY
A Harcourt Health Sciences Company

The Curtis Center
Independence Square West
Philadelphia, Pennsylvania 19106-3399

Library of Congress Cataloging-in-Publication Data

Kanel, Gary C.
    Liver biopsy evaluation/Gary C. Kanel, Jacob Korula.—1st ed.

        p. ; cm.
    Includes bibliographical references.

    ISBN 0-7216-7692-8

    1. Liver—Biopsy. 2. Liver—Histopathology. I. Korula, Jacob. II. Title.
    [DNLM: 1. Liver—pathology. 2. Biopsy. 3. Liver Diseases—pathology. WI 700 K153L 2000]

    RC847.5.B56 K36 2000

    616.3′62075—dc21   99-059400

Acquisitions Editor: Marc Strauss
Project Manager: Edna Dick
Senior Production Manager: Peter Faber
Illustration Specialist: Peg Shaw

LIVER BIOPSY EVALUATION:
Histologic Diagnosis and Clinical Correlations   ISBN 0–7216–7692–8

Printed in the United States of America.

Last digit is the print number: 9   8   7   6   5   4   3   2   1

The complexity of liver biopsy interpretation relates in part to the numerous histologic parameters that are encountered. Sometimes the clinical diagnosis is available before the review of the biopsy by the pathologist and the clinician, whereby specific histologic features are searched for. An example is a patient with a clinical diagnosis of primary biliary cirrhosis, in which identification of interlobular bile duct damage on biopsy is the key. This approach is not possible when little or no clinical or laboratory information is available, and unfortunately this situation is not uncommon. A history of a patient with "abnormal liver tests" gives no clue as to the diagnosis. Therefore, all histologic parameters must be examined, with differential diagnoses available for each obvious histologic finding. For instance, in a middle-aged woman with "abnormal liver tests," the presence of nonsuppurative destructive duct changes can lead the pathologist and the clinician into a workable differential diagnosis if a list of liver diseases having this histologic parameter is available for reference.

The purpose of this book is to enable the referring physician and the pathologist ample histopathologic diagnostic possibilities by reviewing the hepatic morphology and directing workup—including history, laboratory tests, and in some instances imaging—to allow a definitive diagnosis. The book is divided into five sections:

1. An **introduction,** dealing with an organized histologic approach in reviewing liver biopsies, and how this book in both table format and disease listing can best be used.

2. A chapter on **Tables** of morphology, presenting 35 specific histologic parameters that can be seen in liver biopsy material and the liver diseases that may exhibit those changes. Some of these tables are further subdivided into the frequency by which those changes are seen. In addition, numerous color and black and white photomicrographs are offered as examples.

3. An alphabetical listing of **liver diseases with pathology and pertinent clinical parameters** in column format. The basic histopathology of each disease is listed in the column to the left, and pertinent clinical and laboratory data are listed in the column to the right.

4. A listing of **drugs and toxins** that may produce liver cell injury, which is organized according to the various histologic features that may be seen. Reference is also made to the particular Table that lists the various diseases (besides drugs and toxins) that may cause similar histologic features.

5. Pertinent **references,** listed in numerical order as they appear in superscript in the text.

Our intent is to enable the pathologist and the clinician dealing with liver diseases to use this tool in correlating histology with specific hepatic disorders and their clinical presentation.

We hope that this book will be a useful teaching reference and help in better understanding and integrating the liver pathology with the patient.

Gary C. Kanel
Jacob Korula

CONTENTS

Preface v

1 Introduction 1

2 Morphologic Landmarks in Liver Pathology 7

Abscess Formation 8

Bile Ducts: Inflammation by Neutrophils (Acute Cholangitis) 11

Bile Ducts: Inflammation by Lymphocytes (Nonsuppurative Cholangitis) 13

Bile Ducts: Reduplication/Ectasia and Biliary Concretions 15

Bile Ducts: Periductal Fibrosis 18

Bile Ducts: Paucity (Ductopenia) 19

Calcification and Ossification 22

Cholestasis, Simple 25

Cysts 27

Diagnostic Lesions 29

Extracellular Deposits (Not Collagen) 36

Fatty Change 37

Granulomas 43

Inclusions: Hepatocytes 48

Inclusions: Kupffer Cells and Portal Macrophages 53

Lobular Necrosis with Inflammation 55

Lobular Necrosis with Minimal to Absent Inflammation 61

Lobular Confluent Necrosis 64

Mallory Bodies 66

Mass Lesions: Benign 69

Mass Lesions: Malignant 71

Pigments 73

Portal Lymphocytes Associated with Minimal to Absent Periportal Activity 79

Portal Lymphocytes Associated with Periportal Activity 80

Portal Neutrophils 83

Portal Plasma Cells 84

Portal Eosinophils 86

Portal Fibrosis: Cirrhosis, or Portal Fibrosis with Progression to Cirrhosis on Serial Biopsies 88

Portal Fibrosis without Progression to Cirrhosis 93

Sinusoids: Fibrosis 94

Sinusoids: Dilatation, Congestion, and Hemorrhage 98

Sinusoids: Peliotic Lesions 100

Sinusoids: Red Blood Cell Extravasation (Red Blood Cell–Trabecular Lesion) 102

Sinusoids: Circulating Cells 103

Sinusoids: Extramedullary Hematopoiesis 105

Syncytial Giant Cells 106

Vessels (Excluding Sinusoids): Inflammation 108

Vessels (Excluding Sinusoids): Thrombosis and Occlusion 111

3 Liver Diseases: Pathology and Clinical Considerations 115

4 Drug-Induced and Toxic Liver Cell Injury 217

5 References 225

Index 245

CHAPTER 1

Introduction

Numerous texts have been written on liver biopsy interpretation[1–12] describing both the major and minor histologic features that may be seen in various liver diseases. Texts that focus on the more pertinent histologic features provide a useful practical approach. When the pathologist recognizes classic morphologic changes, the liver disease may be apparent. For instance, in a patient with fatty change, abundant sinusoidal collagen deposition, and numerous Mallory bodies, a diagnosis of acute alcoholic hepatitis (acute sclerosing hyaline necrosis) is probable; however, it would be errant for the final readout to include that diagnosis without clinical and laboratory information. If the patient with the aforementioned liver biopsy result does *not* drink, then other diagnoses must be considered. The pathologist should then have a ready reference tool by which to look up a list of liver diseases that have Mallory bodies, fatty change, and sinusoidal collagen and determine what other liver diseases best fit the clinical picture. For instance, if the patient is obese or diabetic, a diagnosis of nonalcoholic steatohepatitis would be more appropriate.

Liver Biopsy Assessment

Before discussing an organized framework in which a table format of morphologic parameters can be useful, it is important to review a summary of liver histology. The initial interpretation of the liver biopsy should be approached by the pathologist in organized segments.

The first feature to assess is the *overall lobular architecture,* and whether it is intact or distorted. Portal tracts can be of normal size, expanded by inflammatory cells, or fibrotic without disturbance of the architectural arrangement, in that the relationship of the portal tracts and the terminal hepatic venules (central venules) can still be identified. When bridging fibrosis occurs, however, the architecture becomes distorted. Bridging can occur between portal tracts and between terminal hepatic venules. When bridging fibrosis entirely surrounds liver cells, forming regenerative nodules, then *cirrhosis* is present. It is important not to confuse true fibrosis with lobular collapse. For example, in untreated autoimmune hepatitis, the degree of lobular inflammation and necrosis can be marked, with collapse of the reticulin framework, which appears as fibrosis on hematoxylin-eosin stain; however, on trichrome stain the areas of collapse stain a light pale blue (reticulin fibers) instead of the dark intense blue of mature collagen, a helpful distinguishing feature.

The *portal tracts* should then be evaluated, or if cirrhosis is present, the *fibrous bands* are examined. While reviewing a liver biopsy, it is important to mention whether the portal changes are diffuse and uniformly involve all portal tracts, or whether the features are focal. For instance, in acute viral hepatitis, portal lymphocytic infiltration is prominent and diffusely involves all portal tracts, whereas in chronic viral hepatitis the degree of portal inflammatory infiltrates can vary, at times significantly, from one portal tract to the next. Portal tracts have five basic histologic features to assess: *bile ducts, hepatic arterioles, portal veins, inflammatory cells,* and the *fibrous framework.*

- Normally there are one to two *interlobular bile ducts* in a portal tract. Bile duct proliferation should therefore include greater than two bile ducts per portal tract. Bile ducts not only may be increased in number but also may be dilated (ectatic). The presence of periductal fibrosis, cytologic duct atypia, or inflammatory cells directly oriented to ducts should be noted. In addition, mention must be made of the type of inflammatory cells oriented to ducts; for example, neutrophils warrant the diagnosis of acute cholangitis and are most frequently seen in infections (e.g., ascending cholangitis), whereas the presence of mononuclear cells, chiefly lymphocytes, leads to a diagnosis of nonsuppurative cholangitis, which often leads to duct loss (ductopenia), as seen in primary biliary cirrhosis. Interlobular bile ducts should be distinguished from *cholangioles,* the latter originating from transformed or metaplastic hepatocytes, because cholangioles may be present and even proliferate in liver diseases associated with loss of the interlobular ducts (e.g., primary biliary cirrhosis). Cholangioles occur at the junction of the portal tracts and parenchyma, whereas interlobular ducts are located near the hepatic arterioles, from which they directly receive their blood supply.

- The *hepatic arterioles and small arteries* should be assessed in relation to their thickness, whether there is luminal occlusion, and whether inflammatory cells are directly oriented to the endothelium and wall. It should be noted, however, that in vasculitis, with the exception of humeral (hyperacute) rejection in liver transplant patients, the small to medium-sized hepatic arteries and *not* the arterioles are usually involved.

- *Portal veins* may be increased in number (seen in most examples of portal hypertension) and in some instances may be inflamed (e.g., endothelialitis associated with acute hepatic allograft rejection). In assessing larger portal tracts, note that the larger portal vein will have an identifiable wall. Inflammation involving the endothelium and also the wall is termed *pylephlebitis.*

- An *inflammatory infiltrate* is usually present within the portal tracts. The infiltrate can vary as to its degree and possible variation from one portal tract to another. The predominant cell type should be mentioned, and certainly mixed infiltrates consisting of a variety of different cell types may be present. Also note whether these inflammatory cells are confined to the portal tracts, or spill over into the adjacent periportal regions. Spillover itself is quite common in a variety of liver diseases; however, when the inflammatory cells surround individual and small groups of hepatocytes in the periportal regions, then piecemeal necrosis is present, which implies that the liver disease may have progressive potential.

- The degree of *fibrosis* may be slight, or the fibrosis may connect (bridge) with terminal hepatic venules or other portal tracts, and is assessed initially when the architectural pattern is described.

The *parenchyma* should then be examined. The *architectural structure,* the individual *hepatocytes* with nuclear and cytoplasmic changes and associated inflammation, and the *sinusoids* are assessed. In addition, *pigments,* including bile, and individual *vascular structures* are evaluated.

- The basic *cord-sinusoid pattern* can be intact or distorted. The normal lobule consists of liver cell plates one to two cells thick, lined by endothelial and Kupffer cells. In certain liver diseases, the cords and sinusoids can easily be identified, even if the liver disease is acute. For instance, in acute viral hepatitis secondary to cytomegalovirus (CMV) infection, the structure of the hepatic cords is only minimally disturbed despite the presence of necrosis and inflammation. Severe ballooning degeneration of liver cells is an uncommon finding; however, in acute viral hepatitis secondary to the hepatotropic viruses (e.g., hepatitis B), the cord-sinusoid pattern may be markedly distorted due to variable and sometimes prominent hydropic ballooning change of hepatocytes along with hepatocytolysis and formation of acidophil bodies.

- *Lobular inflammation* should next be assessed. Inflammation with associated necrosis should be graded in relation to its severity, the type of inflammatory cell involved, and the variation of the inflammation from one lobule to the next as well as the zonal distribution of the inflammation. Liver cell injury is predominantly manifested in three ways: *hydropic ballooning* of hepatocytes, *acidophil body* formation (apoptosis), and *cell dropout* with replacement by inflammatory cells and Kupffer cells phagocytizing the damaged liver cells. In some diseases, however, especially in inflammatory disorders of the neonate, *giant cell transformation* of hepatocytes can also occur due to inhibition of mitotic activity and damage with disintegration of cell membranes.

- Lobular inflammation in many liver diseases may form discrete clusters and are termed *granulomas.* They may be composed of compact inflammatory cells of virtually any type ("inflammatory type"), or contain specialized epithelial-type cells (transformation of monocytes to activated macrophages) with abundant eosinophilic cytoplasm and enlarged, relatively clear nuclei with or without multinucleated giant cell formation ("epithelioid type"). The frequency and specific features of granulomas should be carefully examined, since in some instances their presence may be diagnostic for one disease entity (e.g., identification of microorganisms [*Schistosoma* ova] on routine hematoxylin-eosin or special stains).

- The degree of *fatty change* should be qualitatively graded as 1 + (≤25% hepatocytes involved), 2+ (26–50% hepatocytes involved), 3+ (51–75% hepatocytes involved), to 4+ (>75% hepatocytes involved). In addition, the type of fat should be mentioned as *macrovesicular* (fat globules equal to or greater than the size of the nucleus), *microvesicular* (fat globules smaller than the nucleus), or mixed, as well as the zonal distribution of the fat. Fat may also be associated with inflammatory infiltration, with the fat often becoming extracellular and eliciting a histiocytic and rarely a giant cell reaction (lipogranuloma). Much less commonly, fat can also accumulate to variable degrees within portal macrophages.

- Distinct *inclusions* either may be large and involve the nucleus (e.g., CMV) or cytoplasm (e.g., Lafora bodies in myoclonus epilepsy), or may be small, single (e.g., megamitochondria) or multiple (e.g., alpha$_1$-antitrypsin globules). The location of the inclusions may also be important. Lafora bodies, for instance, are usually distributed within the periportal hepatocytes. Although in many instances special histochemical or immunohistochemical stains may be necessary to confirm the exact identity of the inclusions, in some instances the inclusions are diagnostic on hematoxylin-eosin stain (e.g., herpesvirus nuclear inclusions). *Mallory bodies* and *"ground-glass"* cells are particular types of cytoplasmic inclusions and should be assessed in relation to the amount seen and, in the case of Mallory bodies, the zonal distribution.

- *Cholestasis* may be present within dilated canaliculi, liver cell cytoplasm, or Kupffer cells (phagocytosis of damaged hepatocytes that contained bile). Cholestasis may be associated with an inflammatory infiltrate, or may be seen alone (simple cholestasis). In addition, in various liver diseases bile may have a zonal distribution, whereby perivenular bile is characteristic of large bile duct obstruction, while bile within the periportal (periseptal) zone may be present in the advanced stages of primary biliary cirrhosis. It should be noted that when cholestasis is extensive and involves all zones, with prominent periportal bile accumulation, bile may be present within the canals of Hering and within cholangioles, often associated with a neutrophilic infiltrate in and among the cholangioles. This should *not* be confused with acute cholangitis, which involves the interlobular bile ducts.

- The presence of *sinusoidal collagen* deposition should be graded in relation to its intensity and zonal distribution. For instance, extensive perivenular sclerosis is a helpful, although not diagnostic, clue in acute and chronic alcoholic liver disease. The trichrome stain is useful in best identifying thin collagen bands that may be difficult to visualize on hematoxylin-eosin stain. The sinusoidal collagen should always be distinguished from the *noncollagen extracellular deposits* seen in some liver diseases, which usually consists of fibrin or amyloid, and can be confirmed on special stains (phosphotungstic acid–hematoxylin stain for fibrin, Congo red for amyloid).

- One of the most common *pigments* is lipochrome (wear and tear pigment), and it is seen to some degree in normal livers, especially as a function of age. Lipochrome may on hematoxylin-eosin stain resemble hemosiderin and bile; however, these pigments can best be differentiated by their staining characteristics, summarized as follows.

	Hematoxylin-Eosin	Helpful Special Stain
Lipochrome	Finely granular, dark brown	Weakly positive (Ziehl-Neelsen)
Hemosiderin	Coarsely granular, golden brown	Strongly positive (Perls' iron stain)
Bile	Clumped, green-yellow; also seen within adjacent dilated canaliculi	Strongly positive (Hall's bilirubin)

In addition, in noncirrhotic livers, bile and lipochrome tend first to be distributed in the perivenular zone, whereas hemosiderin is seen earliest in the periportal hepatocytes. When a pigment is seen that does not meet the above histologic characteristics, then rarer pigments (e.g., protoporphyrin in erythropoietic protoporphyria) must be considered.

- The *sinusoids* should be assessed for whether they are open and dilated and whether they contain increased numbers of *circulating cells.* Their relationship to blood flow may also be important. *Congestion* and *hemorrhage,* or *red blood cell extravasation* into the space of Disse, may be present. Hemorrhage may also be focal and have a cyst-like pattern, representing *peliosis.* Finally, *extramedullary hematopoiesis* may also be seen within the sinusoids as well as within the portal tracts.
- *Inflammation of hepatic arteries* and *portal veins* have already been mentioned in the discussion of portal tracts. It is important at the same time to assess whether the *hepatic outflow vessels,* from the terminal hepatic (central) venules to the hepatic vein, are also involved, and whether vascular occlusion is present as well.
- Other features that should be noted include *cysts,* whether microscopic or grossly identifiable. Cysts are usually lined by duct epithelium; however, lining cells may not be present, often due to a coexisting inflammatory infiltrate. When cysts are filled with neutrophils, then *abscess* formation is present and may be microscopic or grossly seen. *Calcifications* are usually microscopic but in some instances may be large enough for visualization on imaging (e.g., cystadenoma with mesenchymal stroma, hydatid cyst). Calcifications may often occur in areas of necrosis (e.g., hepatocellular carcinoma). In rare instances, *ossification* may also be seen.

Clinical-Pathologic Correlation

This book is constructed in a table format. A wide variety of liver diseases that are known to demonstrate particular histologic features are listed in each table. After the pathologist assesses the morphologic changes found on the biopsy, he or she can then refer to the tables. A number of scenarios can occur, as described in the list that follows. Note that each of the histologic changes has the corresponding reference table in parenthesis.

- A liver biopsy shows the following features: (1) portal fibrosis with bridging (Table 2–28, Portal Fibrosis); (2) portal mononuclear infiltrates consisting of lymphocytes and abundant numbers of plasma cells (Table 2–26, Portal Plasma Cells); (3) lymphocytes surrounding and invading into interlobular bile ducts (Table 2–3, Bile Ducts: Inflammation by Lymphocytes); (4) Mallory bodies in periportal hepatocytes (Table 2–19, Mallory Bodies); and (5) a mild focal necrosis and hepatocytolysis without cholestasis within the lobule (Table 2–16, Lobular Necrosis with Inflammation). Reviewing the tables for these biopsy findings reveals that numerous liver diseases meet some of the features; however, the pathologist notes that by comparing the listing of portal plasma cells, bile duct inflammation by lymphocytes, and Mallory bodies, the differential diagnosis becomes limited, and that only primary biliary cirrhosis (PBC) and primary sclerosing cholangitis (PSC) are the liver diseases that show all of the described histologic changes. Clinical information related to PBC and PSC are available for review in Chapter 3, Liver Diseases: Pathology and Clinical Considerations, which also includes a summary of the histologic features of each disease. It is noted in the summary that PSC characteristically shows periductal fibrosis, a feature *not* seen in this liver biopsy. Therefore, PBC is the leading diagnosis. The pertinent clinical and laboratory features of PBC can then be assessed, whereby a positive anti-mitochondrial antibody (AMA) and high alkaline phosphatase activity would support a clinical-pathologic diagnosis of PBC.
- When the histology fits nicely into one diagnosis (such as the liver biopsy described previously), then even if the clinical and laboratory features are not entirely supportive, the morphologic diagnosis should still be stated to the clinician. For instance, if the alkaline phosphatase activity in the aforementioned case is normal, PBC should still be considered as a possible diagnosis, since well-documented cases of PBC with normal alkaline phosphatase activity have been reported.
- In a more complicated case the liver biopsy shows portal plasma cells with variable lobular inflammation but without Mallory bodies or lymphocytes attacking ducts. After referring to the appropriate table (Table 2–26, Portal Plasma Cells), the differential diagnosis is seen to be more extensive. However, if the plasma cells are abundant, then the differential diagnosis is more limited (noted in the table as ++), since only a handful of liver diseases (which includes PBC) are associated with striking portal plasma cells.
- Too often the histology may not fit into one disease entity only. For example, if the biopsy shows features characteristic for acute sclerosing hyaline necrosis (e.g., abundant sinusoidal collagen deposition with numerous Mallory bodies) in a known alcoholic, but also shows numerous intracytoplasmic inclusions that are periodic acid–Schiff-positive after diastase digestion in periportal hepatocytes, then a

diagnosis of acute sclerosing hyaline necrosis in a patient with alpha₁-antitrypsin deficiency should be entertained, which then would be supported if the inclusions were positive on immunoperoxidase staining for alpha₁-antitrypsin.

- Not infrequently the biopsy is not characteristic of any single or small group of liver diseases, and thus the differential diagnoses are quite numerous. An example is a liver biopsy that shows portal fibrosis, mild portal lymphocytic infiltration with the presence of normal interlobular ducts, and minimal lobular inflammation. Although many liver diseases may cause these features as the pathologist will note when referring to the tables, at least certain diagnoses can be ruled out. For instance, if the physician suspects a clinical diagnosis of PBC, then the presence of portal plasma cells, bile ducts attacked by lymphocytes, or bile duct depletion are some of the features the pathologist would search for to confirm that diagnosis. The fact that the liver biopsy on that patient does *not* show any of those features would rule out PBC. On the other hand, if the patient is known to be anti–hepatitis C virus-positive and is on interferon therapy, the histologic changes seen on the biopsy are then supportive of chronic hepatitis C with response to therapy.

- Finally, a few liver diseases are diagnostic for one disease entity alone, regardless of the clinical and laboratory data, and are listed in Table 2–10, Diagnostic Lesions. For instance, if the liver biopsy shows hepatocytes having an increased nuclear-cy-

toplasmic ratio, forming cords four to six cells thick lined by endothelial cells, then hepatocellular carcinoma is present. If the clinician states that the alpha-fetoprotein is normal and there is no suspected mass lesion, then the pathologist can recommend further workup and review of the imaging. Similarly, the presence of eosinophilic amorphous material in the sinusoids that stains positive on Congo red stain and exhibits apple-green birefringence under polarized light is diagnostic for amyloidosis, although the patient's clinical signs and symptoms may be secondary to a coexisting liver disease that may also be present on histologic examination (e.g., amyloidosis in a patient with chronic hepatitis C).

It should be noted that drug-induced hepatotoxicity can cause virtually any histologic feature seen in liver biopsies. It is imperative when making a diagnosis of drug- or toxin-induced liver cell injury that all other diagnoses are ruled out, and that the time sequence of how long the patient was on medication fits the clinical-pathologic diagnosis. For instance, if a biopsy shows changes similar to acute viral hepatitis but the patient is serologically negative for all the hepatotropic viruses, and has been on isoniazid (INH) for 4 months, then INH-induced hepatotoxicity is likely. Discontinuance of INH with rapid resolution of the liver tests to normal would support that diagnosis; however, if the patient had been on INH for only 1 week or for many years, then INH-induced hepatotoxicity could be ruled out.

CHAPTER 2

Morphologic Landmarks in Liver Pathology

Abscess Formation

An *abscess* is characterized by aggregates of inflammatory cells that are chiefly neutrophils. Sometimes these lesions are large and well demarcated; however, small microscopic clusters of neutrophils can also be seen in various conditions either within the portal tracts or the parenchyma, and are termed *microabscesses* (Table 2–1). Most frequently, hepatic abscesses arise either directly from the hepatic artery due to systemic bacteremia, or from the biliary tree secondary to partial bile duct obstruction with ascending cholangitis. Less commonly, abdominal infection may initiate inflammation of the portal vein and its radicals (*pylephlebitis*) with secondary abscess formation. Some diseases may at first form microabscesses (e.g., early phase of extrahepatic biliary obstruction), but coalescence of these lesions may eventually occur, forming abscesses that can be identified on ultrasound or other imaging techniques. It must be emphasized that in biopsies taken at the time of laparotomy, neutrophilic clusters are not uncommon, are most often seen toward the capsule and terminal hepatic outflow vessels, and are most frequent after long surgical procedures. These aggregates are secondary to repeated manipulation of the liver with resultant localized impaired blood flow, focal acute liver ischemia, and secondary neutrophilic infiltration (*surgical hepatitis*). It is also important to note that acute sclerosing hyaline necrosis (acute alcoholic hepatitis) is characteristically associated with numerous neutrophils within the lobules; however, they arise primarily from a chemotactic response to Mallory bodies, and are not true microabscesses.

Figures 2–1 through 2–7 demonstrate various examples of abscess formation.

TABLE 2–1
Abscess Formation

	Microabscess	Abscess That May Be Visualized on Imaging
Actinomycosis	++	+
Adult polycystic disease	++	
Allograft, ischemia secondary to hepatic artery thrombosis	++	+
Amebiasis (early stage)	++*	
Amebiasis (well developed)		++*
Bacterial sepsis	++	+
Blastomycosis	++	
Brucellosis	++	
Candidiasis	++	+
Caroli's disease	++	+
Cat-scratch disease	++	
Choledochal cyst	++	+
Chronic granulomatous disease of childhood	++	+
Congenital hepatic fibrosis	++	
Crohn's disease	+	++
Cytomegalovirus infection (post transplant)	++	
Extrahepatic biliary obstruction, early	++	+
Extrahepatic biliary obstruction, late (months)	++	+
Extrahepatic biliary obstruction, late (years)	++	+
Listeriosis	++	
Melioidosis	++	+
Nocardiosis	++	+
Pylephlebitis	+	++
Pyogenic abscess		++
Recurrent pyogenic cholangiohepatitis	+	++
Surgical hepatitis	++	

+ = Occasionally seen; ++ = predominantly seen.

*Although amebiasis commonly is associated with hepatic "abscess" formation, neutrophils are usually seen in the early developing stage. When the lesion is enlarged and well developed, the inflammatory infiltrate is usually sparse and when present consists chiefly of lymphocytes and plasma cells with only rare neutrophils; however, in some instances bacterial superinfection occurs, whereby neutrophils are then frequent.

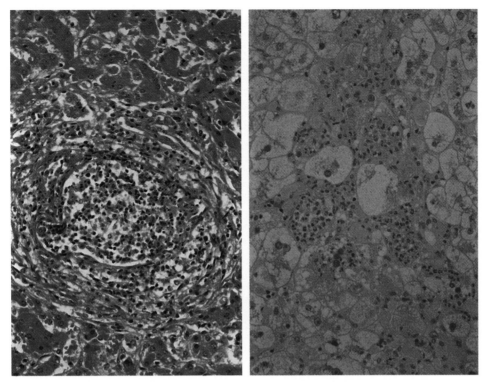

Figures 2–1, 2–2 Bacterial Sepsis (Fig. 2–1, *left*) Ascending cholangitis led to total damage of the duct epithelium, with microabscess formation within the portal tract. (Fig. 2–2, *right*) Numerous microabscesses are seen in the perivenular zone. The neutrophils can also be identified infiltrating into damaged liver cell cytoplasm.

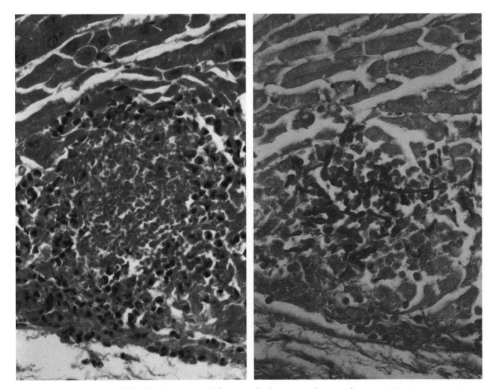

Figures 2–3, 2–4 Candidiasis (Fig. 2–3, *left*) A small abscess with central necrosis is present in a liver biopsy 18 years post transplant. A suggestion of yeast forms is seen at its center. (Fig. 2–4, *right*) A periodic acid–Schiff (PAS) stain after diastase digestion confirms the presence of budding pseudohyphae, characteristic of *Candida albicans* infection.

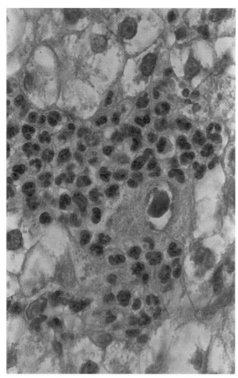

Figure 2–5 Cytomegalovirus Infection A microabscess surrounding a liver cell with a prominent viral nuclear inclusion characteristic of cytomegalovirus is seen in a liver biopsy 8 weeks post transplant.

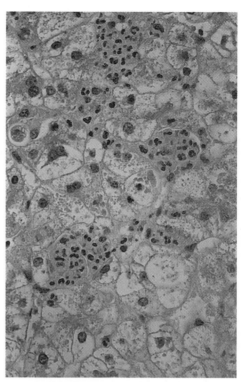

Figure 2–7 Surgical Hepatitis Clusters of neutrophils are present within the lobule. Although the adjacent hepatocytes are swollen, there is no evidence of hepatocellular necrosis, with the neutrophils predominantly confined to the sinusoids. This photomicrograph is taken from a wedge biopsy performed at the time of cholecystectomy. Liver tests were normal, and there were no clinical signs or symptoms of sepsis.

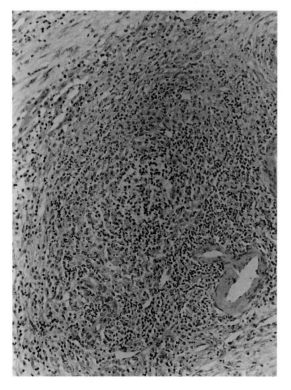

Figure 2–6 Recurrent Pyogenic Cholangiohepatitis An abscess secondary to acute cholangitis is seen within a portal tract.

Bile Ducts

Inflammation by Neutrophils

(Acute Cholangitis)

The process whereby bile ducts are surrounded and infiltrated by neutrophils is termed *acute cholangitis* (Table 2–2). The most common cause is biliary tract obstruction with resultant ascending cholangitis. Characteristically, the ducts are dilated and often show variable and in some instances prominent reduplication (refer to Table 2–4, Bile Ducts: Replication/Ectasia and Biliary Concretions). Associated cholangiolar proliferation is often seen as well, these bile ducts often surrounded by neutrophils. Repeated bouts of acute cholangitis secondary to biliary tract obstruction seldom lead to duct depletion. It is important to distinguish acute cholangitis from acute cholangiolitis, the former representing inflammation of the *interlobular bile ducts,* the latter representing inflammation of the *cholangioles* and *metaplastic ducts* (periportal hepatocytes transformed into duct-like structures that express cytokeratins 7 and 19 characteristic of bile duct epithelium). Acute cholangiolitis is associated not only with bile duct obstruction but also may be seen in any liver disease related to prominent cholestasis that also involves the periportal zones. A helpful clue in distinguishing between these duct structures relates to the hepatic microcirculation: the hepatic arteriole divides to follow a spiral course around the interlobular ducts and hence can be visualized within the portal tracts near the interlobular ducts, while the cholangioles and metaplastic ducts derive their oxygen supply from the peribiliary plexus as it drains into the sinusoids and do not abut against the arterioles.

Figures 2–8 through 2–13 demonstrate various examples of acute cholangitis.

TABLE 2–2

Bile Ducts: Inflammation by Neutrophils

Adjacent to space-occupying lesions
Allograft, acute (cellular) rejection
Allograft, ischemia secondary to hepatic artery thrombosis
Ascariasis
Bacterial sepsis
Caroli's disease
Choledochal cyst
Congenital hepatic fibrosis
Cystic fibrosis
Drugs/toxins (refer to Table 4–6)
Extrahepatic biliary atresia
Extrahepatic biliary obstruction, early
Extrahepatic biliary obstruction, late (months)
Fascioliasis
Heat stroke
Hydatid cyst
Hyperpyrexia
Infantile microcystic disease
Kawasaki disease
Primary biliary cirrhosis
Primary sclerosing cholangitis
Pyogenic abscess
Recurrent pyogenic cholangiohepatitis
Salmonellosis
Syphilis, secondary
Toxic shock syndrome
Tuberculosis

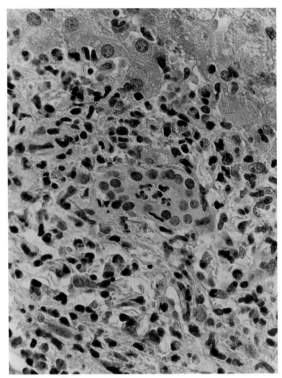

Figure 2–8 Allograft, Acute (Cellular) Rejection This portal tract shows a mixed inflammatory infiltrate consisting of lymphocytes, eosinophils, and neutrophils. Neutrophils can also be seen within the lumen of an interlobular bile duct, suggestive of bile duct obstruction; however, the cholangiogram showed no evidence of duct obstruction or stricture, and there was no evidence of sepsis.

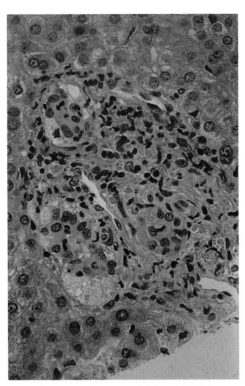

Figure 2–10 Drug-induced Damage (Chlorothiazide) Neutrophils are present surrounding and infiltrating into ducts, which also show hydropic change and variable cytologic damage.

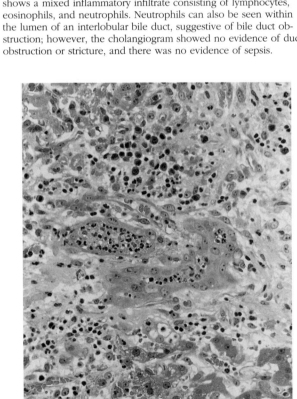

Figure 2–9 Bacterial Sepsis Neutrophils are seen within these dilated interlobular bile ducts, which also show periductal edema. The liver from this patient also exhibited in other fields acute inflammation of the portal venous radicals (pylephlebitis) and abscess formation.

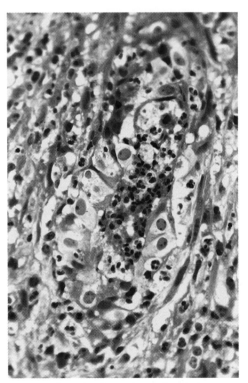

Figure 2–11 Extrahepatic Biliary Obstruction, Early Neutrophils can be seen surrounding and infiltrating into interlobular duct epithelium, with clusters also present within the duct lumen.

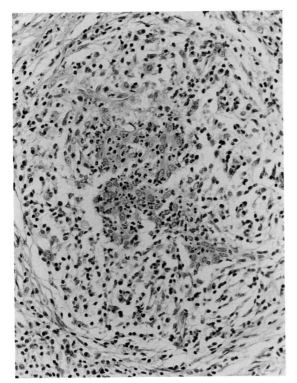

Figure 2–12 Extrahepatic Biliary Obstruction, Late (Months)
Neutrophils infiltrate into duct epithelium and lumen, with prominent duct damage and periductal edema.

Bile Ducts

Inflammation by Lymphocytes
(Nonsuppurative Cholangitis)

Various liver diseases are associated with interlobular bile ducts surrounded and infiltrated by lymphocytes (*nonsuppurative cholangitis*) (Table 2–3). The bile duct epithelium shows variable cytologic atypia, consisting of hydropic change, nuclear pyknosis, and in some instances reactive epithelial hyperplasia. In many of the diseases listed in Table 2–3, depletion of ducts may eventually result (refer to Table 2–6, Bile Ducts: Paucity), and is often, but not always, associated with biliary cirrhosis. Nonsuppurative cholangitis may be diffuse, involving the majority of portal tracts (e.g., severe acute cellular rejection), or focal (e.g., early stages of primary biliary cirrhosis). As in duct paucity, the mechanism is multifactorial, and relates to host immune responses against infectious agents, autoantigens, and alloantigens.

Figures 2–14 through 2–18 demonstrate various examples of nonsuppurative cholangitis.

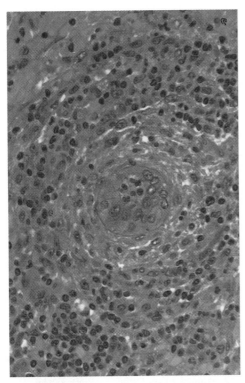

Figure 2–13 Recurrent Pyogenic Cholangiohepatitis Clusters of neutrophils are present within the duct lumen. Mild periductal fibrosis and edema are also seen.

TABLE 2–3
Bile Ducts: Inflammation by Lymphocytes

Allograft, acute (cellular) rejection
Autoimmune hepatitis (cholangiopathy)
Cytomegalovirus infection
Drugs/toxins (refer to Table 4–7)
Epstein-Barr virus infection
Graft-versus-host disease
Human immunodeficiency virus–associated cholangiopathy
Hydatid cyst
Idiopathic adulthood ductopenia
Langerhans' cell histiocytosis
Lymphoma, Hodgkin's
Paucity of intrahepatic ducts, syndromatic
Primary biliary cirrhosis
Primary sclerosing cholangitis
Sarcoidosis
Ulcerative colitis
Viral hepatitis, acute, type C
Viral hepatitis, chronic, type C

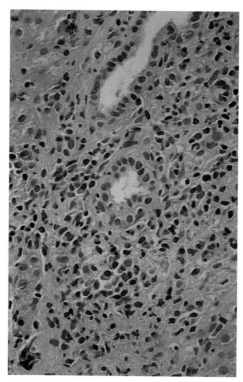

Figure 2–14 Autoimmune Hepatitis The portal infiltrate consists of lymphocytes and plasma cells. The interlobular duct is partially infiltrated by lymphocytes.

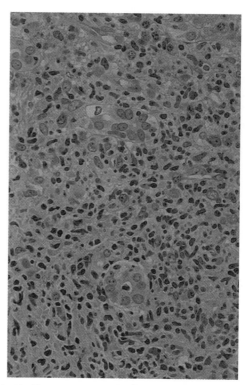

Figure 2–16 Human Immunodeficiency Virus–associated Cholangiopathy The interlobular bile ducts show prominent cytologic atypia, and are infiltrated by lymphocytes.

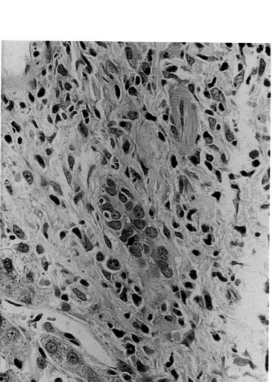

Figure 2–15 Epstein-Barr Virus Infection The liver from this patient with infectious mononucleosis and high alkaline phosphatase activity exhibits an interlobular bile duct with lymphocytes infiltrating beneath the duct basement membrane.

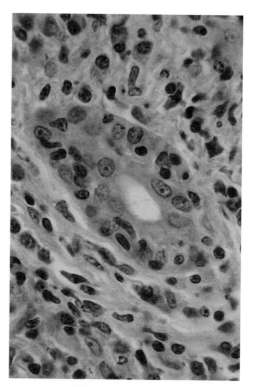

Figure 2–17 Primary Biliary Cirrhosis This interlobular bile duct is slightly hyperplastic, and exhibits lymphocytes within the duct wall.

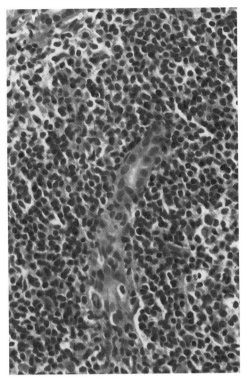

Figure 2–18 Viral Hepatitis, Chronic, Type C The portal tract shows a lymphoid aggregate with a centrally located interlobular bile duct focally infiltrated by lymphocytes. Variable cytologic atypia of the duct epithelium is also present, but this latter feature is relatively mild.

Bile Ducts

Reduplication/Ectasia and Biliary Concretions

Proliferation and dilatation (ectasia) of both interlobular bile ducts and cholangioles can be seen in most conditions that impede bile flow, whether this obstruction is secondary to lesions in the biliary tree (e.g., bile duct obstruction due to stones) or intrahepatic cholestatic disorders (e.g., bacterial sepsis) (Table 2–4). Neutrophilic infiltration of cholangioles may also be present when the associated cholestasis is severe; in addition, sometimes the cholangioles are markedly dilated and filled with biliary concretions (inspissated bile). Proliferation of ductules may also be seen in certain hepatic mass lesions (e.g., focal nodular hyperplasia), and is quite striking adjacent to large intrahepatic ducts containing *Clonorchis sinensis* (liver fluke). All the liver diseases listed in Table 2–4 often show bile duct reduplication and ectasia; in addition, those disorders that also may exhibit biliary concretions are noted in the adjacent column.

Figures 2–19 through 2–26 depict various examples of bile duct reduplication.

TABLE 2–4

Bile Ducts: Replication/Ectasia and Biliary Concretions

	Associated Biliary Concretions		Associated Biliary Concretions
Adenoma, bile duct		Galactosemia	+
Adjacent to space-occupying lesions		Heat stroke	
Adult polycystic disease		Hereditary fructose intolerance	+
Allograft, harvesting (preservation) injury (severe)	+	Hyperalimentation, infants	+
Allograft, ischemia secondary to hepatic artery thrombosis		Hyperpyrexia	
		Infantile hemangioendothelioma	
Bacterial sepsis	+	Infantile microcystic disease	
Biliary hamartoma	+	Mesenchymal hamartoma	
Caroli's disease	+	Primary biliary cirrhosis	
Choledochal cyst	+	Primary sclerosing cholangitis	+
Clonorchiasis		Progressive familial intrahepatic cholestasis	
Congenital hepatic fibrosis	+	Recurrent cholestasis with lymphedema	
Cystic fibrosis	+	Recurrent pyogenic cholangiohepatitis	+
Extrahepatic biliary atresia	+	Viral hepatitis, acute, classic type	
Extrahepatic biliary obstruction, early	+	Viral hepatitis, acute, type E	+
Extrahepatic biliary obstruction, late (months)	+	Viral hepatitis, acute, with bridging necrosis	+
Extrahepatic biliary obstruction, late (years)	+	Viral hepatitis, acute, with impaired regeneration	+
Focal nodular hyperplasia		Viral hepatitis, acute, with panacinar necrosis	+

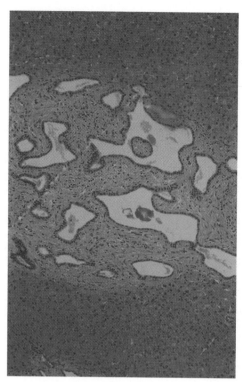

Figure 2–19 Biliary Hamartoma These discrete, predominantly portal lesions exhibit dilated duct structures that over half the time contain variable inspissated bile.

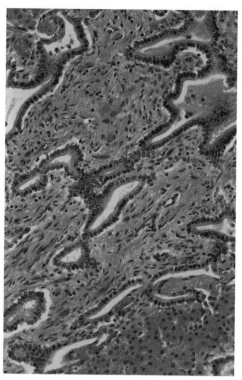

Figure 2–21 Congenital Hepatic Fibrosis All portal tracts exhibit dilated anastomosing duct structures.

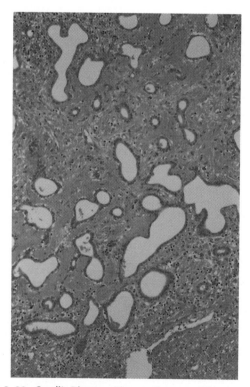

Figure 2–20 Caroli's Disease The portal tracts exhibit numerous dilated and ectatic interlobular bile ducts and cholangioles.

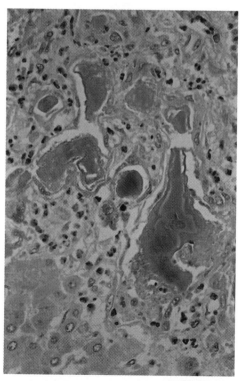

Figure 2–22 Cystic Fibrosis The bile ducts and cholangioles are dilated and contain abundant inspissated biliary concretions.

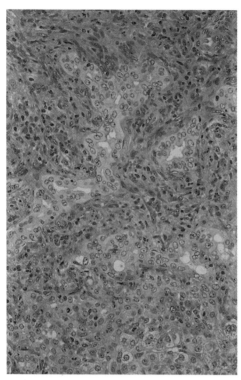

Figure 2–23   Extrahepatic Biliary Atresia   Although extrahepatic bile ducts are hypoplastic or atretic in this condition, the intrahepatic bile ducts shown in this photomicrograph characteristically show prominent proliferation.

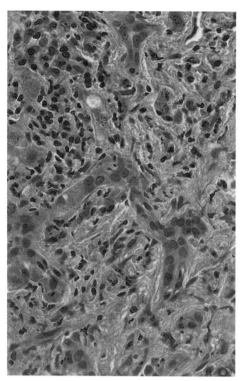

Figure 2–25   Primary Biliary Cirrhosis   As primary biliary cirrhosis progresses into the fibrotic stage, atypical proliferating cholangioles may be present toward the edge of the portal tracts, the cholangioles having no lumen and composed of flattened duct epithelium proliferating in a serpentine pattern.

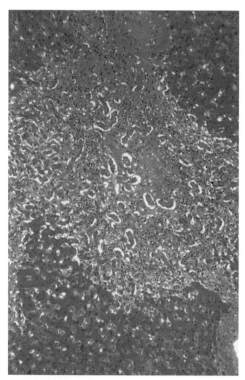

Figure 2–24   Extrahepatic Biliary Obstruction, Early and Late Phases   Bile duct proliferation is seen in all phases of extrahepatic biliary tract obstruction, and is often associated with intermittent acute cholangitis.

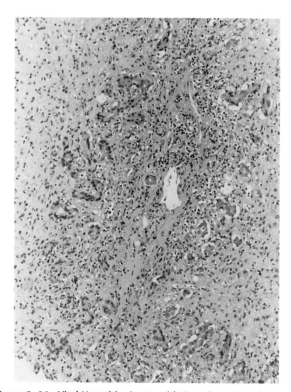

Figure 2–26   Viral Hepatitis, Acute, with Panacinar Necrosis   Striking cholangiolar proliferation is seen at the border of a portal tract and lobule, the latter in this case showing complete liver cell dropout and lobular collapse.

Bile Ducts
Periductal Fibrosis

Intermittent inflammation of bile duct epithelium may in some instances elicit a reactive process from the adjacent fibrous stroma. This is manifested by thin fibrous bands repeatedly laid down next to and surrounding the duct epithelium, and is morphologically similar to scar formation (Table 2–5). The inflammatory exudate, when present, is usually neutrophilic. With repeated duct damage, the fibrous bands become progressively thicker. This type of lesion can be seen involving both the medium-sized and small interlobular bile ducts. The most common cause of this lesion is extrahepatic or large-duct intrahepatic biliary tract obstruction. Depending on the site of obstruction (e.g., gallstone within the common bile duct), the larger extrahepatic ducts may also be histologically involved. Periductal fibrosis usually is a striking feature in primary sclerosing cholangitis. In this disease, correlation with other morphologic features (e.g., duct loss as the disease progresses) and findings on imaging studies (e.g., intermittent strictures and beading of the ducts on endoscopic retrograde cholangiopancreatography) is necessary for a more definitive diagnosis.

Figures 2–27 to 2–29 show various examples of periductal fibrosis.

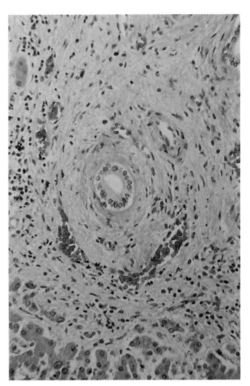

Figure 2–27 Extrahepatic Biliary Obstruction, Late (Months to Years) Periductal fibrosis is present. Although not demonstrated in this photomicrograph, acute cholangitis may also intermittently be seen.

TABLE 2–5
Bile Ducts: Periductal Fibrosis

Caroli's disease
Choledochal cyst
Cryptococcosis
Cryptosporidiosis
Cytomegalovirus infection
Drugs/toxins (refer to Table 4–8)
Extrahepatic biliary obstruction, early
Extrahepatic biliary obstruction, late (months)
Extrahepatic biliary obstruction, late (years)
Human immunodeficiency virus–associated cholangiopathy
Hydatid cyst
Idiopathic adulthood ductopenia
Langerhans' cell histiocytosis
Microsporidiosis
Primary sclerosing cholangitis
Recurrent pyogenic cholangiohepatitis
Ulcerative colitis

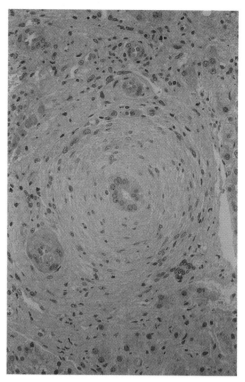

Figure 2-28 Primary Sclerosing Cholangitis Periductal fibrosis is striking, with fibro-obliterative "onion-skinning" a common feature. Eventually duct depletion occurs.

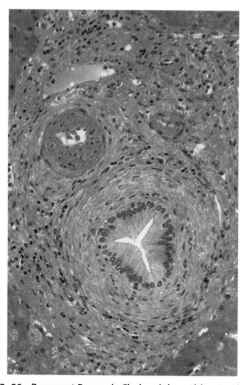

Figure 2-29 Recurrent Pyogenic Cholangiohepatitis Periductal fibrosis is common due to intrahepatic biliary concretions obstructing bile flow.

Bile Ducts

Paucity

(Ductopenia)

When interlobular bile ducts are attacked by inflammatory cells (chiefly lymphocytes), their destruction may eventually result in duct loss (*ductopenia*) (Table 2–6). The etiologies are often multifactorial and include enhanced expression of major histocompatibility complex (MHC) class I antigens and aberrant expression of MHC class II antigens on bile duct epithelium in various conditions such as primary biliary cirrhosis, primary sclerosing cholangitis, and chronic transplantation rejection. In cases of intermittent biliary tract obstruction (e.g., repeated passage of gallstones), duct regeneration occurs, with duct loss uncommon; however, when duct damage is diffuse and persistent, duct depletion may then be seen, usually after many years. In many instances, portal fibrosis is also present and may eventually lead to biliary cirrhosis; however, in some cases (e.g., chronic transplantation rejection), there may be minimal portal fibrosis. A helpful special stain in instances in which duct depletion is suspected is the *orcein* stain, which stains *copper-binding protein*. Chronic cholestatic disorders and disorders associated with duct loss often have increase in copper-binding protein in periportal or periseptal hepatocytes as the disease progresses, although these pigments may be seen in earlier stages as well. This protein represents polymerized metallothionein that accumulates within lysozomes and is dark brown to black and coarsely granular. An increase in hepatic *copper* is also seen in many of these conditions and can be demonstrated by the *rubeanic acid* stain as granular, dark blue-green pigment within the cytoplasm; however, the orcein stain is quicker to perform, and more reliable in early-stage lesions. (Refer to Table 2–22, Pigments, for other causes of increase in copper and copper-binding protein).

Figures 2–30 through 2–36 show various examples of ductopenia.

TABLE 2-6

Bile Ducts: Paucity (Ductopenia)

Allograft, chronic (ductopenic) rejection
Allograft, ischemia secondary to hepatic artery thrombosis
Alpha$_1$-antitrypsin deficiency (childhood onset)
Autoimmune hepatitis (cholangiopathy)
Cryptosporidiosis
Cystic fibrosis
Cytomegalovirus
Down syndrome
Drugs/toxins (refer to Table 4–7)
Extrahepatic biliary atresia
Extrahepatic biliary obstruction, late (years)
Graft-versus-host disease
Human immunodeficiency virus–associated cholangiopathy
Idiopathic adulthood ductopenia
Infantile microcystic disease
Langerhans' cell histiocytosis
Lymphoma, Hodgkin's
Microsporidiosis
Niemann-Pick disease
Paucity of intrahepatic ducts, syndromatic and nonsyndromatic
Primary biliary cirrhosis
Primary sclerosing cholangitis
Progressive familial intrahepatic cholestasis
Recurrent cholestasis with lymphedema
Rubella virus infection
Sarcoidosis
Viral hepatitis, chronic, type C
Zellweger's syndrome

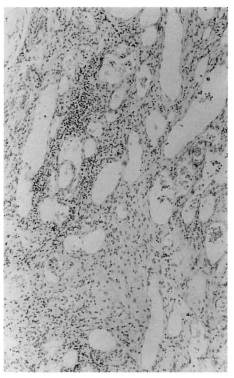

Figure 2–31 Cystic Fibrosis The fibrous band shows numerous increased portal venous radicals and lymphatic channels, with mild lymphocytic infiltration. No interlobular bile ducts are seen.

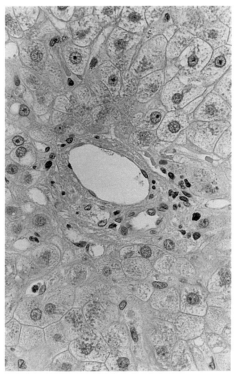

Figure 2–30 Allograft, Chronic (Ductopenic) Rejection The portal tract exhibits a portal vein and two hepatic arteriole segments; however, there is no interlobular bile duct.

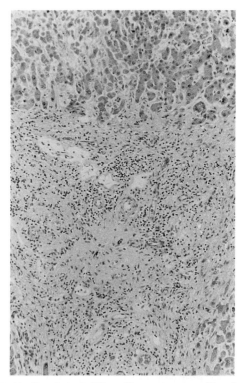

Figure 2–32 Extrahepatic Biliary Obstruction, Late (Years) The fibrous band in this example of secondary biliary cirrhosis shows numerous vascular channels, scattered hepatic arterioles, and a lymphocytic infiltrate; however, no interlobular bile ducts are present.

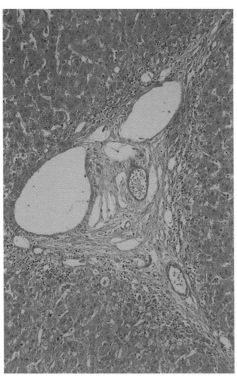

Figure 2–33 Paucity of Intrahepatic Ducts, Syndromatic (Alagille's Syndrome) Increased vascular channels are seen, but interlobular bile ducts are absent.

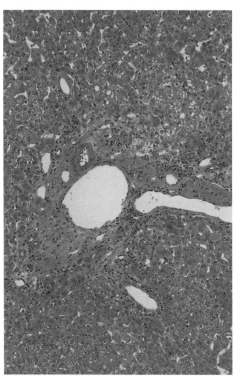

Figure 2–35 Primary Sclerosing Cholangitis The fibrotic portal tract shows increased numbers of portal venous radicals and a slightly thickened arteriole; however, interlobular bile ducts are absent.

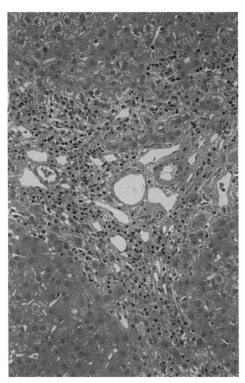

Figure 2–34 Primary Biliary Cirrhosis The fibrotic portal tract exhibits an increase in vascular channels (suggestive of portal hypertension) and moderate lymphocytic infiltration. There are no interlobular bile ducts.

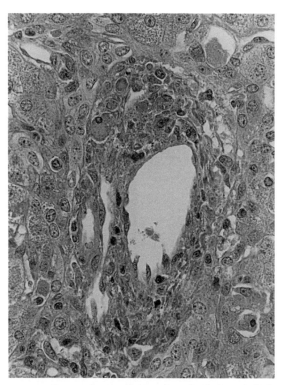

Figure 2–36 Progressive Familial Intrahepatic Cholestasis (Byler's Syndrome) The portal tract is normal in size in this early-stage disease; portal vein segments and a hepatic arteriole are seen, but there are no interlobular bile ducts.

Calcification and Ossification

Calcium deposits can occur in damaged tissue; the calcium is derived from the circulation and interstitium rather than directly from the injured cells (*dystrophic calcification*). The calcified lesions are usually microscopic, but in some instances (e.g., cavernous hemangioma) may be demonstrated on imaging and gross examination (Table 2–7). *Metastatic calcification* refers to abnormal calcium metabolism with associated hypercalcemia, and does not require preexisting liver injury. Calcium deposits may also be a component of the liver disorder itself (e.g., hepatoblastoma). In some instances differentiation into newly woven bone (*ossification*) may also be present.

Figures 2–37 through 2–46 demonstrate various examples of calcification and ossification.

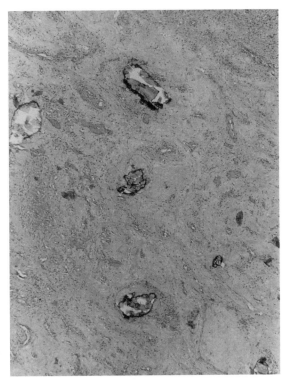

Figure 2–37 Cavernous Hemangioma   Cavernous hemangiomas often may have central sclerosis; when present, calcification can occur, as seen in this case.

TABLE 2–7

Calcification and Ossification

Calcification	Ossification
Adenoma, bile duct	Hepatoblastoma
Adenoma, liver cell	Hepatocellular carcinoma,
Adult polycystic disease	trabecular, acinar, duc-
Amyloidosis	tular type
Brucellosis	Histoplasmosis
Budd-Chiari syndrome, chronic	
Cavernous hemangioma	
Cholangiocarcinoma	
Cystadenoma with or without	
mesenchymal stroma	
Epithelioid hemangioendothelioma	
Focal nodular hyperplasia	
Gaucher's disease	
Heart failure, left-sided with hypo-	
tension	
Hepatoblastoma	
Hepatocellular carcinoma, fibrola-	
mellar type	
Hepatocellular carcinoma, trabec-	
ular, acinar, ductular type	
Histoplasmosis	
Hydatid cyst	
Peliosis hepatis	
Pentastomiasis	
Schistosomiasis	
Solitary nonparasitic cyst	
Syphilis, tertiary	
Tuberculosis	

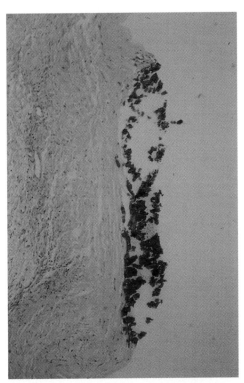

Figure 2–38 Cystadenoma with or without Mesenchymal Stroma   A calcified nodule is seen involving the inner aspect of the fibrous capsule. A mesenchymal component is not present in this case.

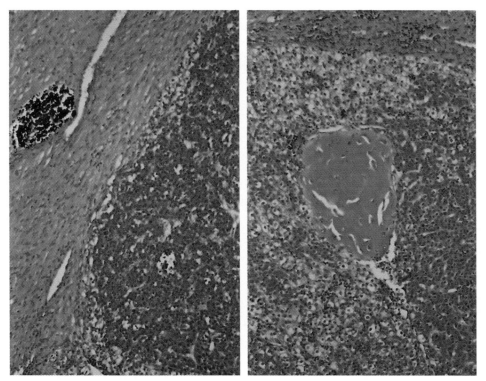

Figures 2–39, 2–40   Hepatoblastoma   (Fig. 2–39, *left*) The epithelial component consisting of small hepatocytes forming thickened cords is present. The adjacent stroma shows focal calcification. (Fig. 2–40, *right*) Ossification is present within the epithelial component.

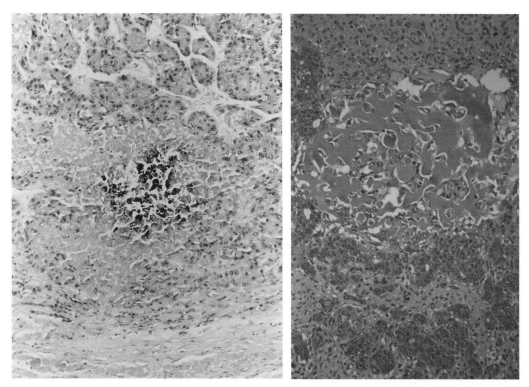

Figures 2–41, 2–42   Hepatocellular Carcinoma, Trabecular Type   (Fig. 2–41, *left*) Calcification may occur in areas of tumor necrosis. (Fig. 2–42, *right*) Ossification may also be seen within the fibrous stroma, although this feature is relatively uncommon.

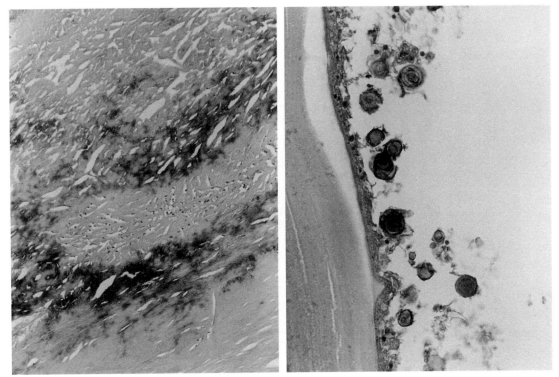

Figures 2–43, 2–44 Hydatid Cyst (Fig. 2–43, *left*) Calcification is often seen within the outer laminated capsule. (Fig. 2–44, *right*) Calcification also may be identified adjacent to the germinal membrane or within the amorphous granular sediment, and sometimes represents calcified dead protoscolices.

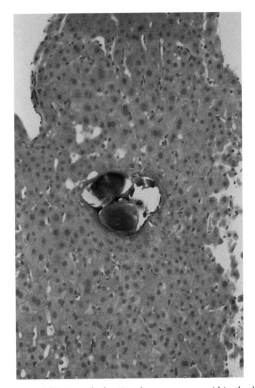

Figure 2–45 Schistosomiasis Dead ova are seen within the lobule, and are totally calcified.

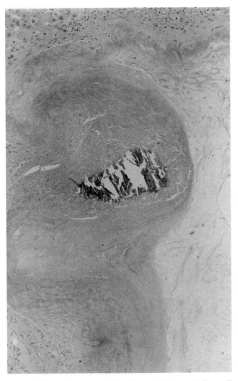

Figure 2–46 Solitary Nonparasitic Cyst This partially collapsed simple cyst shows a focus of calcification within the thickened wall.

Cholestasis, Simple

Cholestasis is an accumulation of bile visualized on histologic sections, the bile located within liver cell cytoplasm as well as dilated biliary canaliculi. Most frequently cholestasis involves the perivenular zone (zone 3), but may extend throughout all zones (Table 2–8). Cholestasis may be subdivided into two general etiologic categories: (1) *extrahepatic,* whereby bile flow is impeded by lesions causing mechanical obstruction of the large intrahepatic ducts or extrahepatic biliary tree (e.g., gallstones within the common bile duct); and (2) *intrahepatic,* in which the cause relates to damage to hepatocytes or biliary canaliculi (e.g., drugs and toxins). Cholestasis may also be seen in well-differentiated primary hepatic neoplasms, in which liver cells synthesize bile that cannot be excreted. Although cholestasis may exhibit a coexisting inflammatory infiltrate within the parenchyma, sometimes the degree of lobular inflammation can be bland or absent (*simple cholestasis*). It is important to note that many liver diseases (e.g., early phase of bile duct obstruction) may exhibit either simple cholestasis or cholestasis with variable degrees of lobular inflammation (refer to Table 2–16, Lobular Necrosis with Inflammation).

Figures 2–47 through 2–53 show various examples of simple cholestasis.

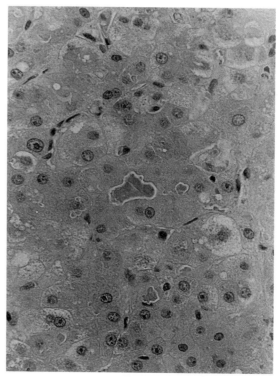

Figure 2–47 Allograft, Harvesting (Preservation) Injury The bile plugs may be perivenular or diffuse. Some hydropic change (ballooning) of occasional hepatocytes is also present, but in this case is relatively mild.

TABLE 2–8

Cholestasis, Simple

Acute fatty liver of pregnancy	Heart failure, left-sided without hypotension
Adenoma, liver cell	Heart failure, right-sided
Adjacent to space-occupying lesions	Heat stroke
Alcoholic foamy degeneration	Hepatoblastoma
Allograft, harvesting (preservation) injury	Hepatocellular carcinoma, fibrolamellar type
Amyloidosis	Hepatocellular carcinoma, trabecular, acinar, ductular type
Benign postoperative intrahepatic cholestasis	Hyperpyrexia
Benign recurrent intrahepatic cholestasis	Inspissated bile syndrome
Biliary hamartoma	Nodular regenerative hyperplasia
Budd-Chiari syndrome, acute	Polyarteritis nodosa
Congenital hepatic fibrosis	Progressive familial intrahepatic cholestasis
Crigler-Najjar syndrome	Recurrent cholestasis with lymphedema
Drugs/toxins (refer to Table 4–5)	Recurrent intrahepatic cholestasis of pregnancy
Extrahepatic biliary obstruction, early	Recurrent pyogenic cholangiohepatitis
Focal nodular hyperplasia	Veno-occlusive disease, acute
Heart failure, left-sided with hypotension	

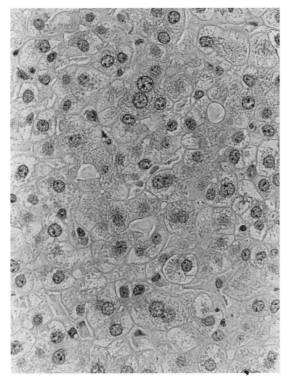

Figure 2–48 Benign Recurrent Intrahepatic Cholestasis Bile plugs are present within dilated canaliculi.

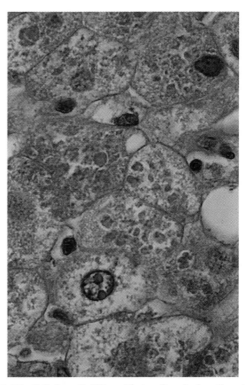

Figure 2–50 Extrahepatic Biliary Obstruction, Early Abundant, coarsely granular to globular intracellular bile can be seen.

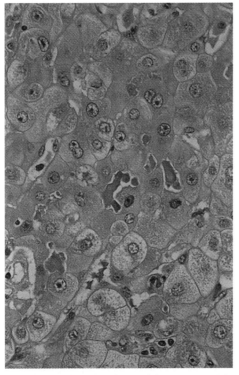

Figure 2–49 Drug-induced (Methimazole) Numerous bile plugs are seen within dilated canaliculi.

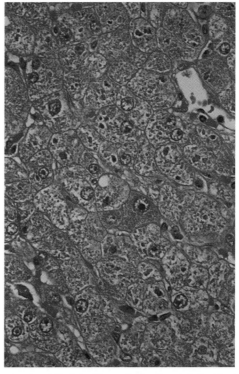

Figure 2–51 Focal Nodular Hyperplasia Intracellular bile is abundant in this example.

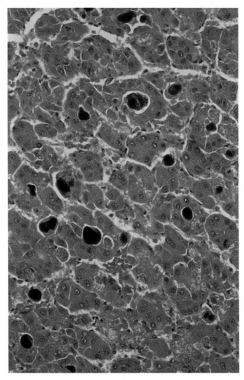

Figure 2–52 Hepatocellular Carcinoma, Trabecular, Acinar Type Bile plugs are present within canalicular (acinar) channels in this well-differentiated neoplasm. Bile is also present within the cytoplasm of many of the tumor cells.

Cysts

Hepatic cysts may be of various sizes, from microscopic (e.g., infantile microcystic disease) to large distinct lesions (e.g., solitary unilocular [nonparasitic] cyst). They generally arise from the biliary system, and can be developmental, secondary to infection, or neoplastic (Table 2–9). The cyst lining is composed of simple cuboidal to flattened duct epithelium, but may also be ciliated or show squamous differentiation. In some instances, however, no distinct lining is visualized in biopsy specimens. The cysts sometimes demonstrate an adjacent fibrous capsule, although in bile duct cystadenomas, mesenchymal differentiation may also be present. The cysts can be incidental findings at autopsy, symptomatic multilocular single cysts, or multiple cysts. It is important to note that some of the cysts have potential for malignant transformation, most notably cystadenomas; therefore, multiple tissue sections from these lesions should be reviewed before final interpretation.

Figures 2–54 to 2–56 demonstrate various examples of hepatic cysts.

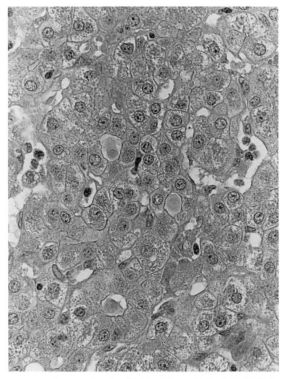

Figure 2–53 Progressive Familial Intrahepatic Cholestasis (Byler's Syndrome) The intracanalicular bile plugs show no inflammatory reaction. In early-stage disease, the bile has a perivenular (zone 3) accentuation; however, bile accumulates predominantly within the periseptal zone in the cirrhotic stage.

TABLE 2–9

Cysts

Lined by Biliary Epithelium	Nonepithelial Lined
Adult polycystic disease	Amebiasis
Caroli's disease	Peliosis hepatis
Choledochal cyst	Pentastomiasis
Ciliated hepatic foregut cyst	Toxoplasmosis (microscopic)
Clonorchiasis	
Cystadenoma with or without mesenchymal stroma	
Fascioliasis	
Hydatid cyst	
Infantile microcystic disease	
Mesenchymal hamartoma	
Recurrent pyogenic cholangiohepatitis	
Solitary nonparasitic cyst	

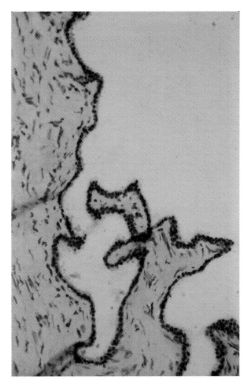

Figure 2–54   Adult Polycystic Disease   This high-power photomicrograph demonstrates the cyst lining composed of simple cuboidal duct epithelium.

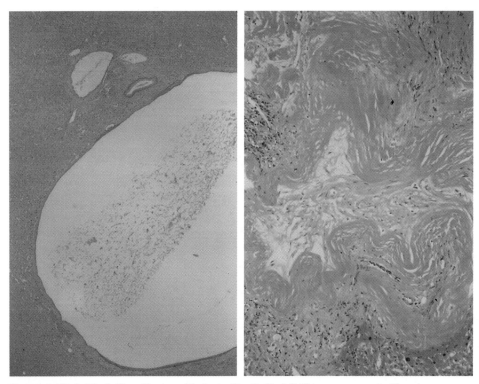

Figures 2–55, 2–56   Solitary Nonparasitic Cyst   (Fig. 2–55, *left*) This cyst was an incidental finding at autopsy, and is present immediately adjacent to a portal tract. (Fig. 2–56, *right*) The cysts may collapse, whereby the center becomes fibrotic. Eventually, these lesions resemble a small scar.

Diagnostic Lesions

Table 2–10 lists various liver diseases that are diagnostic either by routine histologic examination or use of special histochemical or immunoperoxidase stains. In instances in which the hematoxylin-eosin stain alone is not diagnostic (e.g., acute hepatitis suspicious for viral etiology), correlation with laboratory tests (e.g., hepatitis B surface antigen [HBsAg]–positive, anti-delta IgM–positive) should lead to further histologic evaluation for *diagnostic* interpretation (e.g., immunoperoxidase stains negative for HBsAg but positive for delta antigen leading to a diagnosis of acute viral hepatitis type B plus delta).

Figures 2–57 through 2–77 show various examples of diagnostic lesions.

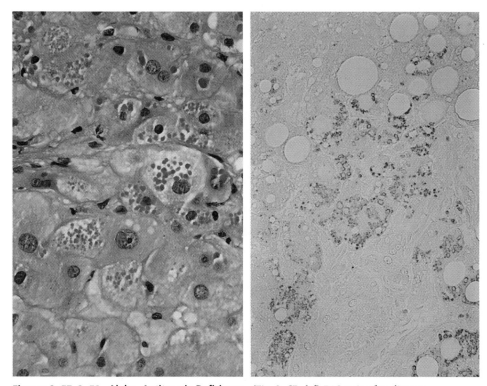

Figures 2–57, 2–58 Alpha₁-Antitrypsin Deficiency (Fig. 2–57, *left*) PAS stain after diastase digestion shows numerous discrete cytoplasmic inclusions in periportal hepatocytes. (Fig. 2–58, *right*) These inclusions can be confirmed as alpha₁-antitrypsin deposits on immunoperoxidase stain. Note that some of the larger globules in the center of the field have peripheral staining with central sparing, characteristic of alpha₁-antitrypsin bodies.

TABLE 2-10
Diagnostic Lesions

Disease	Diagnostic Features
Alpha$_1$-antitrypsin deficiency	Numerous small round eosinophilic cytoplasmic inclusions in periportal or periseptal hepatocytes that are PAS-positive after diastase digestion, confirmed on immunoperoxidase stain as alpha$_1$-antitrypsin inclusions
Amyloidosis	Sinusoidal, portal, vascular deposits of amorphous linear or globular acellular material, Congo red–positive with apple-green birefringence on polarized light
Angiomyolipoma	Intermixed smooth muscle, vascular spaces, fat, and hematopoietic elements within a distinct mass lesion
Angiosarcoma	Anaplastic endothelial cells lining markedly dilated sinusoids, these cells containing factor VIII–associated antigen confirmed by immunoperoxidase stain
Biliary hamartoma	Ectatic benign duct elements sometimes containing bile, embedded within a fibrous stroma, forming relatively small distinct lesions
Cavernous hemangioma	Fibrous honeycombed network of dilated vascular channels often containing red blood cells, these channels lined by benign endothelial cells
Clonorchiasis	Parasites (liver flukes) within large dilated ducts with prominent adjacent ductular hyperplasia
Coccidioidomycosis	Epithelioid granulomas containing spherules 20 to 200 μm in diameter (positive on methenamine silver stain) with endospores (2 to 5 μm) or granular eosinophilic material
Cystadenoma with mesenchymal stroma	Cyst lined by cuboidal epithelium with underlying cellular spindle cell elements
Cystinosis	Kupffer cells and portal macrophages containing hexagonal to cylindrical cystine crystals that under polarized light are brightly silver and birefringent
Cytomegalovirus infection (immunocompromised patient)	Distinct large basophilic nuclear inclusions within hepatocytes, Kupffer cells, and duct epithelium; sometimes smaller cytoplasmic inclusions are seen; confirmed on immunoperoxidase stain
Epithelioid hemangioepithelioma	Dendritic and epithelial neoplastic components, confirmed on immunoperoxidase stain as containing factor VIII–associated antigen
Erythropoietic protoporphyria	Dark brown pigment (protoporphyrin) in hepatocytes, bile ducts, and Kupffer cells, with intense red autofluorescence on frozen section
Fibrinogen storage disease	Round to oval eosinophilic PTAH-positive globules within hepatocytes
Focal nodular hyperplasia	Central fibrous scars containing lymphocytes and lined by atypical ducts in a distinct mass lesion
Hepatoblastoma	Mixed trabecular and stromal malignant neoplastic components in a primary hepatic mass lesion
Hepatocellular carcinoma, fibrolamellar	Large eosinophilic polygonal cells sometimes containing cytoplasmic inclusions ("pale bodies"), the cells surrounded by acellular fibrous parallel bands
Hepatocellular carcinoma, trabecular type	Hepatocytes with increased nuclear-cytoplasmic ratio forming cords greater than two cells thick, the cords lined by endothelial cells
Herpes simplex virus infection	Distinct intranuclear inclusions that are eosinophilic with peripheral halo, or basophilic with peripheral chromatin rim, confirmed on immunoperoxidase stain
Hydatid cyst (*Echinococcus* species)	Hyalinized laminated membrane with attached protoscolices
Lymphoma, Hodgkin's	Mixed cellular infiltrates containing Reed-Sternberg cells
Malaria (*Plasmodium falciparum*)	Dark brown pigment (hemozoin) in hypertrophic Kupffer cells along with parasitized circulating red blood cells
Pneumocystis carinii infection	Frothy eosinophilic exudative material that on methenamine silver stain demonstrates oval or cup-shaped cysts
Porphyria cutanea tarda	Needle-shaped birefringent cytoplasmic inclusions (uroporphyrin) within hepatocytes, with intense red autofluorescence on frozen section
Schistosomiasis	Characteristic eggs with or without a granulomatous reaction, the eggs sometimes calcified
Syphilis, congenital	Focal lobular necrosis containing abundant spirochetes demonstrated by Warthin-Starry stain
Viral hepatitis	
Acute, type B + delta	Delta antigen demonstrated on immunoperoxidase stain within liver cell nuclei; HBsAg, HBcAg not present; associated histologic changes of acute viral hepatitis
Chronic, type B	"Ground-glass" hepatocytes that are positive on orcein stain, confirmed as HBsAg on immunoperoxidase stain; HBcAg may be present within nuclei on immunoperoxidase stain; delta antigen not present; associated histologic changes of chronic viral hepatitis
Chronic, type B + delta	"Ground-glass" hepatocytes that are positive on orcein stain, confirmed as HBsAg on immunoperoxidase stain; delta antigen within liver cell nuclei (usually HBcAg-negative) on immunoperoxidase stain; associated histologic changes of chronic viral hepatitis

HBcAg = Hepatitis B core antigen; HBsAg = hepatitis B surface antigen; PAS = periodic acid–Schiff stain; PTAH = phosphotungstic acid–hematoxylin stain.

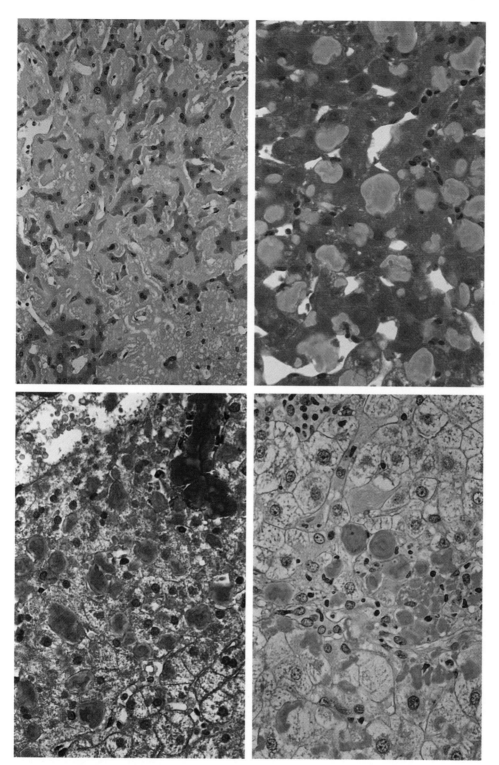

Figures 2–59 to 2–62 Amyloidosis   (Fig. 2–59, *upper left*) Acellular amorphous eosinophilic material is seen within the space of Disse and sinusoids (*sinusoidal amyloid*), compressing the adjacent hepatocytes. (Fig. 2–60, *upper right*) Amyloid also may form round to
oval discrete inclusions (*globular amyloid*) within the sinusoids (seen in this photomicrograph) and portal tracts. (Fig. 2–61, *lower left*) Amyloid nicely stands out on trichrome stain,
as these well-demarcated sinusoidal globules demonstrate. (Fig. 2–62, *lower right*) Both
sinusoidal and globular amyloid can be confirmed by positive Congo red staining, as seen in
this example. Apple-green birefringence of these Congo red–positive deposits under polarized light is diagnostic. Immunohistochemical staining for amyloid P component is also
helpful.

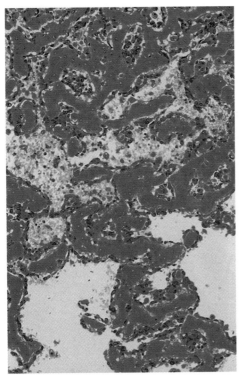

Figure 2–63   Angiosarcoma   The dilated sinusoids are lined by multilayered malignant endothelial cells. These cells can be confirmed as having an endothelial origin by positive immunoperoxidase staining for factor VIII–associated antigen.

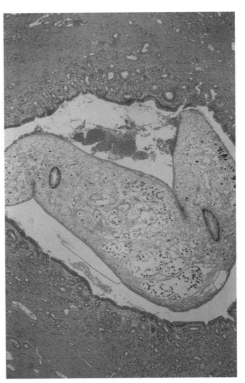

Figure 2–65   Clonorchiasis   The liver fluke (*Clonorchis sinensis*) is present within a major intrahepatic bile duct. Note that prominent adjacent ductular proliferation ("adenomatous ductular hyperplasia") is characteristically seen in this disorder.

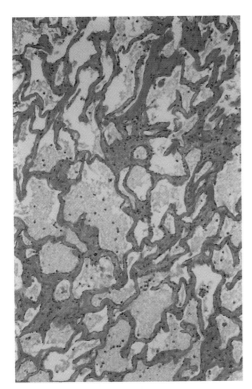

Figure 2–64   Cavernous Hemangioma   Dilated vascular spaces are lined by flattened single-layered endothelial cells, with variable degrees of interstitial fibrosis between the vascular spaces.

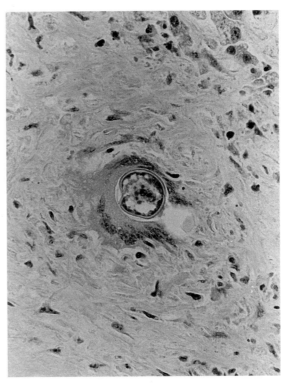

Figure 2–66   Coccidioidomycosis   A large spherule with a thickened wall is seen within a multinucleated giant cell. These spherules contain numerous *Coccidioides immitis* endospores.

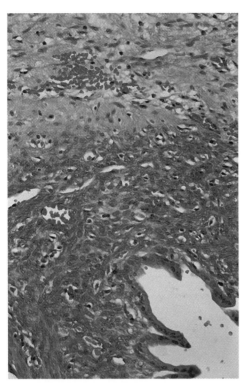

Figure 2–67 Cystadenoma with Mesenchymal Stroma The cyst lining is composed of cuboidal to slightly columnar benign duct epithelium. The underlying stroma is composed of cellular spindle (mesenchymal) cells. Malignant transformation of the duct epithelium may occur in up to 25% of cases.

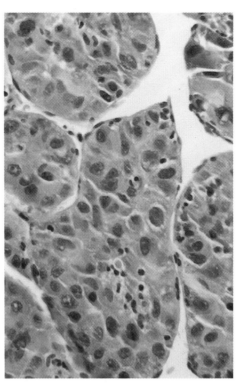

Figure 2–69 Hepatocellular Carcinoma, Trabecular Type Hepatocytes having hyperchromatic nuclei and increased nuclear-cytoplasmic ratio are seen forming thickened trabecular cords lined by flattened endothelial cells.

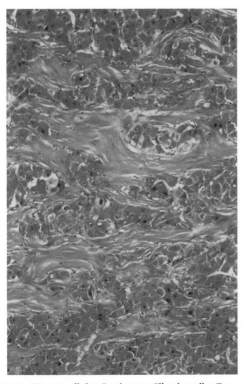

Figure 2–68 Hepatocellular Carcinoma, Fibrolamellar Type Large eosinophilic tumor cells are present with interspersed fibrous bands laid down in a parallel (fibrolamellar) fashion.

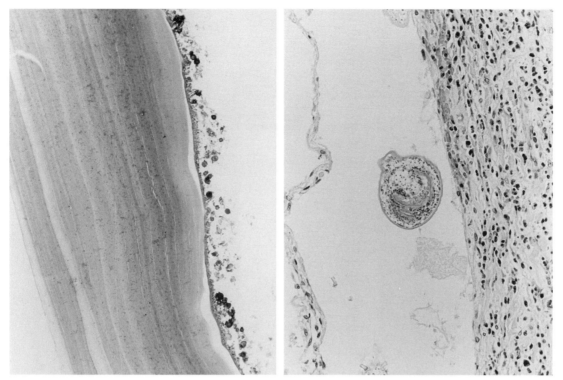

Figures 2–70, 2–71 Hydatid Cyst (Fig. 2–70, *left*) The acellular laminated membrane is characteristic for hydatid cyst. In this example, focal areas of calcification are also seen along the inner germinal membrane. (Fig. 2–71, *right*) High power adjacent to the inflamed cyst wall demonstrates an *Echinococcus* protoscolex with a refractile hooklet.

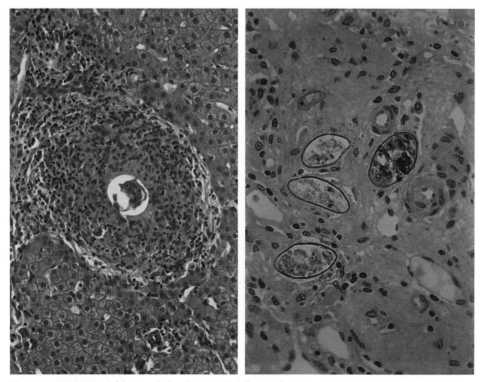

Figures 2–72, 2–73 Schistosomiasis (Fig. 2–72, *left*) A well-demarcated granuloma in a patient with early-stage disease is present within a portal tract, the granuloma consisting of lymphocytes and macrophages with a central schistosome ova (*Schistosoma mansoni*). (Fig. 2–73, *right*) In older lesions of schistosomiasis, the dead eggs are often partially calcified and do not usually elicit an inflammatory response; however, variable degrees of portal fibrosis are often present surrounding these ova.

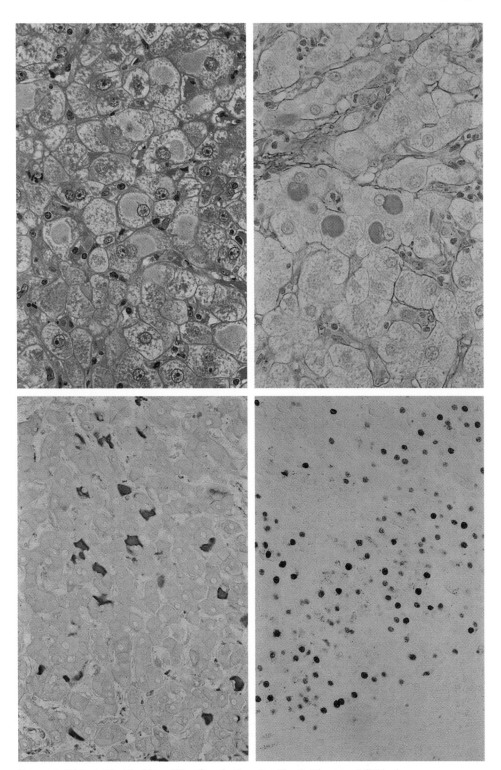

Figures 2–74 to 2–77 Viral Hepatitis, Chronic, Type B (Fig. 2–74, *upper left*) The hematoxylin-eosin (H & E) stain shows discrete intracytoplasmic inclusions having a finely granular "ground-glass" appearance, with peripheral cytoplasmic clearing. This staining characteristic represents proliferation of the smooth endoplasmic reticulin synthesizing the hepatitis B surface antigen (HBsAg) particles. (Fig. 2–75, *upper right*) The ground-glass cells themselves are not diagnostic of HBsAg inclusions on H & E stain alone; however, positive staining of these inclusions with orcein stain is diagnostic of HBsAg, and is demonstrated in this photomicrograph. (Fig. 2–76, *lower left*) The ground-glass cells can also be confirmed as HBsAg particles with immunoperoxidase stain for the surface antigen, which shows strong cytoplasmic but not nuclear uptake. (Fig. 2–77, *lower right*) Positive nuclear staining for hepatitis B core antigen (HBcAg) on immunoperoxidase stain is often seen when there is active viral replication.

Extracellular Deposits

(Not Collagen)

Although the most common extracellular (sinusoidal) deposit is collagen (refer to Table 2–29, Sinusoids: Fibrosis), a variety of liver diseases also exhibit histologically similar substances on examination of biopsies by routine hematoxylin-eosin stain (Table 2–11). Some of the deposits form globules (e.g., eosinophilic hyaline globules in perivenular sinusoids in heart failure) while others form dense bands that may fill the entire sinusoid (e.g., typical amyloid). Special stains are often helpful in better identifying these substances. Note that Mallory bodies may also be seen in an extracellular location in instances in which the liver cell originally containing the Mallory body is damaged.

Figures 2–78 to 2–80 demonstrate various examples of extracellular (non-collagen) deposits.

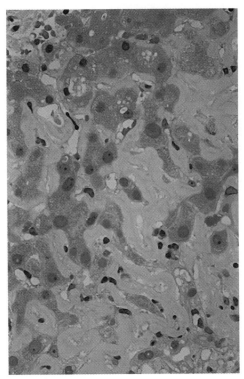

Figure 2–78 Amyloidosis The amyloid is deposited within the sinusoidal space of Disse, often compressing the adjacent hepatic cords.

TABLE 2–11

Extracellular Deposits (Not Collagen)

	Substance (Helpful Special Stain)
Acute fatty liver of pregnancy	Fibrin located within the sinusoids (PTAH-positive)
Amyloidosis	Amyloid within the sinusoids, portal tracts, and vessels (Congo red–positive)
Heart failure, left-sided with hypotension	Eosinophilic hyaline globules within the perivenular sinusoids
Heart failure, right-sided	Eosinophilic hyaline globules within the perivenular sinusoids
Hemolysis, elevation of liver enzymes, low platelet (HELLP) syndrome	Fibrin located within the sinusoids (PTAH-positive)
Light chain disease	Eosinophilic deposits within sinusoids and portal tracts (DiPAS-positive; light chains confirmed on immunoperoxidase stain)
Mallory bodies (associated diseases)	(Refer to Table 2–19, Mallory Bodies)
Multiple myeloma	Amyloid within sinusoids, portal tracts, and vessels (Congo red-positive)
Q fever	Granuloma with a central vacuole surrounded by a fibrin ring (PTAH-positive)
Sickle cell anemia	Fibrin within sinusoids admixed with clumped red blood (sickle) cells (PTAH-positive)
Toxemia of pregnancy	Fibrin within sinusoids and portal veins (PTAH-positive)
Waldenström's macroglobulinemia	Amyloid within sinusoids, portal tracts, and vessels (Congo red–positive) Nonamyloid deposits within sinusoids (confirmed as light chains on immunoperoxidase stain)

DiPAS = periodic acid–Schiff–positive after diastase digestion; PTAH = phosphotungstic acid–hematoxylin stain.

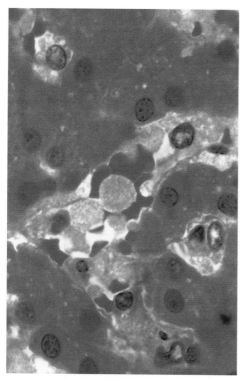

Figure 2–79 Heart Failure, Right-sided, and Left-sided with Hypotension Eosinophilic acellular globules can be seen within the sinusoids, and most likely represent cytoplasmic extrusions from damaged hepatocytes.

Fatty Change

Fat accumulation in hepatocytes (*steatosis*) appears as round, well-circumscribed clear spaces within the cytoplasm. Although fat cannot be directly demonstrated on hematoxylin-eosin stain after routine processing, Oil Red O stain on frozen sections sharply demonstrates the lipid. Fat is predominantly composed of neutral triglycerides. Its classification in the liver can be subdivided into *macrovesicular* (fat globules equal to or greater than the size of the liver cell nucleus) and *microvesicular* (fat globules smaller than the liver cell nucleus). Often both macrovesicular and microvesicular fat can be seen within the same cell, although usually one type predominates. In some instances, the fat deposition may have a zonal distribution (e.g., perivenular [zone 3] in alcoholic liver disease), while in others the fat is randomly distributed throughout all zones (e.g., nonalcoholic steatohepatitis). A subdivision of microvesicular fat includes *foamy change,* although on hematoxylin-eosin stain the small fat droplets may not be appreciated (the cells may appear hydropic). Table 2–12 lists liver diseases associated with fatty change, and denotes whether the fat accumulation is significant (>50% of liver cells involved) or modest (≤50% of liver cells involved). In addition, Table 2–12 shows whether the fatty change that is present is predominantly macrovesicular or microvesicular, or whether both types are equally present. Although many of the liver diseases have associated inflammation (e.g., neutrophils in acute sclerosing hyaline necrosis, lymphocytes in chronic viral hepatitis type C), Table 2–12 relates only to the fatty change. For liver diseases associated with inflammation, refer to Table 2–16, Lobular Necrosis with Inflammation.

Figures 2–81 through 2–93 demonstrate disorders associated with fatty change.

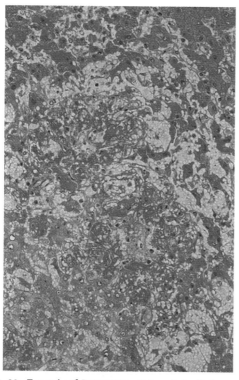

Figure 2–80 Toxemia of Pregnancy Extracellular fibrin can be seen among ischemically damaged liver cells.

TABLE 2–12

Fatty Change

Disorders Associated with Prominent Fatty Change (>50% of Liver Cells Involved)

	Macrovesicular	Microvesicular		Macrovesicular	Microvesicular
Abetalipoproteinemia	++	+	Heat stroke		++
Acute fatty liver, alcoholic etiology	++		Hereditary fructose intolerance	++	+
Acute fatty liver of pregnancy	+	++	Homocystinuria	++	
Acute sclerosing hyaline necrosis (acute alcoholic hepatitis)	++	+	Hyperpyrexia		++
Alcoholic cirrhosis (active drinker)	++		Kwashiorkor (early stage)		++
Alcoholic fatty liver	++		Kwashiorkor (later stage)	++	
Alcoholic foamy degeneration	+	++	Long/medium chain acyl-CoA dehydrogenase deficiency	++	+
Alpers' disease		++	Nonalcoholic steatohepatitis	++	+
Cholesterol ester storage disease	+	++	Perivenular fibrosis, alcoholic etiology	++	
Drugs/toxins*			Progressive perivenular alcoholic fibrosis	++	
Focal fatty change	++		Q fever	++	
Galactosemia	+	+	Reye's syndrome		++
Glycogen storage disease types I, II, and VI	++		Systemic carnitine deficiency	++	+
			Weber-Christian disease	++	
			Wolman's disease	+	++

Disorders Associated with Moderate Fatty Change (≤50% of Liver Cells Involved)

	Macrovesicular	Microvesicular		Macrovesicular	Microvesicular
Adenoma, liver cell	++		Leishmaniasis	++	
Adenomatous hyperplasia	++		Lyme disease		++
Alpha$_1$-antitrypsin deficiency	++		Lymphoma, Hodgkin's	++	
Amebiasis	++		Malaria	++	
Bacterial sepsis	++	+	Mannosidosis		++
Budd-Chiari syndrome, acute	+	+	Marasmus	++	
Chronic granulomatous disease of childhood	++		Nonspecific reactive hepatitis	++	
Crohn's disease	++		Polymyalgia rheumatica	++	
Cystic fibrosis	++	+	Porphyria cutanea tarda	++	
Cytomegalovirus infection	++	+	Primary sclerosing cholangitis	++	
Drugs/toxins*			Rheumatoid arthritis	++	
Epstein-Barr virus infection	++	+	Rubeola virus infection	++	+
Focal nodular hyperplasia	++		Salmonellosis		++
Hemochromatosis	++		Sickle cell anemia	++	
Hemolysis, elevation of liver enzymes, low platelet (HELLP) syndrome	++		Systemic lupus erythematosus	++	
Hepatocellular carcinoma, trabecular, acinar, ductular type	++	+	Toxic shock syndrome		++
Human immunodeficiency virus infection	+	+	Tuberculosis	++	
Hyperalimentation, adult	++		Tyrosinemia	++	
Hyperthyroidism	++		Ulcerative colitis	++	
Indian childhood cirrhosis (early stage)	++	+	Viral hepatitis, acute, type B + delta		++
			Viral hepatitis, chronic, type B + delta		++
			Viral hepatitis, chronic, type C	++	
			Wilson's disease	++	+
			Yellow fever		++

*Drugs and toxins that produce both prominent and moderate fatty change are listed together (refer to Table 4–10) but are subdivided in that table into macrovesicular versus microvesicular fat.

+ = Occasional type of fat seen; ++ = predominant type of fat seen; CoA = coenzyme A.

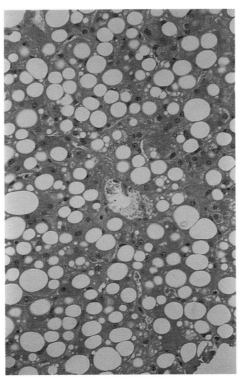

Figure 2–81 Alcoholic Fatty Liver The majority of hepatocytes show a macrovesicular fatty change in an active alcoholic.

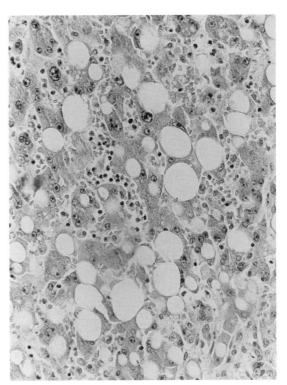

Figure 2–83 Bacterial Sepsis Macrovesicular fatty change is usually seen. The numerous neutrophils present within the sinusoids correspond to the patient's leukocytosis.

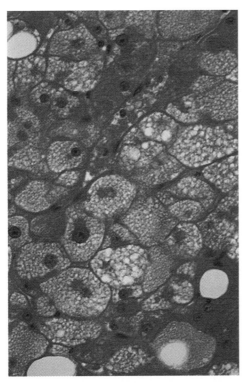

Figure 2–82 Alcoholic Foamy Degeneration The hepatocytes show abundant microvesicular fat, and have a characteristic "foamy" appearance.

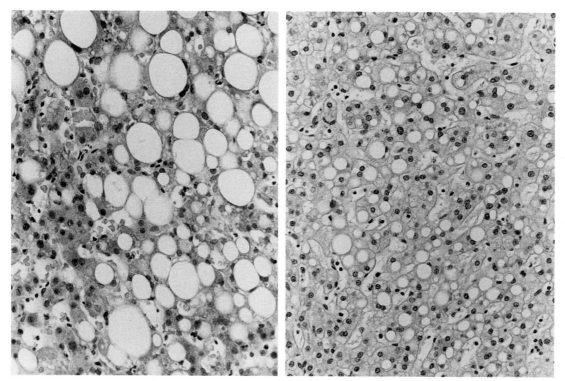

Figures 2–84, 2–85 Crohn's Disease *(left).* **Ulcerative Colitis** *(right).* Both of these variants of inflammatory bowel disease may demonstrate a macrovesicular fatty change.

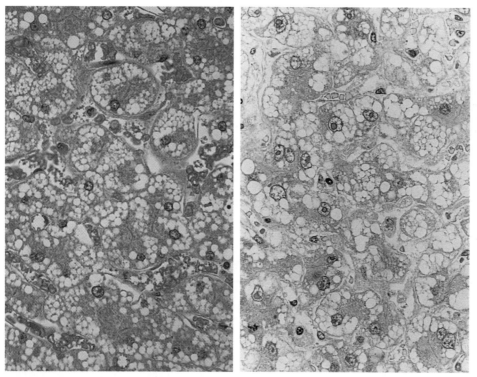

Figures 2–86, 2–87 Drug-induced Fatty Change (Tetracycline and Cocaine) (Fig. 2–86, *left*) Tetracycline, when given intravenously, may demonstrate a diffuse microvesicular fatty change. (Fig. 2–87, *right*) Cocaine hepatotoxicity may show a predominantly periportal fatty change, the fat usually microvesicular, although macrovesicular fat is also present in this photomicrograph.

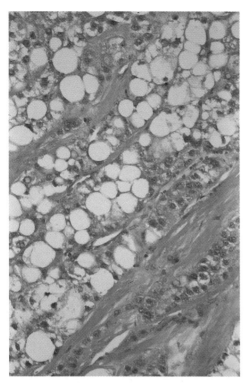

Figure 2–88 Hepatocellular Carcinoma, Trabecular, Acinar, Ductular Type Well-differentiated tumors may show fatty change, which is usually macrovesicular.

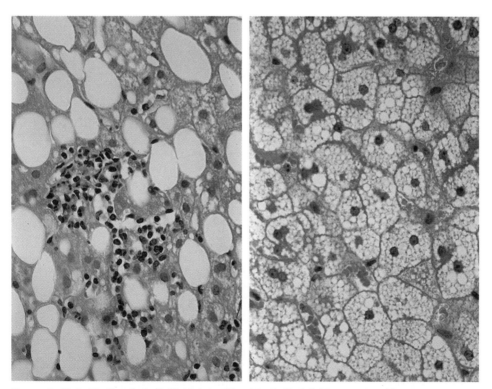

Figures 2–89, 2–90 Nonalcoholic Steatohepatitis (Fig. 2–89, *left*) The majority of liver cells show a macrovesicular fatty change associated with variable degrees of necroinflammatory change. (Fig. 2–90, *right*) Microvesicular fat may also be present, and when seen is usually focal. Inflammation is not present in this photomicrograph, but was identified in other fields.

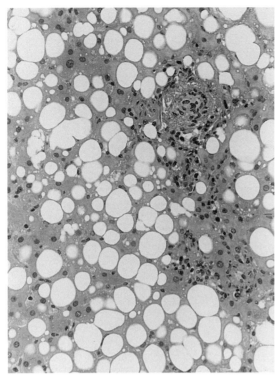

Figure 2–91 Q Fever Fatty change is usually seen. A characteristic fibrin-ring granuloma is present toward the upper field.

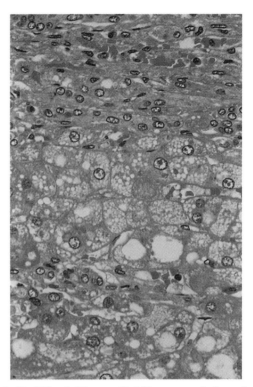

Figure 2–93 Wilson's Disease Variable macrovesicular and occasional microvesicular fat is seen.

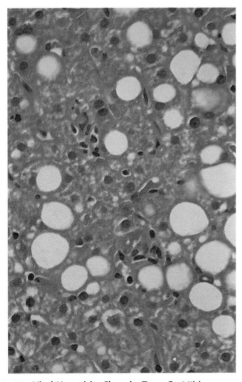

Figure 2–92 Viral Hepatitis, Chronic, Type C Mild macrovesicular fatty change is usually present.

Granulomas

Granulomas are loosely defined as collections of inflammatory cells (Table 2–13). *Epithelioid* granulomas are well defined and are composed of a variable number of lymphocytes, occasional plasma cells, and prominent numbers of activated macrophages that have round to indented clear nuclei and abundant eosinophilic cytoplasm (*epithelioid cells*). Multinucleated giant cells are often but not always seen. *Inflammatory* granulomas are usually smaller than the epithelioid type, and are composed of a mixed inflammatory infiltrate consisting of lymphocytes, macrophages, and occasional plasma cells, neutrophils, and eosinophils. These granulomas may or may not be poorly defined. Although occasional multinucleated giant cells can be seen, they are much less frequent than in the epithelioid granulomas. A combination of both epithelioid and inflammatory granulomas may be seen within the same biopsy specimen. Granulomas may occur anywhere within the liver. Although in some instances they may be more prominent within the portal tracts (e.g., primary biliary cirrhosis), in other disorders they are seen more commonly within the lobules (e.g., drug induced); however, many liver disorders (such as primary biliary cirrhosis) may demonstrate granulomas within the portal tracts and lobules. Some granulomas have unusual histologic features very characteristic of one disease entity (e.g., schistosomiasis with pipestem granuloma having a central schistosome ova). Special stains may at times be helpful (e.g., Ziehl-Neelsen or periodic acid–Schiff [PAS] in *Mycobacterium avium-intracellulare* infection), although in immunocompetent patients, granulomas secondary to an infectious process (especially mycobacteria) are more often negative on special stains. In addition, some liver diseases may exhibit granulomas that coalesce (e.g., sarcoidosis), forming distinct mass lesions that may be visualized on imaging (refer to Table 2–20, Mass Lesions, Benign).

Figures 2–94 through 2–109 demonstrate examples of granulomas in various diseases.

TABLE 2–13

Granulomas

Actinomycosis	Leprosy
Adenoma, liver cell	Leukemia, hairy cell
Alcoholic fatty liver	Listeriosis
Ascariasis	Lymphoma, Hodgkin's and
Bacterial sepsis	non-Hodgkin's
Blastomycosis	Melioidosis
Boutonneuse fever	Mucolipidosis II
Brucellosis	*Mycobacterium avium-intra-*
Candidiasis	*cellulare* infection
Capillariasis	Nocardiosis
Cat-scratch disease	Nonalcoholic steatohepatitis
Chronic granulomatous	(secondary to jejunoileal
disease of childhood	bypass)
Coccidioidomycosis	Nonspecific reactive hepatitis
Crohn's disease	Paracoccidioidomycosis
Cryptococcosis	Penicilliosis
Cytomegalovirus infection	Polyarteritis nodosa
Drugs/toxins*	Polymyalgia rheumatica
Enterobiasis	Primary biliary cirrhosis
Eosinophilic gastroenteritis	Q fever
Epstein-Barr virus infection	Rheumatoid arthritis
Farber's lipogranulomatosis	Salmonellosis
Fascioliasis	Sarcoidosis
Foreign body giant cell re-	Schistosomiasis
action†	Strongyloidiasis
Hepatocellular carcinoma,	Syphilis, congenital, second-
fibrolamellar type	ary and tertiary
Histoplasmosis	Systemic lupus erythemato-
Hydatid cyst	sus
Idiopathic granulomatous	Toxoplasmosis
hepatitis	Tuberculosis
Inflammatory pseudotumor	Visceral larva migrans
Langerhans' cell histiocyto-	Whipple's disease
sis	Zygomycosis
Leishmaniasis	

*For drugs and toxins causing granulomas, refer to Table 4–15.

†Foreign body giant cell granulomas are most frequently seen in patients who have had previous hepatobiliary surgery. Although intravenous drug users may have polarizable talc-like injectant within portal tracts, this foreign material seldom elicits a giant cell reaction. Foreign body granulomas are not included in Chapter 3, Liver Diseases: Pathology and Clinical Considerations.

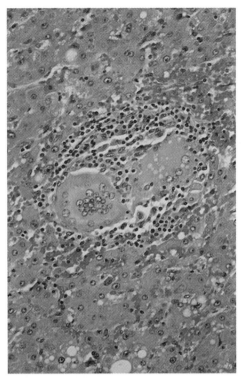

Figure 2–94   Adenoma, Liver Cell   Although uncommon, small granulomas sometimes containing multinucleated giant cells may be seen within the tumor.

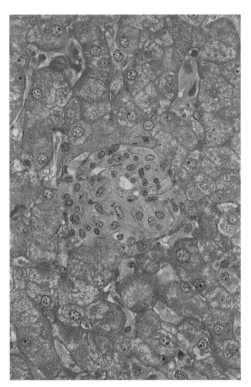

Figure 2–96   Brucellosis   The granulomas are composed of lymphocytes and histiocytes without a giant cell reaction.

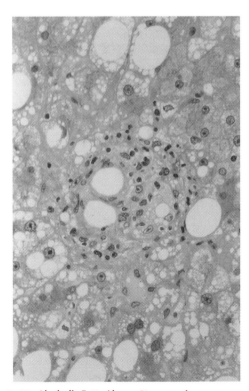

Figure 2–95   Alcoholic Fatty Liver   *Lipogranulomas* composed of histiocytes containing lipid are sometimes seen.

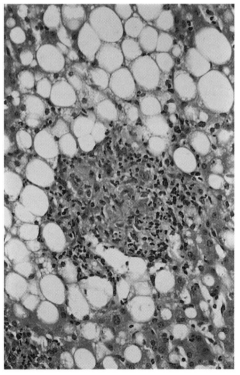

Figure 2–97   Crohn's Disease   The granulomas are well demarcated and may or may not elicit a giant cell reaction.

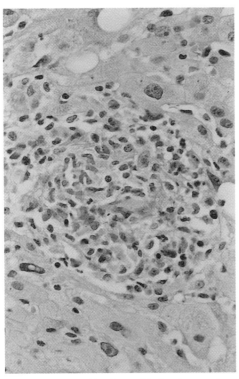

Figure 2–98 Drug-induced (Sulfonamides) The granulomas are poorly defined, and exhibit a mixed inflammatory infiltrate. Multinucleated giant cells may be seen, but are not frequent, and are not present in this example.

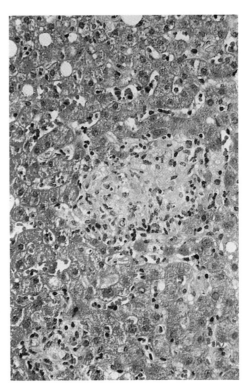

Figure 2–100 Leishmaniasis Well- to poorly-formed granulomas can be seen within the lobules.

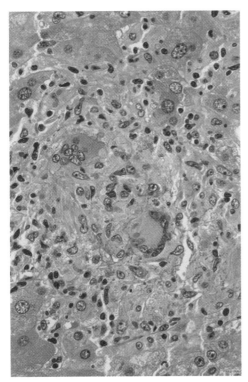

Figure 2–99 Histoplasmosis The granulomas are composed of histiocytes and multinucleated cells containing the microorganisms, which are best demonstrated by methenamine silver stain.

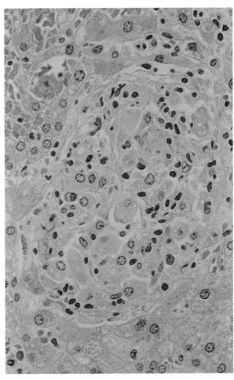

Figure 2–101 Leprosy This well-circumscribed granuloma is composed of numerous epithelioid cells.

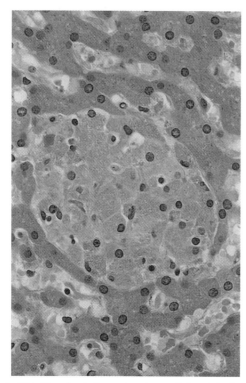

Figure 2–102 *Mycobacterium avium intracellulare* **Infection** The granulomas in immunocompromised patients, particularly those with AIDS, show clusters of histiocytes without lymphocytic or giant cell reaction. These granulomas also contain abundant organisms on acid-fast stain.

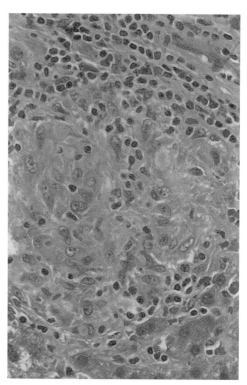

Figure 2–104 **Primary Biliary Cirrhosis** The granulomas are often seen within portal tracts but may also be present within the lobules.

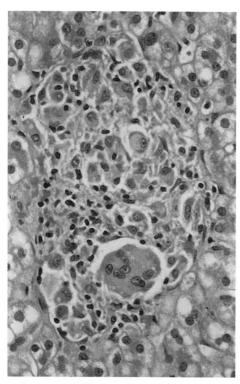

Figure 2–103 **Nonalcoholic Steatohepatitis (Status Post Jejunoileal Bypass)** In approximately 7% of cases, epithelioid granulomas may be seen within the lobules.

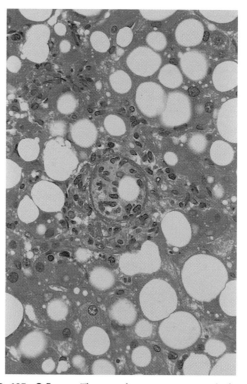

Figure 2–105 **Q Fever** The granulomas are composed of mixed inflammatory cells with a central empty space resembling fat, with a rim of fibrin ("doughnut" lesion).

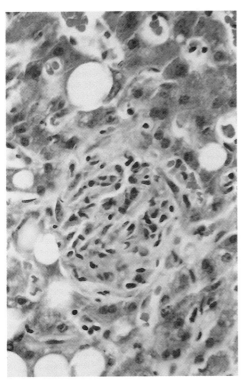

Figure 2–106 Salmonellosis The granulomas are composed of clusters of mixed inflammatory cells without giant cell reaction.

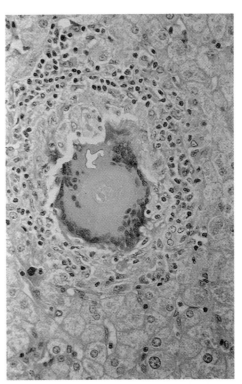

Figure 2–108 Schistosomiasis In early-stage disease, the organisms (not seen in this photomicrograph) may elicit a granulomatous response, sometimes with multinucleated giant cells.

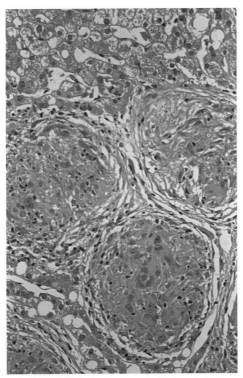

Figure 2–107 Sarcoidosis The well-circumscribed granulomas frequently show a perigranulomatous fibrous reaction. These clusters of granulomas often form by fibrous subdivision of a larger single granuloma.

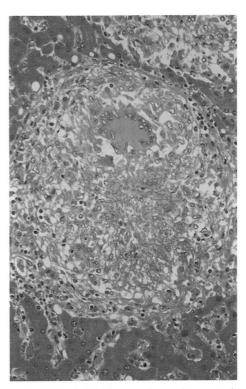

Figure 2–109 Tuberculosis The granulomas show central caseous necrosis with multinucleated giant cell reaction.

Inclusions

Hepatocytes

Inclusions within liver cells may be subdivided into *nuclear* and *cytoplasmic* (Table 2–14). The inclusions may be seen as single, well-demarcated, round cytoplasmic globules (e.g., megamitochondria in acute fatty liver, alcoholic etiology) or may be numerous within the same cell (e.g., alpha$_1$-antitrypsin globules in periportal hepatocytes). Inclusions may also diffusely involve the cytoplasm and have a finely granular to smooth appearance ("ground glass–like"). Special stains can at times be helpful in classifying the etiology of the inclusions (e.g., orcein stain identifying the HBsAg particles of the "ground-glass" cells in chronic hepatitis B virus [HBV] infection). *Glycogenated nuclei* are enlarged liver cell nuclei that are clear on hematoxylin-eosin stain, the glycogen best demonstrated on PAS stain using frozen section material. Although hepatocytes containing these nuclei tend to be periportal, in some liver diseases (e.g., Wilson's disease) they may be focal or diffuse. A Mallory body is a specific type of cytoplasmic inclusion that is discussed and demonstrated separately (refer to Table 2–19).

Figures 2–110 through 2–121 demonstrate examples of nuclear and cytoplasmic inclusions.

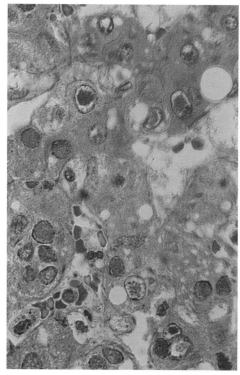

Figure 2–111 Herpes Simplex Infection The nuclear inclusions may be seen as (1) large and eosinophilic, with a peripheral halo (Cowdry type A), and (2) basophilic, taking up the entire nucleus, with a peripheral rim of chromatin (Cowdry type B).

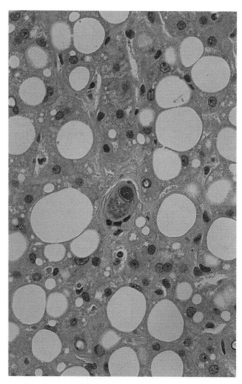

Figure 2–110 Cytomegalovirus Infection Discrete large nuclear inclusions are characteristic of cytomegalovirus infection in the immunocompromised patient; finely to coarsely granular cytoplasmic inclusions may also be seen. Both types of inclusions in a liver cell are shown in this photomicrograph.

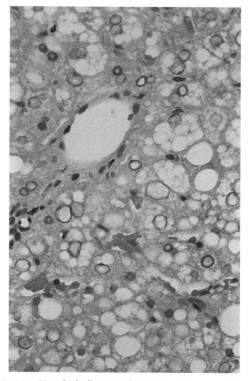

Figure 2–112 Nonalcoholic Steatohepatitis Glycogenated nuclei are seen within periportal hepatocytes.

TABLE 2–14

Hepatocytes, Inclusions

Nuclear Inclusions

Viral	Glycogenated
Adenovirus infection	Glycogen storage disease types I, III, and VI
Cytomegalovirus infection (immunocompromised host)*	Hemochromatosis
Drugs/toxins (viral-like)†	Hepatocellular carcinoma, trabecular, acinar, ductular type
Herpes simplex virus infection	Nonalcoholic steatohepatitis
Herpes zoster virus infection	Viral hepatitis, chronic, type C
Rubeola virus infection	Wilson's disease
Yellow fever	

Cytoplasmic Inclusions

	Type of Inclusion
Acute fatty liver, alcoholic etiology	Megamitochondria‡
Acute fatty liver of pregnancy	Megamitochondria‡
Acute sclerosing hyaline necrosis (acute alcoholic hepatitis)	Megamitochondria‡
Alcoholic cirrhosis	Packed mitochondria (oncocytes)
Alcoholic foamy degeneration	Megamitochondria‡
Alpha$_1$-antichymotrypsin deficiency	Eosinophilic globules (alpha$_1$-antichymotrypsin)
Alpha$_1$-antitrypsin deficiency*	Eosinophilic globules (alpha$_1$-antitrypsin)
Cytomegalovirus infection (immunocompromised host)*	Cytoplasmic and/or nuclear viral inclusions
Drugs/toxins†	"Ground-glass"–like appearance
Fibrinogen storage disease (fibrinogen)	Eosinophilic globules
Glycogen storage disease type IV	Amylopectin-like material
Heart failure, left-sided with hypotension	Eosinophilic globules
Heart failure, right-sided	Eosinophilic globules
Hepatocellular carcinoma, fibrolamellar type	Pale bodies; DiPAS-positive inclusions
Hepatocellular carcinoma, trabecular, acinar, ductular type	DiPAS-positive inclusions; fibrinogen
Mannosidosis	PAS-negative vacuoles
Metachromatic leukodystrophy*	Metachromatic granules
Mucopolysaccharidoses*	Vacuolated cytoplasm
Myoclonus epilepsy	Mucopolysaccharide inclusions
Nonalcoholic steatohepatitis	Megamitochondria‡
Porphyria cutanea tarda	Needle-shaped birefringent
Reye's syndrome	Irregular eosinophilic (distorted mitochondria)
Viral hepatitis, chronic, classic type	Packed mitochondria (oncocytes)
Viral hepatitis, chronic, type B	"Ground-glass" (HBsAg particles)

* Inclusions may also be present in bile duct epithelium.
† Refer to Table 4–17 for hepatocyte inclusions caused by drugs and toxins.
‡ The megamitochondria that are round and discrete are characteristic of alcoholic liver disease; however, thin spindle-shaped mitochondria can be seen in both alcoholic and nonalcoholic liver diseases.

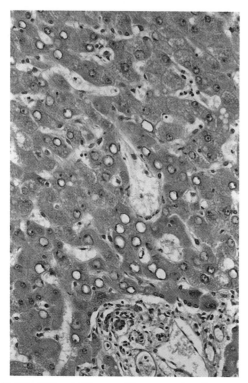

Figure 2–113   Wilson's Disease   Glycogenated nuclei may be seen diffusely or in clusters.

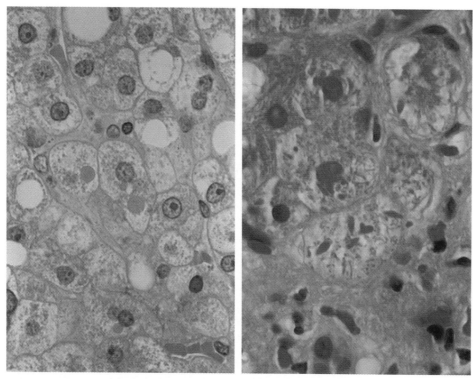

Figures 2–114, 2–115   Alcoholic Fatty Liver   (Fig. 2–114, *left*) *Megamitochondria* may be seen in a minority of cases, and are well-circumscribed eosinophilic cytoplasmic globules, which usually occur singly within the cytoplasm. These globules are negative on PAS after diastase digestion, to help differentiate from alpha₁-antitrypsin inclusions. (Fig. 2–115, *right*) Sometimes spindly mitochondria may also be seen.

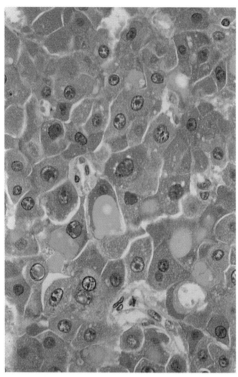

Figure 2–116 Hepatocellular Carcinoma, Fibrolamellar Type
Large eosinophilic cytoplasmic inclusions ("pale bodies") are often
seen and represent microvilli on electron microscopy.

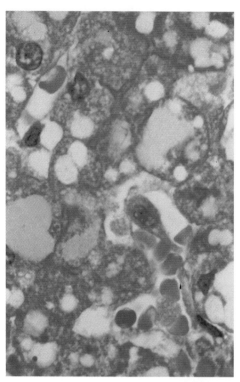

Figure 2–118 Myoclonus Epilepsy (LaFora's Disease) The discrete
eosinophilic cytoplasmic inclusions are seen predominantly within
periportal hepatocytes.

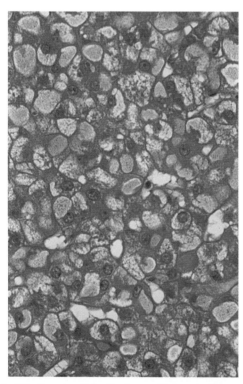

Figure 2–117 Hepatocellular Carcinoma, Trabecular Type Distinct
cytoplasmic inclusions may occasionally be seen and usually represent fibrinogen deposits. Although these resemble the "ground-glass"
cells seen in chronic hepatitis B virus infection, the inclusions do *not*
represent proliferating smooth endoplasmic reticulin and HBsAg particles.

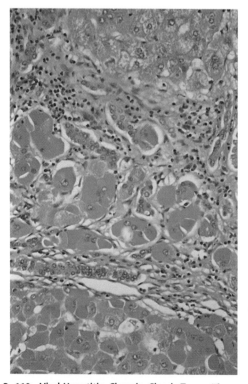

Figure 2–119 Viral Hepatitis, Chronic, Classic Type The cytoplasmic inclusions in periportal or periseptal hepatocytes sometimes are
strongly eosinophilic and finely granular and take up the entire
cytoplasm. These represent closely packed mitochondria (onco-
cytes). Although these cells may be seen in chronic viral hepatitis,
they may also be noted in alcoholic cirrhosis.

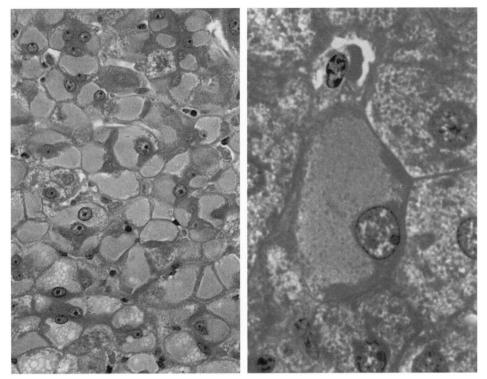

Figures 2–120, 2–121 Viral Hepatitis, Chronic, Type B (Fig. 2–120, *left*) "Ground-glass" cells usually occur singly or in small clusters; however, sometimes these cells may be quite abundant. (Fig. 2–121, *right*) High power shows the finely granular nature of the cytoplasm, which represents proliferating smooth endoplasmic reticulum synthesizing the HBsAg particles.

Inclusions

Kupffer Cells and Portal Macrophages

The *Kupffer cell* is the hepatic component of the mononuclear phagocyte, whereby blood monocytes originating from bone marrow macrophage stem cells are deposited along the sinusoids of the liver as well as in other organs such as the spleen and lungs. These cells can be activated by certain stimuli and function as a host defense against bacteria, parasites, viruses and tumor cells, and also function in clearing endotoxins from the circulation. Activation of Kupffer cells may also induce liver cell injury by the release of cytokines and proteases. Kupffer cells can be seen as hyperplastic in a wide variety of inflammatory conditions in the liver (e.g., acute viral hepatitis), and in that way are not diagnostically helpful and not included in Table 2–15; however, certain liver diseases may demonstrate characteristic distinct deposits within Kupffer cells and occasionally within portal macrophages. For instance, the striated, wrinkled cytoplasmic inclusions within markedly enlarged Kupffer cells are virtually diagnostic of Gaucher's disease.

Figures 2–122 through 2–126 demonstrate examples of inclusions in Kupffer cells and portal macrophages in various diseases.

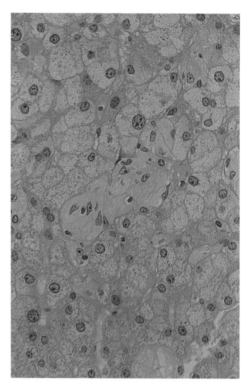

Figure 2–123 Gaucher's Disease These clusters of hypertrophic Kupffer cells have a striated wrinkled cytoplasm characteristic of Gaucher's disease.

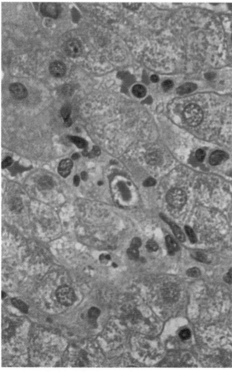

Figure 2–122 Cytomegalovirus Infection A characteristic nuclear inclusion is seen within this Kupffer cell.

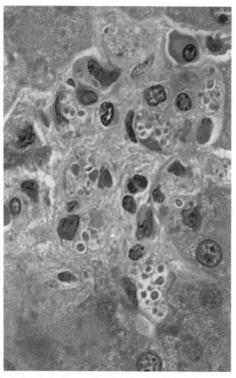

Figure 2–124 Histoplasmosis Encapsulated yeast forms with a surrounding retracted clear ("halo") space are seen within hypertrophic Kupffer cells.

TABLE 2–15

Kupffer Cells and Portal Macrophages, Inclusions

	Type of Inclusion		Type of Inclusion
Angiosarcoma	Erythrophagocytosis; Thorotrast in adjacent nontumor*	Gaucher's disease	Striated wrinkled cytoplasm
		Histoplasmosis	Encapsulated yeast
		Human immunodeficiency virus infection	Erythrophagocytosis
Babesiosis	Ring-shaped parasites		
Benign postoperative intrahepatic cholestasis	Erythrophagocytosis	Leishmaniasis	Oval to rod-shaped parasites
Borreliosis	Erythrophagocytosis	Leptospirosis	Erythrophagocytosis
Cholangiocarcinoma	Thorotrast in adjacent nontumor*	Malaria	Ring-shaped parasites; hemozoin pigment
Cholesterol ester storage disease	Birefringent cholesterol ester crystals	Metachromatic leukodystrophy	Metachromatic granules
Cryptococcosis	Encapsulated budding yeast	Mucolipidoses I and II	Foamy cytoplasm
Cystinosis	Hexagonal, cylindrical crystals	Mucopolysaccharidoses	Vacuolated cytoplasm
		Niemann-Pick disease	Foamy cytoplasm
Cytomegalovirus infection	Cytoplasmic and/or nuclear viral inclusions	Penicilliosis	Nonbudding yeast
		Salmonellosis	Erythrophagocytosis
Drugs/toxins†		Tangier's disease	Foamy cytoplasm; needle-shaped birefringent cholesterol ester crystals
Fabry's disease	Birefringent crystals		
Familial hyperlipoproteinemia	Lipid-laden cytoplasm; crystalline megamitochondria		
		Viral hepatitis, chronic, classic type (IV drug users)	Particulate injectant‡
Gangliosidosis, GM₁	Lipid-laden cytoplasm; PAS-positive (type II)	Whipple's disease	Foamy cytoplasm
Gangliosidosis, GM₂	PAS-positive, Luxol–fast blue-positive cytoplasmic granules	Wolman's disease	Birefringent cholesterol ester crystals

*Thorotrast (thorium dioxide), a colloid arteriographic solution extensively used from 1930 to 1953, is well associated with angiosarcoma and even cholangiocarcinoma many years after exposure. This pigment is seen in Kupffer cells as a finely to coarsely granular gray-green deposit (refer to Figure 2–182 for a photomicrographic example), which emits alpha, beta, and gamma radiation.

†Refer to Table 4–18 for Kupffer cell and portal macrophage inclusions with a drug or toxin etiology.

‡This foreign material is generally seen free within portal tracts, and is best visualized under polarized light.

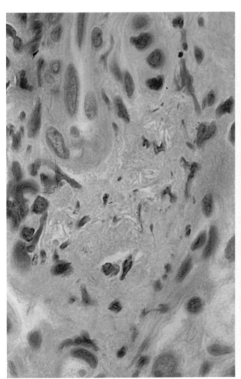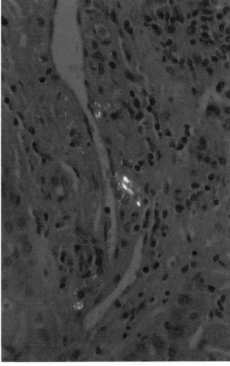

Figures 2–125, 2–126   Viral Hepatitis, Chronic, Classic Type (Intravenous Drug Users)
(Fig. 2–125, *left*) Particulate injectant is seen on high power and is free within a portal tract.
(Fig. 2–126, *right*) Polarized light easily demonstrates these inclusions.

Lobular Necrosis with Inflammation

This section is subdivided into the type of inflammatory cells involved (lymphocytes versus neutrophils) and whether or not cholestasis is a frequent associated feature (Table 2–16). In all the conditions listed in Table 2–16, a portal inflammatory infiltrate is also present and may be predominantly lymphocytic, neutrophilic, or mixed. The PAS stain after diastase digestion (DiPAS) is often helpful in determining the degree of necroinflammatory change, since the areas of focal necrosis often demonstrate increased lysosomal activity which is DiPAS-positive. Granulomas represent specific types of inflammation and are dealt with separately (refer to Table 2–13); however, some liver diseases that characteristically cause granuloma formation may also be associated with variable lobular necrosis and inflammation (e.g., sarcoidosis, cytomegalovirus infection) and are also listed in Table 2–16.

Figures 2–127 through 2–142 show examples of lobular necrosis with inflammation in various diseases.

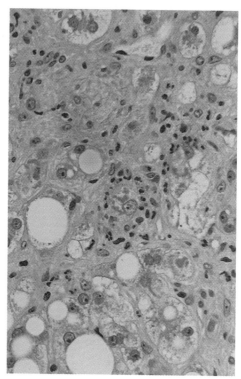

Figure 2–128   Acute sclerosing hyaline necrosis (acute alcoholic hepatitis)   Fatty change and prominent sinusoidal collagen deposition are seen. The hepatocyte in the center of the field contains Mallory bodies, which typically elicit a neutrophilic infiltrate.

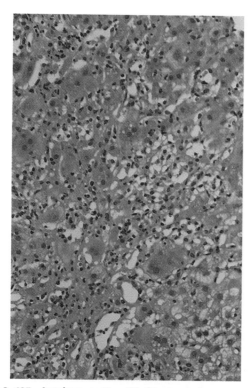

Figure 2–127   Autoimmune Hepatitis (Nontreated)   In patients with this liver disease who are not on steroid therapy, the degree of inflammation and necrosis can be diffuse and marked.

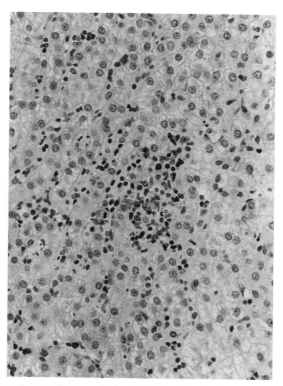

Figure 2–129   Cytomegalovirus Infection   The focal necrosis and inflammation is usually mild, with associated lymphocytosis.

TABLE 2–16

Lobular Necrosis with Inflammation

	Inflammatory Cell				Inflammatory Cell		
	Lymphocyte	Neutrophil	Cholestasis		Lymphocyte	Neutrophil	Cholestasis
Acute fatty liver, alcoholic etiology	+		*	Idiopathic adulthood ductopenia	+		*
Acute sclerosing hyaline necrosis (acute alcoholic hepatitis)		++	*	Indian childhood cirrhosis	+	+	
Alcoholic foamy degeneration	+		*	Leptospirosis	+		*
Allograft, acute (cellular) rejection	+		*	Lymphoma, Hodgkin's	+		*
Allograft, acute graft failure		+	*	Neonatal hepatitis	++	+	*
Allograft, chronic (ductopenic) rejection	+		*	Niemann-Pick disease (neonate)	+/++		*
Allograft, fibrosing cholestatic hepatitis	+		*	Nonalcoholic steatohepatitis	+	+	
Allograft, hyperacute (humoral) rejection		+	*	Nonspecific reactive hepatitis	+		
Alper's disease	+			Paucity of intrahepatic ducts, syndromatic and nonsyndromatic	+		*
Alpha₁-antitrypsin deficiency (neonate)	++		*	Polymyalgia rheumatica	+		
Alpha₁-antitrypsin deficiency (adult)	+			Porphyria cutanea tarda	+		
Autoimmune hepatitis (untreated)	++		*	Primary biliary cirrhosis (early phase)	+		
Bacterial sepsis	+	+	*	Primary biliary cirrhosis (late phase)	+		*
Benign recurrent intrahepatic cholestasis	+		*	Primary sclerosing cholangitis	+		*
Borreliosis	+			Progressive familial intrahepatic cholestasis	+		*
Boutonneuse fever	+			Pyogenic abscess		++	
Brucellosis	+			Q fever	+		
Caroli's disease (associated bile duct obstruction)		+/++	*	Recurrent cholestasis with lymphedema	+		*
Choledochal cyst (associated bile duct obstruction)		+/++	*	Recurrent intrahepatic cholestasis of pregnancy	+		*
Clonorchiasis (associated bile duct obstruction)		+/++	*	Recurrent pyogenic cholangiohepatitis		++	*
Crohn's disease	+			Rheumatoid arthritis	+		
Cystic fibrosis (associated bile duct obstruction)		+/++	*	Rubella virus infection	+/++		*
Cytomegalovirus infection	+			Rubeola virus infection	+		
Cytomegalovirus infection (allograft)	+	++		Salmonellosis	+		
Drugs/toxins†				Sarcoidosis	+		*
Epstein-Barr virus infection	+			Surgical hepatitis		++	
Erythropoietic protoporphyria	+		*	Syphilis, congenital	+		*
Extrahepatic biliary atresia	+		*	Systemic lupus erythematosus	+		
Extrahepatic biliary obstruction, early and late (months–years)	+	+/++	*	Toxic shock syndrome	+	+	*
Graft-versus-host disease	+		*	Toxoplasmosis (neonate)	+/++		*
Group B coxsackievirus infection	+	+	*	Tyrosinemia	+		*
Hemochromatosis	+/++		*	Ulcerative colitis	+		
Hemochromatosis, neonatal variant	++		*	Viral hepatitis, acute, classic type	++		*
Hemolysis, elevation, of liver enzymes, low platelet (HELLP) syndrome	+			Viral hepatitis, acute, with impaired regeneration	++		*
Hereditary fructose intolerance	+		*	Viral hepatitis, acute, with bridging necrosis	++		*
Hyperalimentation, adults and infants	+		*	Viral hepatitis, acute, with panacinar necrosis	++		*
Hyperthyroidism	+			Viral hepatitis, chronic, classic type	+/++		
				Viral hepatitis, chronic, classic type (with reactivation)	++		*
				Weber-Christian disease	+/++	+/++	
				Wilson's disease (untreated)	+/++		*
				Yellow fever	+		
				Zellweger's syndrome	+		*

†Refer to Tables 4–2 and 4–4 for drug and toxin etiologies for lobular necrosis with inflammation, and cholestasis with inflammation, respectively.

Degree of inflammation: + = Mild; ++ = Moderate to marked.

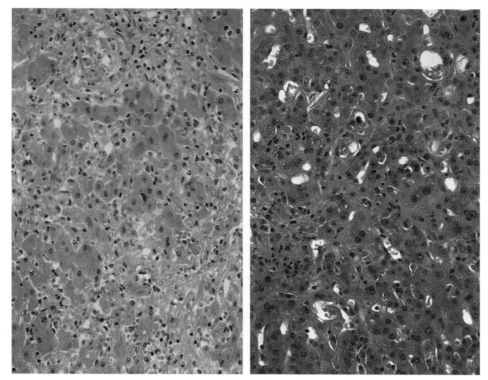

Figures 2–130, 2–131 Drug-induced Necroinflammatory Change (Isoniazid and Chlorpromazine) (Fig. 2–130, *left*) Isoniazid typically causes a diffuse necroinflammatory change resembling acute viral hepatitis. (Fig. 2–131, *right*) Chlorpromazine shows not only focal necrosis and hepatocytolysis but also prominent cholestasis.

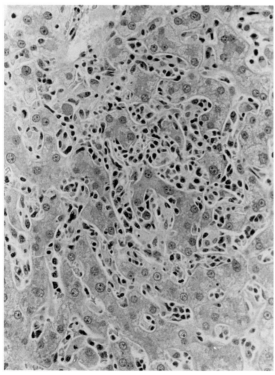

Figure 2–132 Epstein-Barr Virus Infection Focal necroinflammatory change is seen with associated lymphocytosis, the lymphocytes relatively large and "atypical."

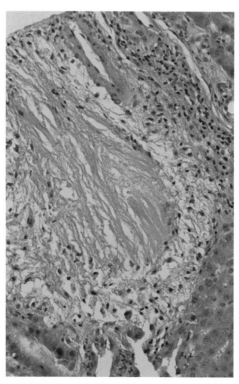

Figure 2–133 Extrahepatic Biliary Obstruction, Late (Months) Liver cell necrosis and extravasation of bile within the lobule may elicit a surrounding histiocytic reaction; this feature is termed "bile infarct."

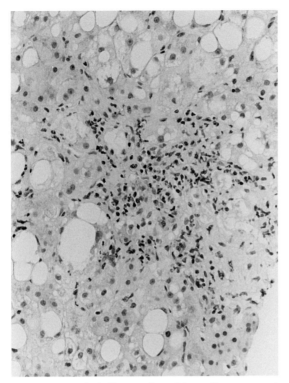

Figure 2–134   Nonalcoholic Steatohepatitis   Diffuse macrovesicular fatty change is present as well as focal necrosis and inflammatory infiltrates, the inflammatory cells consisting of both lymphocytes and neutrophils.

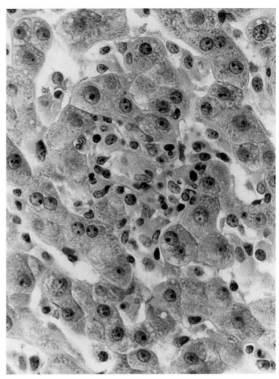

Figure 2–135   Salmonellosis   Focal necroinflammatory change is present, but overall is relatively mild. Enlarged hypertrophic Kupffer cells are also noted.

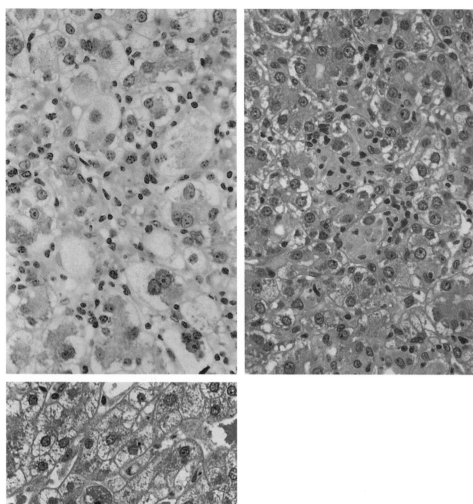

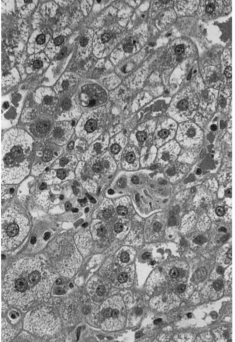

Figures 2–136 to 2–138   Viral Hepatitis, Acute, Classic Type   All three photomicrographs show a moderate degree of liver cell swelling, focal necrosis, and hepatocytolysis, with the inflammatory infiltrate consisting chiefly of lymphocytes. (Fig. 2–136, *upper left*) The inflammatory infiltrate has a perivenular accentuation, which is typically seen in the early phase of acute viral hepatitis. (Fig. 2–137, *upper right*) Focal necroinflammatory changes are also present within the other zones of the lobule. (Fig. 2–138, *lower left*) One type of necrosis seen in this field, whereby the liver cell becomes shrunken and markedly eosinophilic with pyknotic nuclei, is the "acidophil" (Councilman) body, a characteristic feature in both acute and chronic viral hepatitis and also seen in a variety of nonviral inflammatory conditions.

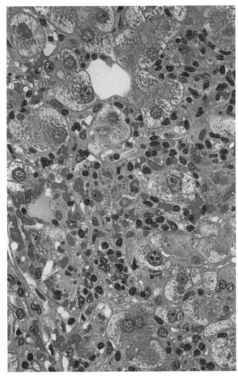

Figure 2–139 Viral Hepatitis, Acute, Type B The inflammation and necrosis is most pronounced in the perivenular zone and midzone in this photomicrograph. Ground glass cells are *not* a feature of acute viral hepatitis type B.

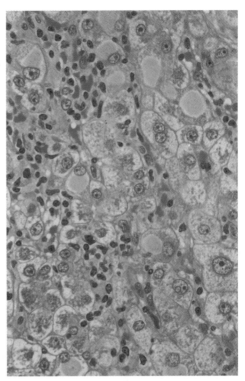

Figure 2–141 Viral Hepatitis, Chronic, Type B Inflammation and focal necrosis are seen with scattered "ground glass" cells containing the HBsAg; ground glass cells are seen in 50% to 75% of cases of chronic HBV infection.

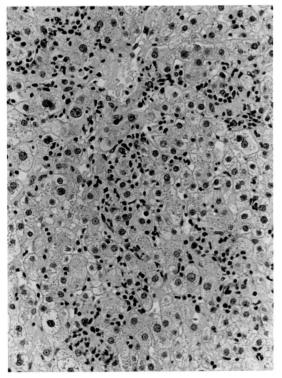

Figure 2–140 Viral Hepatitis, Acute, Type C Diffuse necroinflammatory change is present. In addition, increase in circulating lymphocytes is seen in acute HCV infection as well, more so than in acute hepatitis secondary to the other hepatotropic viruses.

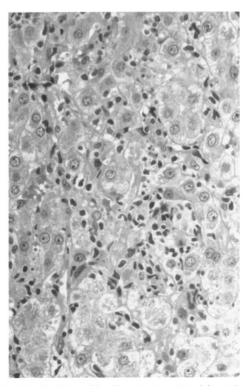

Figure 2–142 Viral Hepatitis, Chronic, Type B + delta The degree of inflammation and necrosis is usually more prominent than in chronic HBV infection alone.

Lobular Necrosis with Minimal to Absent Inflammation

Although inflammation is a frequent finding when there is liver cell necrosis, in some liver diseases the degree of inflammation is minimal to absent (Table 2–17). In many instances the associated liver diseases have some degree of vascular compromise. For example, in liver transplant patients, hyperacute (humoral) rejection is associated with sinusoidal red blood cell sludging and severe necrotizing endothelial damage of small arteries and arterioles, the end result being severe ischemic (coagulative) necrosis of hepatocytes. Similarly, vasculitis in nontransplant patients (e.g., rheumatoid arthritis, systemic lupus erythematosus) may be associated with vascular thrombosis and liver cell ischemia. It must be noted that neutrophilic infiltration may be seen as a secondary response to ischemic necrosis. Interestingly, certain viral infections (e.g., adenovirus) elicit only a minimal inflammatory response when compared with acute viral hepatitis from the more common hepatotropic viruses.

Figures 2–143 to 2–148 demonstrate examples of lobular necrosis with minimal to absent inflammation in various diseases.

TABLE 2–17

Lobular Necrosis with Minimal to Absent Inflammation

Adenovirus infection
Allograft, acute graft failure
Allograft, harvesting (preservation) injury
Allograft, hyperacute (humoral) rejection
Allograft, ischemia secondary to hepatic artery thrombosis
Amebiasis
Aspergillosis
Babesiosis
Budd-Chiari syndrome, acute
Cirrhosis (any etiology) with severe esophageal variceal bleeding*
Dengue fever
Drugs/toxins (refer to Table 4–1)
Ebola virus infection
Heart failure, left-sided with hypotension
Heat stroke
Herpes simplex virus infection
Herpes zoster virus infection
Hyperpyrexia
Lassa fever
Marburg virus infection
Myeloproliferative disorders
Pneumocystis carinii infection
Polyarteritis nodosa
Recurrent pyogenic cholangiohepatitis
Rheumatoid arthritis
Sickle cell anemia
Spontaneous rupture in pregnancy
Systemic lupus erythematosus
Toxemia of pregnancy
Veno-occlusive disease, acute

* In instances in which extensive esophageal variceal hemorrhage occurs, the regenerative nodules within a *cirrhotic* liver may undergo severe ischemic necrosis. This feature is usually focal, with viable regenerative nodules often immediately adjacent to the necrotic nodules.

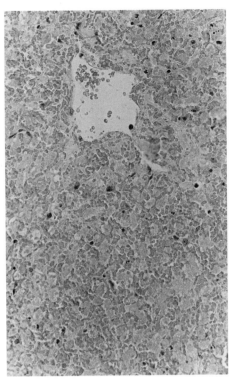

Figure 2-143   Allograft, Acute Graft Failure   The perivenular and midzonal hepatocytes show extensive ischemic necrosis and dropout, with acute hemorrhage. No inflammatory infiltrate is present.

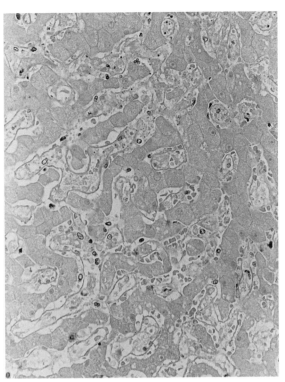

Figure 2-145   Allograft, Ischemia Secondary to Hepatic Artery Thrombosis   The hepatocytes show an intact cord-sinusoid pattern but severe ischemic necrosis, best demonstrated by virtual absence of nuclear staining on hematoxylin.

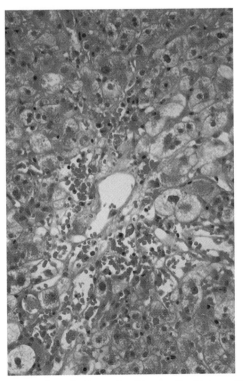

Figure 2-144   Allograft, Harvesting (Preservation) Injury   The perivenular hepatocytes show ballooning, with mild liver cell necrosis, dropout, and acute hemorrhage.

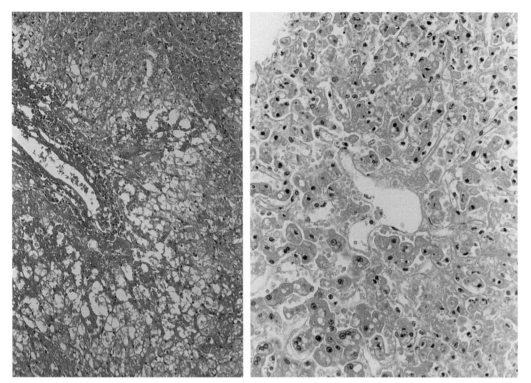

Figures 2–146, 2–147   Drug-induced Liver Cell Injury (Ferrous Sulfate and Acetamino-phen)   Drug-induced liver cell injury without an inflammatory infiltrate may have a zonal predominance. (Fig. 2–146, *left*) Ferrous sulfate induces liver cell necrosis with ballooning predominantly within the periportal zone (zone 1). (Fig. 2–147, *right*) In acetaminophen hepatotoxicity, the perivenular liver cells (zone 3) show coagulative necrosis.

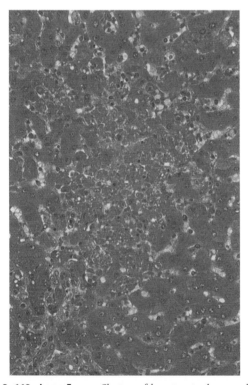

Figure 2–148   Lassa Fever   Clusters of hepatocytes have undergone coagulative necrosis. The area of necrosis as well as the adjacent hepatic cords show no inflammatory infiltrate.

Lobular Confluent Necrosis

Certain liver diseases may be associated with lobular necrosis that is severe, and may become confluent, with extensive liver cell dropout and associated lobular collapse of the reticulin framework (Table 2–18). The inflammatory infiltrates may be striking (e.g., autoimmune hepatitis) or minimal (e.g., hyperacute allograft rejection). These changes may be focal and not evenly distributed throughout all lobules, as in adenovirus infection, or may be diffuse, as seen in acute graft failure. In addition, the lobular necrosis may be zonal, an example being the perivenular and midzones in left-sided heart failure with hypotension.

Figures 2–149 to 2–153 demonstrate examples of liver diseases with lobular confluent necrosis.

TABLE 2–18

Lobular Confluent Necrosis

Adenovirus infection
Allograft, acute (cellular) rejection (severe)
Allograft, acute graft failure
Allograft, chronic (ductopenic) rejection (severe)
Allograft, fibrosing cholestatic hepatitis
Allograft, hyperacute (humoral) rejection
Allograft, ischemia secondary to hepatic artery thrombosis
Alpers' disease
Autoimmune hepatitis (untreated)
Dengue fever
Drugs/toxins (refer to Table 4–3)
Ebola virus infection
Heart failure, left-sided with hypotension
Hemochromatosis, neonatal variant
Herpes simplex virus infection
Herpes zoster virus infection
Lassa fever
Marburg virus infection
Rubella virus infection
Toxemia of pregnancy
Viral hepatitis, acute, with bridging necrosis
Viral hepatitis, acute, with impaired regeneration
Viral hepatitis, acute, with panacinar necrosis
Viral hepatitis, chronic, classic form, with reactivation
Wilson's disease

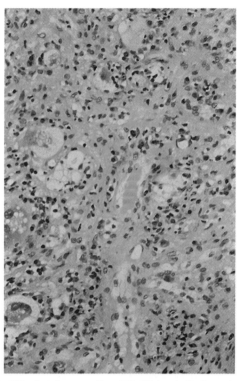

Figure 2–149 Autoimmune Hepatitis (Untreated) In patients not on steroid therapy, the liver cell necrosis can be severe. This field shows variable hydropic hepatocytes, prominent infiltration by lymphocytes and occasional plasma cells, and areas of liver cell dropout and collapse.

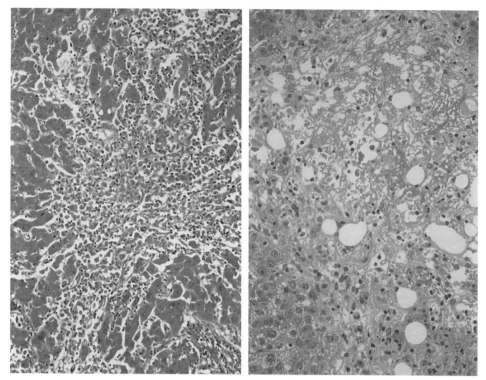

Figures 2–150, 2–151   Drug-induced Liver Cell Injury (Halothane and Niacin)   (Fig. 2–150, *left*) With halothane hypersensitivity reaction, there is prominent perivenular and midzonal liver cell dropout. (Fig. 2–151, *right*) Niacin hepatotoxicity may elicit severe liver cell dropout with fibrin deposition.

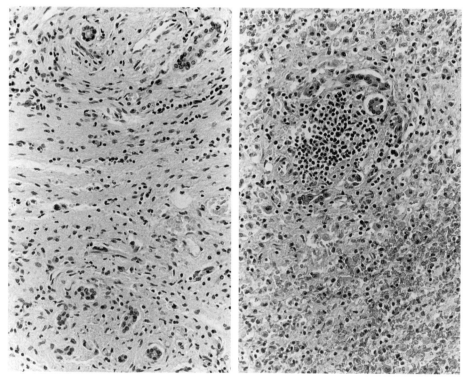

Figures 2–152, 2–153   Viral Hepatitis, Acute, with Panacinar Necrosis   Both examples show total liver cell necrosis and dropout. (Fig. 2–152, *left*) This case of acute hepatitis A virus infection shows two portal tracts at the top and bottom of the field, with extensive collapse of the lobular framework between the portal tracts. Note how close the portal tracts now are to each other. (Fig. 2–153, *right*) This is a case of acute hepatitis B virus infection. The portal tract shows characteristic lymphocytic infiltration; however, the adjacent parenchyma shows total dropout of hepatocytes, with variable acute hemorrhage.

Mallory Bodies

Mallory bodies are cytoplasmic inclusions within hepatocytes that have a characteristic eosinophilic "ropy" appearance on hematoxylin-eosin stain (Table 2–19). These inclusions are composed in part of aggregates of intermediate filaments that are either laid down in a parallel manner or randomly deposited, and may also be seen as granular to amorphous material. In some instances neutrophils can be seen abutting the cell membrane of hepatocytes containing Mallory bodies (*satellitosis*), and occasionally the neutrophils infiltrate into the liver cell cytoplasm itself. On trichrome stain these inclusions may stain either dark blue or red. Mallory bodies are a sign of irreversible liver cell injury, but the deposits may be seen in liver cell cytoplasm for extended periods of time. For instance, in a patient with acute sclerosing hyaline necrosis (acute alcoholic hepatitis) who stops drinking, the Mallory bodies may still be identified up to 4 months after abstinence. Mallory bodies are present in a number of chronic cholestatic conditions, and their deposition can be caused by numerous drugs and toxins. Mallory bodies are also identified in certain primary liver cell neoplasms and may be a helpful clue in differentiating these tumors from metastatic lesions.

Figures 2–154 through 2–163 demonstrate Mallory bodies in various diseases.

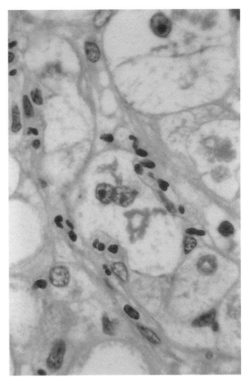

Figure 2–154 Acute Sclerosing Hyaline Necrosis (Acute Alcoholic Hepatitis) The Mallory body is surrounded by neutrophils (satellitosis).

TABLE 2–19

Mallory Bodies

	Occurrence
Abetalipoproteinemia	+
Acute sclerosing hyaline necrosis (acute alcoholic hepatitis)	+++
Adenoma, liver cell	+
Adenomatous hyperplasia	+
Alcoholic cirrhosis, active drinker	++/+++
Alpha-1-antitrypsin deficiency	+
Drugs/toxins*	
Extrahepatic biliary atresia	+
Extrahepatic biliary obstruction, late (months–years)	+
Focal nodular hyperplasia	+
Glycogen storage disease type Ia	++
Hepatocellular carcinoma, fibrolamellar type	+
Hepatocellular carcinoma, trabecular, acinar, ductular type	+
Hyperalimentation, adult	+
Indian childhood cirrhosis	+++
Kwashiorkor	+
Nonalcoholic steatohepatitis	++
Primary biliary cirrhosis	++
Primary sclerosing cholangitis	+
Weber-Christian disease	+
Wilson's disease	++

*Refer to Table 4–20 for drug and toxin etiologies of Mallory bodies.

+ = Rare; ++ = occasional; +++ = common.

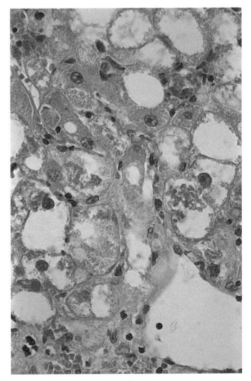

Figure 2–155 Adenoma, Liver Cell Although uncommon, Mallory bodies can be seen in this benign hepatic neoplasm; however, their occurrence is more frequent in the adenoma with malignant transformation to hepatocellular carcinoma.

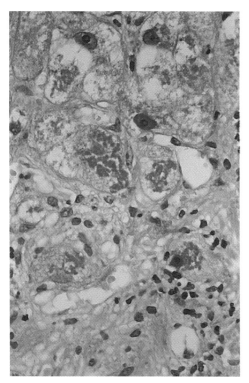

Figure 2–156 Drug-induced (Amiodarone) This antiarrhythmic agent may cause Mallory body deposition.

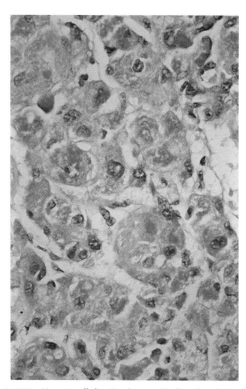

Figure 2–158 Hepatocellular Carcinoma, Trabecular, Acinar, Ductular Type Mallory bodies can be seen in up to 12% of cases of this primary hepatic neoplasm.

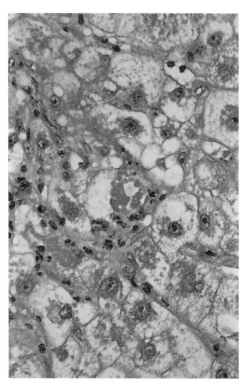

Figure 2–157 Extrahepatic Biliary Obstruction, Late (Months to Years) The Mallory body in the center of the photomicrograph is partially surrounded by neutrophils (satellitosis). This is an example of a patient with a hilar mass lesion and concomitant bile duct obstruction.

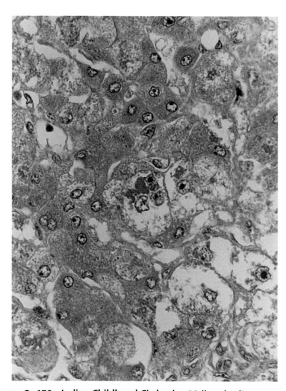

Figure 2–159 Indian Childhood Cirrhosis Mallory bodies are commonly seen in this liver disease.

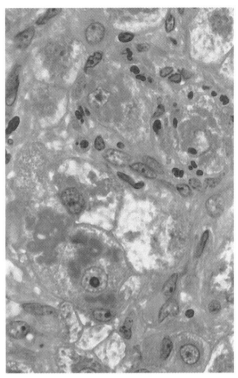

Figure 2–160 Nonalcoholic Steatohepatitis Some of the Mallory bodies exhibit pericellular neutrophils, while others are not eliciting an inflammatory reaction.

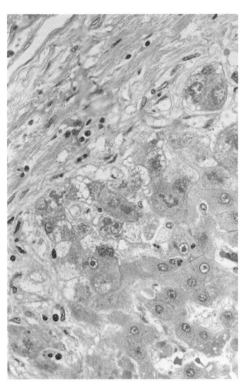

Figure 2–162 Primary Sclerosing Cholangitis As in primary biliary cirrhosis, Mallory bodies are seen in this cholestatic liver disease in the more advanced stages, and are usually situated in periportal or periseptal hepatocytes.

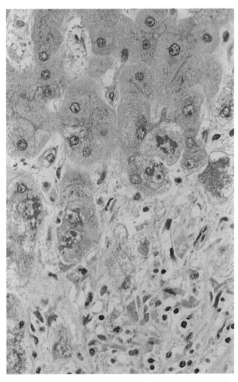

Figure 2–161 Primary Biliary Cirrhosis The Mallory bodies seen in this disorder are usually located in periportal or periseptal hepatocytes, and are seen in up to one fourth of patients in the severely fibrotic and cirrhotic stages.

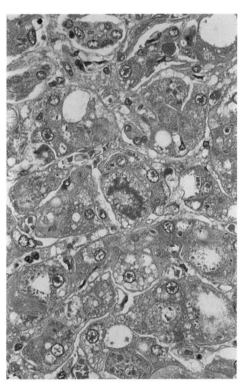

Figure 2–163 Wilson's Disease Mallory bodies may be seen in periportal hepatocytes, and are more common as the disease progresses.

Mass Lesions

Benign

Discrete mass lesions visualized on ultrasound, computed tomography (CT), or magnetic resonance imaging (MRI) may on fine-needle aspirate (FNA) yield only cytologically benign hepatocytes, duct epithelium, vascular channels, or inflammatory cells (Table 2–20). A number of conditions must be kept in mind in the differential diagnoses. It is imperative that the physician performing the biopsy is confident that the biopsy was indeed from the lesion, as certainly a misdiagnosis could be drastic (e.g., diagnosing liver cell adenoma when the FNA missed the mass lesion and consisted only of benign hepatocytes, and repeat biopsy at a later time demonstrated hepatocellular carcinoma). The conditions listed in Table 2–20 are subdivided into their basic morphologic characteristics.

Figures 2–164 through 2–169 demonstrate examples of various benign mass lesions.

TABLE 2–20

Mass Lesions, Benign

Hepatocytes

Adenoma, liver cell*
Adenomatous hyperplasia
Focal fatty change
Focal nodular hyperplasia*
Galactosemia
Nodular regenerative hyperplasia*
Partial nodular transformation

Duct Epithelium

Adenoma, bile duct
Biliary hamartoma
Focal nodular hyperplasia*
Mesenchymal hamartoma

Vascular Channels

Angiomyolipoma
Cavernous hemangioma
Infantile hemangioendothelioma
Lymphangioma
Mesenchymal hamartoma
Peliosis hepatis

Inflammatory Cells

Inflammatory pseudotumor
Pyogenic abscess
Sarcoidosis

Inflammatory Cells and Microorganisms

Enterobiasis
Fascioliasis
Pyogenic abscess
Tuberculosis (tuberculoma)
Visceral larva migrans

*For drug and toxin etiologies of benign mass lesions, refer to Table 4–16.

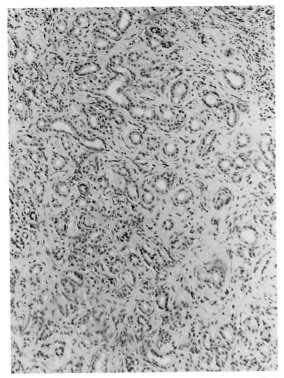

Figure 2–164   Adenoma, Bile Duct   The tumor is composed of cytologically benign bile ducts.

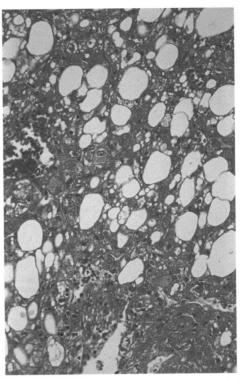

Figure 2–166   Angiomyolipoma   The tumor is composed of a mixture of fat, smooth muscle, hematopoietic elements, and vascular channels.

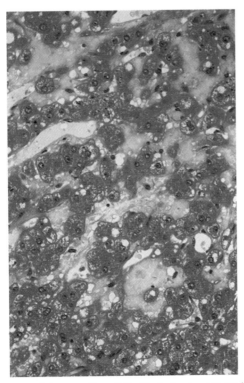

Figure 2–165   Adenoma, Liver Cell   The lesion is composed entirely of benign hepatocytes forming cords no greater than two cells thick.

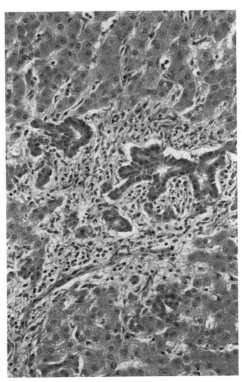

Figure 2–167   Focal Nodular Hyperplasia   This lesion is composed of benign hepatocytes forming a discrete mass having a central radiating scar containing lymphocytes and atypical duct epithelium.

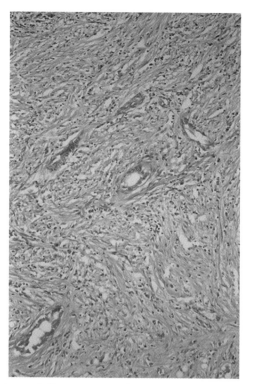

Figure 2–168 Inflammatory Pseudotumor This neoplasm is composed of spindle cells, vascular channels, and scattered benign ducts.

Mass Lesions
Malignant

When discrete mass lesions reveal malignant cells, the diagnosis may be straightforward. For example, thickened hepatic cords are characteristic of hepatocellular carcinoma of trabecular type, whereas acellular fibrous bands laid down in a parallel fashion and interspersed between malignant hepatocytes having abundant eosinophilic cytoplasm are characteristic of fibrolamellar hepatocellular carcinoma (refer to Table 2–10, Diagnostic Lesions). The diagnosis becomes more difficult when dealing with adenocarcinomas and poorly differentiated malignant neoplasms, in which statistically metastatic disease is much more frequent than primary neoplasms. In these instances, immunoperoxidase staining can be most helpful (e.g., prostate-specific antigen for metastatic prostate adenocarcinoma). Table 2–21 includes only *primary* hepatic malignancies.

Figures 2–170 to 2–172 show examples of primary hepatic malignant lesions.

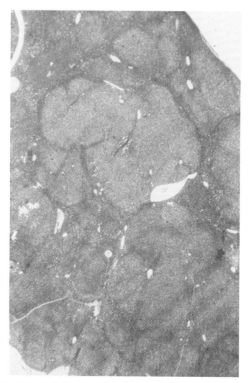

Figure 2–169 Nodular Regenerative Hyperplasia The lesions are multiple and composed of bulging small nodules of regenerating hepatocytes.

TABLE 2–21

Mass Lesions, Malignant

Hepatocytes

Hepatoblastoma
Hepatocellular carcinoma, fibrolamellar type
Hepatocellular carcinoma, trabecular, acinar, ductular type*

Duct Epithelium

Cholangiocarcinoma*
Cystadenoma with or without mesenchymal stroma, with malignant transformation (cystadenocarcinoma)

Vascular Channels

Angiosarcoma*
Epithelioid hemangioendothelioma

Hematopoietic

Lymphoma, non-Hodgkin's
Multiple myeloma

* For drug and toxin etiologies of malignant mass lesions, refer to Table 4–16.

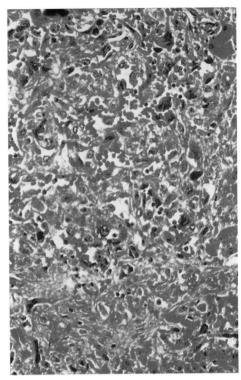

Figure 2–170 Angiosarcoma This tumor is usually multifocal, can be cystic and hemorrhagic or form discrete solid masses, and is composed of proliferating vascular channels lined by malignant endothelial cells.

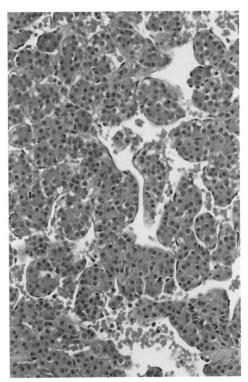

Figure 2–172 Hepatocellular Carcinoma, Trabecular Type The tumor is composed of hepatocytes with increased nuclear-cytoplasmic ratio, forming cords greater than two cells thick, the cords lined by endothelial cells.

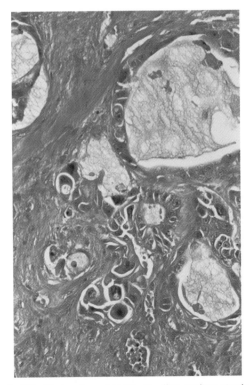

Figure 2–171 Cholangiocarcinoma Small to medium-sized mucin-secreting dilated glands are seen in this example, lined by malignant duct epithelium. Usually there is a coexisting fibrous stroma. At times this neoplasm can be difficult to differentiate from metastatic adenocarcinoma.

Pigments

The most common pigments seen in the liver are lipochrome, hemosiderin, and bile. Bile is discussed in Table 2–8, Cholestasis, Simple, and Table 2–16, Lobular Necrosis with Inflammation. Lipochrome, which overall is the most common pigment, is also known as the wear and tear pigment, and is more prominent in the perivenular and midzonal hepatocytes in the middle-aged to elderly population. This pigment is generally not associated with liver disease, although a similar-type pigment is seen in the Dubin-Johnson syndrome. Hemosiderin may be seen within hepatocytes associated with increase in iron absorption (e.g., hemochromatosis) or within Kupffer cells and portal macrophages in disorders associated with chronic hemolysis. Very often, pigment is seen in both liver cells and Kupffer cells. Copper cannot be visualized on hematoxylin-eosin stain but requires special stains, either directly staining the copper (rubeanic acid) or the copper-binding protein (orcein). This pigment is seen predominantly within liver cell cytoplasm. Both hemosiderin and copper or copper-binding protein are first deposited within periportal hepatocytes, but they can diffusely involve virtually all liver cells in disorders such as Indian childhood cirrhosis (copper or copper-binding protein) and hemochromatosis (hemosiderin). Table 2–22 also lists less common pigments.

Figures 2–173 through 2–188 demonstrate examples of various pigments seen in the liver.

TABLE 2–22

Pigments

Hemosiderin

	Hepatocytes	Kupffer Cells/ Portal Macrophages
Alcoholic cirrhosis	++	
Benign postoperative intrahepatic cholestasis		+
Cystic fibrosis	+/++	
Down syndrome	+/++	
Drugs/toxins*		
Galactosemia	+/++	
Gaucher's disease		++
Hemochromatosis	++	
Hemochromatosis, neonatal variant	++	
Hemosiderosis (secondary iron overload)	+	++
Hyperalimentation, adult	+	+
Inspissated bile syndrome		++
Leukemia	+	++
Lymphoma, Hodgkin's and non-Hodgkin's	+	++
Malaria	+	++
Myeloproliferative disorders	+	++
Neonatal hepatitis	++	
Porphyria cutanea tarda	++	
Sickle cell anemia	+	++
Tyrosinemia	++	
Viral hepatitis, acute, classic type		+
Viral hepatitis, chronic, type C	+/++	
Wilson's disease		+
Zellweger's syndrome	+	+

Table continued on following page

TABLE 2–22

Pigments *Continued*

Copper, Copper-binding Protein

	Pigment within Hepatocytes
Adenoma, liver cell	+
Alpha$_1$-antitrypsin deficiency	+
Congenital hepatic fibrosis	+
Cystic fibrosis	+
Extrahepatic biliary atresia	+/++
Extrahepatic biliary obstruction, late (years)	+/++
Focal nodular hyperplasia	+
Galactosemia	+
Hepatoblastoma	+
Hepatocellular carcinoma, fibrolamellar type	+
Hereditary fructose intolerance	+
Hyperalimentation, adult	+/++
Idiopathic adulthood ductopenia	++
Indian childhood cirrhosis	++
Paucity of intrahepatic ducts, syndromatic and nonsyndromatic	++
Primary biliary cirrhosis	++
Primary sclerosing cholangitis	++
Progressive familial intrahepatic cholestasis	++
Recurrent cholestasis with lymphedema	+/++
Wilson's disease	++

Other Pigments

	Type of Pigment/Material	Location	
		Hepatocyte	Kupffer Cell/ Portal Macrophage
Adenoma, liver cell	Lipochrome	+	
Angiosarcoma	Thorotrast in nontumor		++
Chronic granulomatous disease of childhood	Lipochrome	+	
Cystinosis	Cystine		++
Drugs/toxins*			
Dubin-Johnson syndrome	Lipochrome-like	++	
Erythropoietic protoporphyria	Protoporphyrin	++	++†
Focal nodular hyperplasia	Lipochrome	+	
Gilbert's syndrome	Lipochrome	+	
Hepatoblastoma	Melanin	+	
Malaria	Hemozoin		++
Niemann-Pick disease	Lipochrome	+	
Schistosomiasis	Hemozoin		++
Viral hepatitis, acute, classic type	Lipochrome		+
Viral hepatitis, chronic, classic type	IV particulate material in drug users		+/++‡
Wilson's disease	Lipochrome	+	

* Refer to Table 4–19 for drug and toxin etiologies of hepatic pigments.
† Also seen in bile canaliculi, interlobular bile ducts, and portal collagen.
‡ More often seen free within portal tracts.
+ = Occasionally present; ++ = present and often abundant.

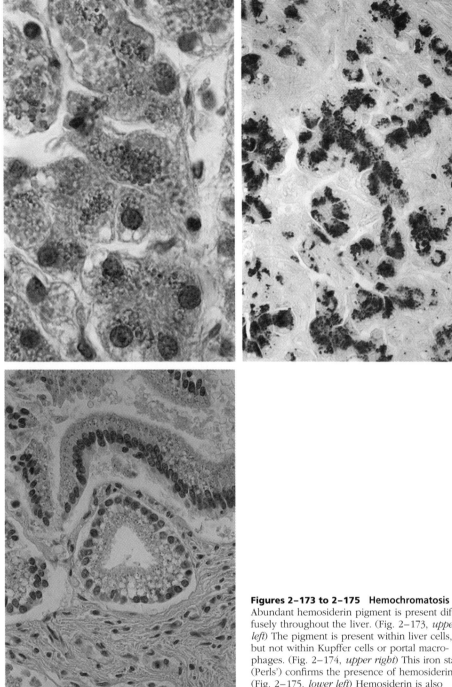

Figures 2–173 to 2–175 **Hemochromatosis**
Abundant hemosiderin pigment is present diffusely throughout the liver. (Fig. 2–173, *upper left*) The pigment is present within liver cells, but not within Kupffer cells or portal macrophages. (Fig. 2–174, *upper right*) This iron stain (Perls') confirms the presence of hemosiderin. (Fig. 2–175, *lower left*) Hemosiderin is also present within duct epithelium, a helpful clue in differentiating hemochromatosis from hemosiderosis secondary to iron overload (refer to Fig. 2–176 for comparison).

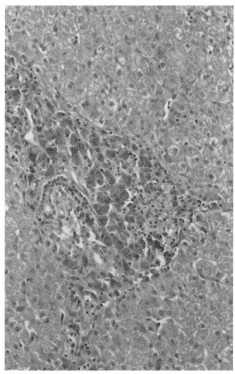

Figure 2–176   Hemosiderosis (Secondary Iron Overload)
Hemosiderin is usually seen not only within Kupffer cells but also within portal macrophages. Note that a bile duct toward the center left of the field contains virtually no pigment (refer to Fig. 2–175 to compare with hemochromatosis).

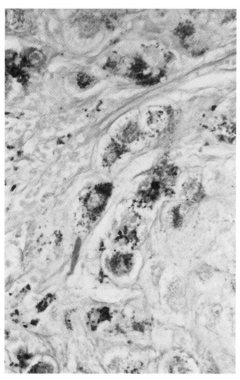

Figure 2–178   Primary Biliary Cirrhosis   Prominent copper-binding protein is present within periportal hepatocytes on orcein stain.

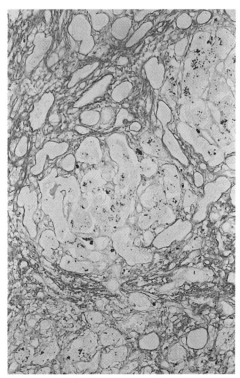

Figure 2–177   Indian Childhood Cirrhosis   Abundant granular, dark brown to black pigment representing copper-binding protein is seen within the liver cells on orcein stain.

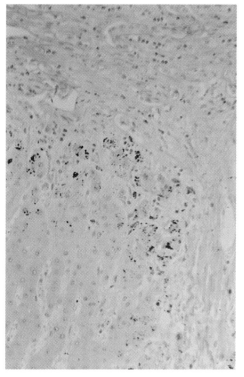

Figure 2–179   Primary Sclerosing Cholangitis   Abundant copper-binding protein is present on orcein stain and is predominantly within periportal hepatocytes.

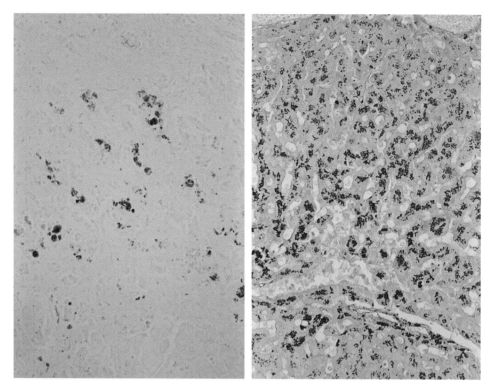

Figures 2–180, 2–181 Wilson's Disease (Fig. 2–180, *left*) Copper is best visualized by rubeanic acid stain, and is coarsely granular and green-black. (Fig. 2–181, *right*) This liver disease also contains abundant copper-binding protein, which is diffusely deposited within hepatocytes on this orcein stain.

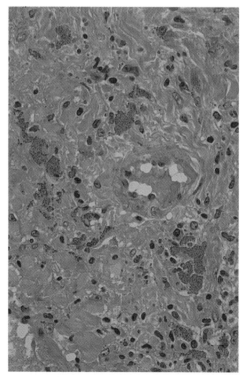

Figure 2–182 Angiosarcoma Thorium dioxide (Thorotrast) pigment is present within macrophages in the liver adjacent to the neoplasm.

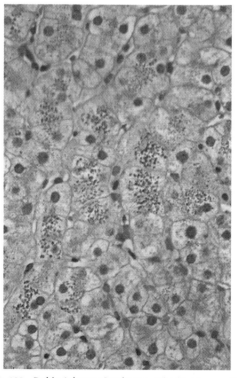

Figure 2–183 Dubin-Johnson Syndrome The lipochrome-like pigment is most prominent within perivenular and midzonal hepatocytes.

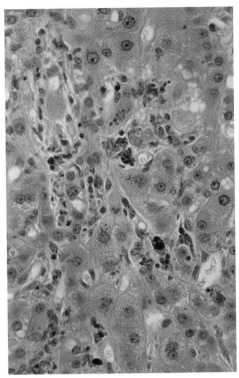

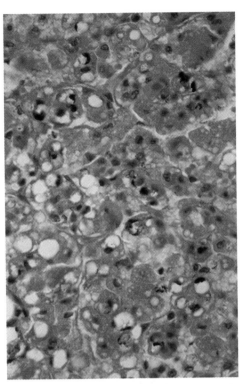

Figure 2–184   Erythropoietic protoporphyria   The dark brown to golden pigment represents protoporphyrin, and is seen in this field predominantly within Kupffer cells.

Figure 2–185   Fatty Change, Alcoholic Etiology   An incidental finding was deposition of formalin pigment, which in this field is predominantly within hepatocytes. This is an artifact of fixation, and *not* related to any liver disease.

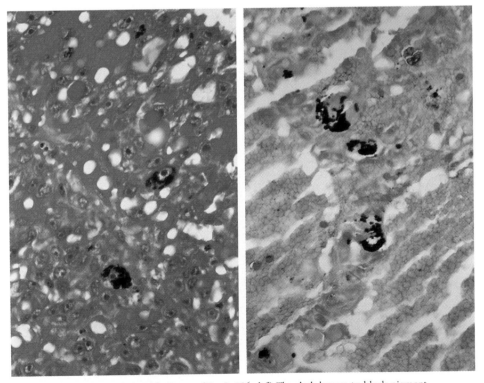

Figures 2–186, 2–187   Hepatoblastoma   (Fig. 2–186, *left*) The dark brown to black pigment represents melanin. (Fig. 2–187, *right*) The black granular pigment on Fontana-Masson stain confirms the pigment as melanin.

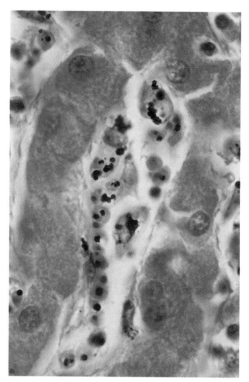

Figure 2–188 Malaria The dark brown to black pigment is seen within Kupffer cells and circulating red blood cells, and represents hemozoin in this example of *Plasmodium falciparum* infection.

Portal Lymphocytes
Associated with Minimal to Absent Periportal Activity

Although liver biopsies exhibiting portal lymphocytic infiltration are numerous and often have some degree of inflammation within the lobules, in some instances periportal activity and lobular inflammatory changes may be minimal to absent (Table 2–23). This is often seen in chronic liver diseases in spontaneous remission or in response to therapy (e.g., autoimmune hepatitis treated with steroids).

Figures 2–189 and 2–190 demonstrate liver biopsies with minimal to absent periportal activity.

TABLE 2–23

Portal Lymphocytes Associated with Minimal to Absent Periportal Activity

Acute fatty liver of pregnancy
Adjacent to space-occupying lesion
Allograft, acute (cellular) rejection, mild
Allograft, post transplant lymphoproliferative disease*
Amyloidosis
Autoimmune hepatitis, treated (in remission)
Extrahepatic biliary obstruction, late (months–years), intermittent
Graft-versus-host disease
Leukemia, lymphocytic*
Lymphoma, non-Hodgkin's*
Polyarteritis nodosa
Primary biliary cirrhosis, early stage
Primary sclerosing cholangitis, early stage
Viral hepatitis, acute, classic type, resolving stage
Viral hepatitis, chronic, classic type, inactive (occult) stage
Viral hepatitis, chronic, classic type, treated (in remission)
Wilson's disease, treated (in remission)

*In cases in which the portal infiltrate is marked, variable spillover of the infiltrate into the adjacent periportal regions may be seen.

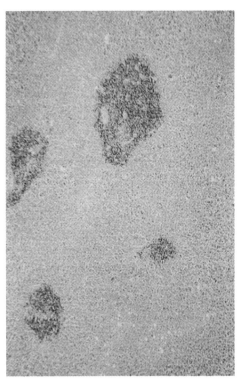

Figure 2–189 Lymphoma, Non-Hodgkin's The portal lymphocytic infiltrates are prominent, and in this case are confined to the portal tracts.

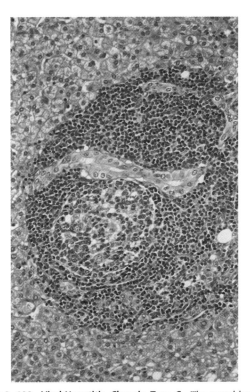

Figure 2–190 Viral Hepatitis, Chronic, Type C The portal lymphocytic infiltrate is prominent, with germinal center formation; however, there is no periportal inflammation. This patient had virtually normal liver tests at the time of biopsy for staging the disease.

Portal Lymphocytes
Associated with Periportal Activity

Spillover of inflammatory cells into the adjacent periportal regions, surrounding individual and small groups of hepatocytes, is termed *piecemeal necrosis*. It is most frequently seen in chronic liver diseases that progress to cirrhosis; however, biopsy specimens may not demonstrate this feature at all times, as (1) the liver disease may be in remission, and (2) piecemeal necrosis may often be focal, involving some but not all portal tracts. In this latter instance, a biopsy may show only portal tracts with minimal periportal activity. The liver diseases listed in Table 2–24 are known to cause piecemeal necrosis; however, rebiopsy, especially if the patient is under therapy, may not show this histologic feature (e.g., chronic viral hepatitis secondary to hepatitis C virus [HCV] responding to interferon therapy).

Figures 2–191 to 2–195 demonstrate liver biopsies with periportal activity.

TABLE 2–24

Portal Lymphocytes Associated with Periportal Activity

Alpers' disease
Alpha₁-antichymotrypsin deficiency
Alpha₁-antitrypsin deficiency
Autoimmune hepatitis, not treated
Cirrhosis, active stage*
Crohn's disease
Erythropoietic protoporphyria
Hypereosinophilic syndrome
Primary biliary cirrhosis
Primary sclerosing cholangitis
Ulcerative colitis
Viral hepatitis, acute, classic type†
Viral hepatitis, chronic, classic type
Wilson's disease, not treated

*Many liver diseases that progress to cirrhosis may at some time during the *active* stage show piecemeal necrosis. "Cirrhosis" in its general sense is not covered in Chapter 3, Liver Diseases: Pathology and Clinical Considerations; refer to Table 2–28, Portal Fibrosis, for a listing of the liver diseases associated with cirrhosis.

†Although spillover and not true piecemeal necrosis is characteristically seen, in some instances piecemeal necrosis can also be present.

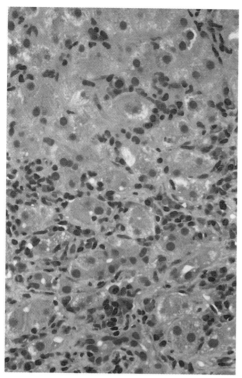

Figure 2–191 Autoimmune Hepatitis (Not on Therapy)
Prominent periportal inflammation is seen, the infiltrates consisting
chiefly of lymphocytes and plasma cells.

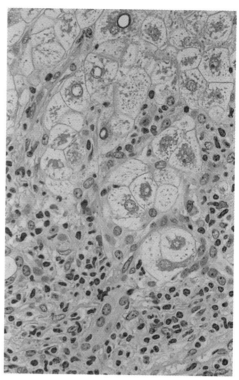

Figure 2–193 Primary Biliary Cirrhosis In approximately 15% of
cases of primary biliary cirrhosis, periportal activity with piecemeal
necrosis can be seen.

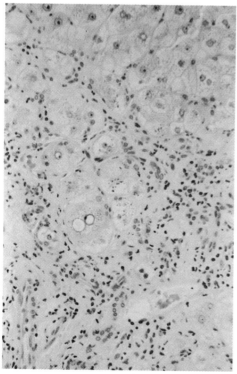

Figure 2–192 Drug-induced Periportal Activity (Methotrexate)
Periportal activity is seen in a biopsy from a patient on long-term
daily low-dose methotrexate for psoriasis.

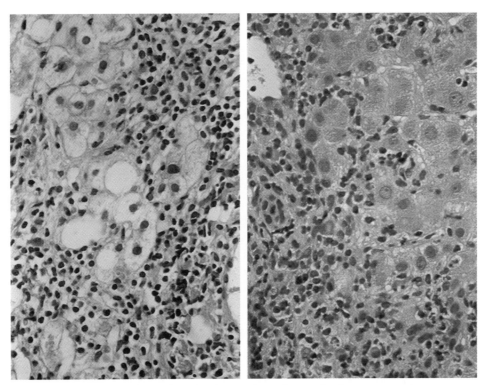

Figures 2–194, 2–195   Viral Hepatitis, Chronic, Type B   Both examples demonstrate peri-portal activity with piecemeal necrosis. (Fig. 2–194, *left*) This biopsy is from a patient who did not respond to interferon therapy. (Fig. 2–195, *right*) This patient had a liver transplant secondary to hepatitis B viral cirrhosis, but developed recurrent chronic hepatitis B viral infection post transplant.

Portal Neutrophils

Neutrophils within portal tracts are most frequently seen in biliary tract obstruction, with the neutrophils oriented to interlobular bile ducts (refer to Table 2–2, Bile Ducts: Inflammation by Neutrophils); however, neutrophils may also be seen scattered throughout the portal tracts and away from duct epithelium on liver biopsy specimens. Although acute cholangitis may clinically be suspected, sometimes portal neutrophils are not seen, as acute cholangitis frequently does not involve all portal tracts equally, and may not be represented in a small biopsy specimen. Nonetheless, some liver diseases (e.g., autoimmune hepatitis) may exhibit portal neutrophils away from duct epithelium and have no clinical or radiologic evidence of bile duct obstruction. Table 2–25 lists disorders in which portal neutrophils may be seen without definite bile duct orientation. Note that many of these diseases (e.g., extrahepatic biliary obstruction) may also exhibit acute cholangitis when multiple tissue sections are examined.

Figures 2–196 to 2–199 demonstrate portal neutrophils in various diseases.

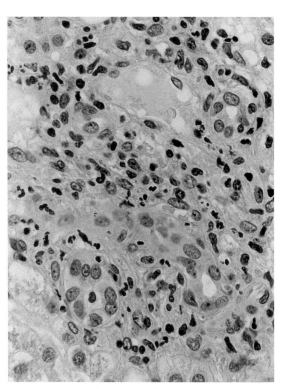

Figure 2–196   Acute Sclerosing Hyaline Necrosis (Acute Alcoholic Hepatitis)   A mixed infiltrate consisting of neutrophils and lymphocytes is present within this portal tract. Some of the neutrophils appear adjacent to bile ducts, while others are scattered.

TABLE 2–25

Portal Neutrophils

	Occurrence
Acute sclerosing hyaline necrosis (acute alcoholic hepatitis)	++
Adjacent to space-occupying lesions	+
Alcoholic foamy degeneration	+
Allograft, acute (cellular) rejection	+
Ascariasis	++
Autoimmune hepatitis	+
Bacterial sepsis	++
Brucellosis	+
Caroli's disease	+
Choledochal cyst	+
Extrahepatic biliary atresia	+
Extrahepatic biliary obstruction, early	++
Extrahepatic biliary obstruction, late (months–years)	+/++
Group B coxsackievirus infection	+
Hyperalimentation, infants	+
Inspissated bile syndrome	+
Nonalcoholic steatohepatitis	+
Polyarteritis nodosa	+
Primary biliary cirrhosis	+
Primary sclerosing cholangitis	+
Pylephlebitis	++
Pyogenic abscess	++
Recurrent pyogenic cholangiohepatitis	+/++
Toxic shock syndrome	+
Tuberculosis (severe)	+
Viral hepatitis, acute, classic type (early stage)	+

+ = Occasionally seen and usually scattered; ++ = frequently seen and often prominent.

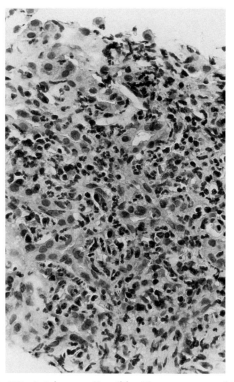

Figure 2–197   Autoimmune Hepatitis   Numerous neutrophils admixed with lymphocytes and plasma cells are seen within the portal tract. Bile ducts are also present without definite evidence of acute cholangitis.

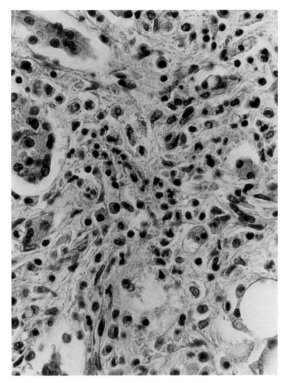

Figure 2–198 Bacterial Sepsis A mixed inflammatory infiltrate consisting of neutrophils, lymphocytes, and occasional plasma cells is seen within the portal tract.

Portal Plasma Cells

Untreated autoimmune hepatitis characteristically shows striking plasma cell infiltrates within the portal tracts and parenchyma; however, other liver diseases in which autoreactivity may play a role (e.g., virus induced) also may demonstrate numerous plasma cells (Table 2–26). These cells may be seen diffusely within the portal regions, but often occur as small localized clusters.

Figures 2–200 through 2–205 demonstrate portal plasma cells in various diseases.

TABLE 2–26

Portal Plasma Cells

	Occurrence
Acute fatty liver of pregnancy	+
Allograft, acute (cellular) rejection	+
Allograft, post transplant lymphoproliferative disease	+
Autoimmune hepatitis (untreated)	++
Chronic granulomatous disease of childhood	+
Epstein-Barr virus infection	+
Human immunodeficiency virus–associated cholangiopathy	+
Hydatid cyst	+
Leishmaniasis	+
Lymphoma, Hodgkin's	+
Malaria	+
Multiple myeloma	++
Nonspecific reactive hepatitis	+
Primary biliary cirrhosis	++
Primary sclerosing cholangitis	+
Q fever	+
Viral hepatitis, acute, type A	++
Viral hepatitis, chronic, type B	++
Viral hepatitis, chronic, type C	+
Waldenström's macroglobulinemia	++
Wilson's disease	+

+ = Occasionally seen, often forming small clusters; ++ = frequently seen and often prominent.

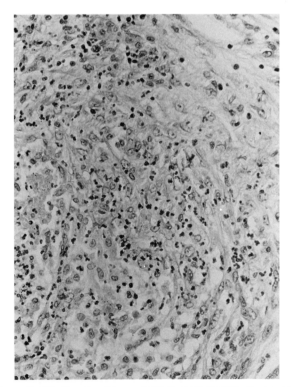

Figure 2–199 Recurrent Pyogenic Cholangiohepatitis Neutrophils can be seen mixed with occasional lymphocytes and numerous histiocytes within the portal tract, which is moderately expanded.

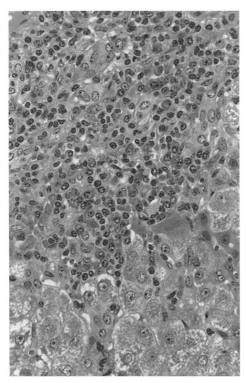

Figure 2–200   Autoimmune Hepatitis A striking portal plasma cell infiltrate is present.

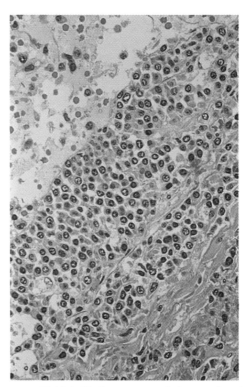

Figure 2–202   Multiple Myeloma A virtual plasma cell "culture" is seen in this markedly expanded portal tract next to a portal vein. This infiltrate rarely can be quite large and visualized on imaging.

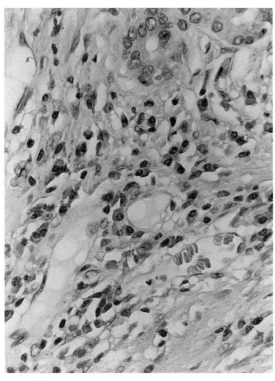

Figure 2–201   Hydatid Cyst A portal tract immediately adjacent to the cyst wall is seen infiltrated by numerous plasma cells.

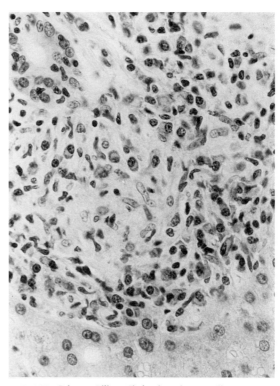

Figure 2–203   Primary Biliary Cirrhosis Plasma cells are seen within this portal tract. An interlobular bile duct infiltrated by lymphocytes, typical for primary biliary cirrhosis, is present at the upper left of the field. Note also that a small cluster of epithelioid cells is present in the center, representing a small granuloma, another feature sometimes seen in this liver disease.

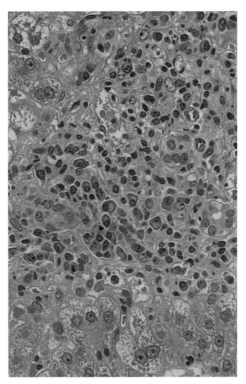

Figure 2–204 Viral Hepatitis, Acute, Type A Prominent numbers of plasma cells can be seen within the portal tract.

Portal Eosinophils

Although the two most common causes of increased numbers of eosinophils within the liver are parasitic infestation and hypersensitivity reactions, in other diseases the liver may be noted to contain increased numbers of eosinophils (Table 2–27). Usually the eosinophils are scattered within the portal tracts, although sometimes they are oriented to specific portal structures (e.g., small and medium-sized hepatic arteries in polyarteritis nodosa). Lobular infiltration can also be seen, especially when there is an associated eosinophilia. Of note is that whenever a liver disease (such as acute and chronic viral hepatitis) is associated with a prominent portal inflammatory infiltrate, eosinophils may occasionally be seen; however, in most cases the eosinophils are generally few in number and not considered for inclusion in Table 2–27 (exceptions are noted with an asterisk).

Figures 2–206 through 2–210 show portal eosinophils in various diseases.

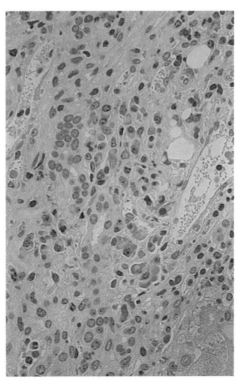

Figure 2–205 Viral Hepatitis, Chronic, Type B Clusters of plasma cells are seen within the center of the portal tract.

TABLE 2–27
Portal Eosinophils

	Occurrence
Acute fatty liver of pregnancy	+
Allograft, acute (cellular) rejection*	++
Ascariasis	++
Capillariasis	++
Clonorchiasis	+/++
Enterobiasis	++
Eosinophilic gastroenteritis	++
Epstein-Barr virus infection*	+
Fascioliasis	++
Hydatid cyst	++
Hypereosinophilic syndrome	++
Lymphoma, Hodgkin's*	+
Nonspecific reactive hepatitis*	+
Polyarteritis nodosa	++
Primary biliary cirrhosis*	+
Primary sclerosing cholangitis*	+
Recurrent pyogenic cholangiohepatitis†	+/++
Schistosomiasis (early)	++
Strongyloidiasis	++
Visceral larva migrans	++

  * Although portal lymphocytes may be numerous in these liver diseases, at times the eosinophils are disproportionately increased.

  † This liver disease is frequently associated with *Clonorchis sinensis* infestation within the large main intrahepatic and extrahepatic bile ducts; the liver fluke is then responsible for the eosinophilic infiltrates.

  + = Occasionally seen and usually scattered; ++ = frequently seen and often prominent.

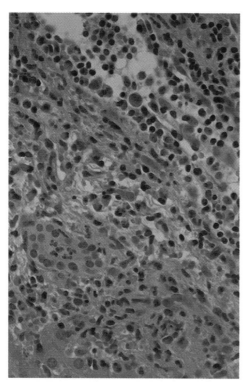

Figure 2–206 Allograft, Acute (Cellular) Rejection A mixed portal infiltrate consisting of small and large (immunoblastic) lymphocytes, macrophages, neutrophils, and numerous eosinophils is seen. Note the endothelialitis, a feature of acute rejection, involving the portal vein.

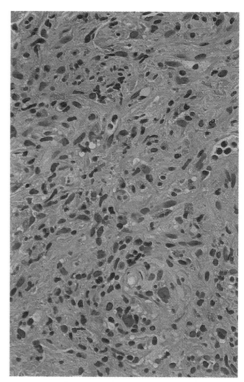

Figure 2–208 Lymphoma, Hodgkin's A mixed portal infiltrate that includes eosinophils can be seen. Note the Reed-Sternberg variant cells in the bottom of the field.

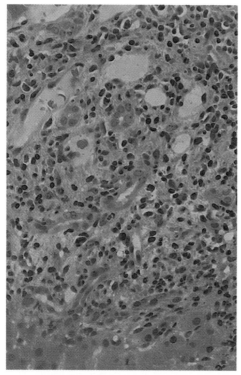

Figure 2–207 Drug-induced Portal Eosinophils (Halothane) Hypersensitivity reactions to numerous drugs, in this case halothane, can induce prominent portal eosinophilic infiltrates.

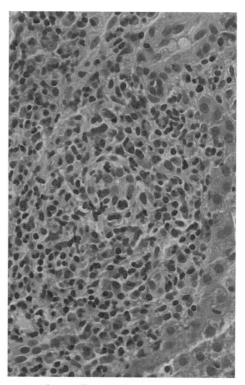

Figure 2–209 Primary Biliary Cirrhosis Although lymphocytes and plasma cells are the usual portal inflammatory infiltrate, at times numerous eosinophils can also be seen.

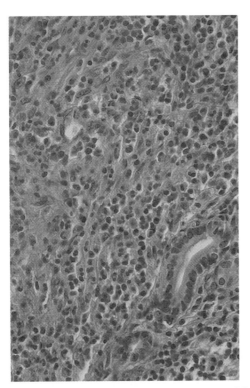

Figure 2–210 Visceral Larva Migrans Prominent eosinophils can be seen within this portal tract. The liver elsewhere showed numerous granulomas with central fibrinoid necrosis.

Portal Fibrosis

Cirrhosis, or Portal Fibrosis with Progression to Cirrhosis on Serial Biopsies

The majority of chronic liver diseases that demonstrate portal fibrosis may eventually lead to *cirrhosis,* defined as fibrous bands with regenerative nodule formation. Depending on their size, the nodules are termed *micronodular* (≤3 mm in diameter) or *macronodular* (>3 mm in diameter). Not infrequently some of the macronodules may subdivide into micronodules as the disease becomes well advanced; hence both macronodules and micronodules (*mixed pattern*) may be seen in the same liver. When cirrhosis is due to biliary tract disorders, the nodules often tend to have a geographic pattern, with the fibrous bands exhibiting collagen laid down in a parallel fashion around the nodules. This type of cirrhosis is termed *biliary,* and the nodules are usually but not always small and micronodular in size. Table 2–28 lists the various etiologies of cirrhosis but is not broken down into macronodular versus micronodular, as there is a tremendous degree of overlap in the type of cirrhosis in many liver diseases. For example, it is often said in the literature that cirrhosis secondary to chronic HBV is macronodular, yet autopsy findings have clearly shown that the nodules can be small (micronodular), especially in the advanced stage. Similarly, the patient with alcoholic cirrhosis who has stopped drinking is said to eventually develop a macronodular cirrhosis; however, in examining explanted livers from alcoholics who have abstained, the nodules may still be small, or the pattern may be mixed.

Figures 2–211 through 2–225 demonstrate examples of liver diseases in which portal fibrosis may progress to cirrhosis.

TABLE 2–28

Portal Fibrosis

Cirrhosis, or Portal Fibrosis with Progression to Cirrhosis on Serial Biopsies

Abetalipoproteinemia
Alcoholic cirrhosis
Allograft, chronic (ducto-penic) rejection
Alpers' disease
Alpha₁-antichymotrypsin deficiency
Alpha₁-antitrypsin deficiency
Autoimmune hepatitis
Budd-Chiari syndrome, chronic
Cholesterol ester storage disease
Chronic granulomatous disease of childhood
Crohn's disease
Cystic fibrosis
Drugs/toxins (refer to Table 4–9)
Erythropoietic protoporphyria
Extrahepatic biliary atresia
Extrahepatic biliary obstruction, late (years)
Fibrinogen storage disease
Galactosemia
Gaucher's disease
Glycogen storage disease types III, IV, and VI
Graft-versus-host disease
Heart failure, right-sided (chronic)
Hemochromatosis
Hereditary fructose intolerance
Hereditary hemorrhagic telangiectasia

Hyperalimentation, infant and adult
Idiopathic adulthood ductopenia
Indian childhood cirrhosis
Langerhans' cell histiocytosis
Long-chain acyl-CoA dehydrogenase deficiency
Mucopolysaccharidoses
Neonatal hepatitis
Niemann-Pick disease
Nonalcoholic steatohepatitis
Paucity of intrahepatic ducts, nonsyndromatic
Porphyria cutanea tarda
Primary biliary cirrhosis
Primary sclerosing cholangitis
Progressive familial intrahepatic cholestasis
Recurrent cholestasis with lymphedema
Sarcoidosis
Tangier's disease
Tyrosinemia
Ulcerative colitis
Veno-occlusive disease, chronic
Viral hepatitis, chronic, classic type
Wilson's disease
Wolman's disease
Zellweger's syndrome

Portal Fibrosis Without Progression to Cirrhosis

Congenital hepatic fibrosis
Drugs/toxins (refer to Table 4–9)
Fascioliasis
Glycogen storage disease types IX and X
Homocystinuria
Hypereosinophilic syndrome
Idiopathic portal hypertension
Infantile microcystic disease
Lymphoma, Hodgkin's and non-Hodgkin's (B cell, high grade)

Malaria
Myeloproliferative disorders
Myoclonus epilepsy
Paracoccidioidomycosis
Paucity of intrahepatic ducts, syndromatic
Schistosomiasis
Syphilis, congenital
Systemic caritine deficiency
Tuberculosis

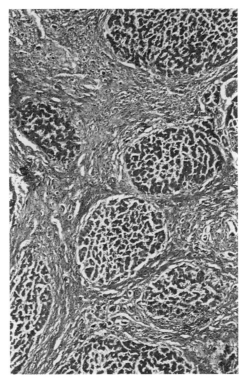

Figure 2–211 Alcoholic Cirrhosis (Trichrome) This photomicrograph is from a liver explant in an alcoholic who stopped drinking 1 year prior to surgery. The regenerative nodules are small (micronodular) but well defined, without any evidence of active disease (e.g., absence of fatty change, sinusoidal collagen, Mallory bodies).

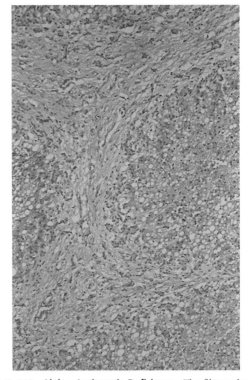

Figure 2–212 Alpha₁-Antitrypsin Deficiency The fibrous bands adjacent to the regenerative nodules have the collagen laid down in a parallel fashion (biliary). Although cholangioles are seen, there is a paucity of interlobular bile ducts. The protease inhibitor type in this 1-year-old child was PiZZ.

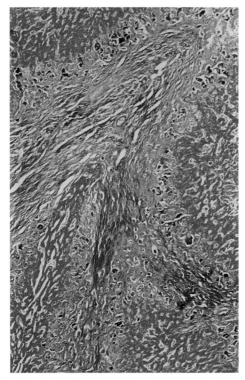

Figure 2–213 Cystic Fibrosis (Trichrome) The fibrous bands are laid down in a parallel fashion (biliary). Numerous bile plugs can also be seen within dilated cholangioles at the border of the fibrous bands and hepatocytes.

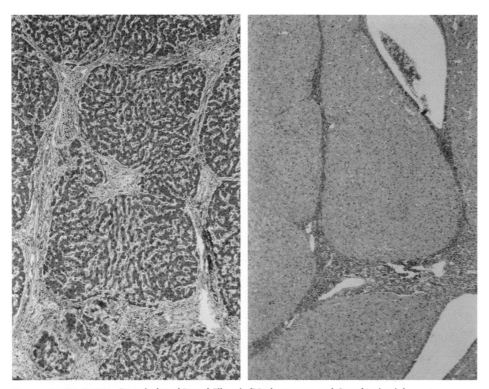

Figures 2–214, 2–215 Drug-induced Portal Fibrosis (Methotrexate and Oxyphenisatin)
(Fig. 2–214, *left*) This is an example of a patient with psoriasis who had taken low-dose methotrexate daily for many years. The methotrexate was stopped after the diagnosis of cirrhosis was made on biopsy. Note that this section of liver taken at autopsy shows a cirrhotic nodule with thin fibrous bands on trichrome stain. (Fig. 2–215, *right*) Oxyphenisatin is known to cause chronic hepatitis, and may eventually lead to cirrhosis, as demonstrated in this photomicrograph, if the medication is not discontinued.

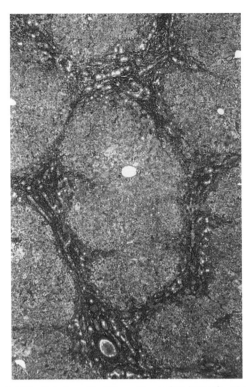

Figure 2-216 Extrahepatic Biliary Atresia (Trichrome) This is a wedge biopsy of liver taken at the time of a Kasai procedure (hepatoportoenterostomy). Small regenerative nodules are seen. Numerous dilated interlobular bile ducts can be identified within the fibrous bands.

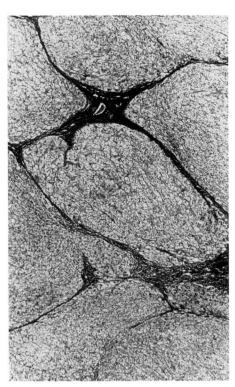

Figure 2-218 Glycogen Storage Disease Type III (Trichrome) Small to medium-sized regenerative nodules are present in this explanted liver.

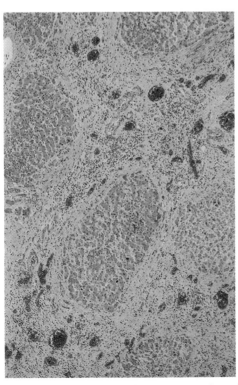

Figure 2-217 Extrahepatic Biliary Obstruction, Late (Years) A micronodular biliary cirrhosis is seen in a patient with chronic pancreatitis and stricture of the common bile duct.

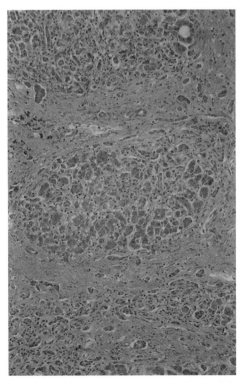

Figure 2-219 Hemochromatosis The regenerative nodules are small. Note that even on low power, pigment representing hemosiderin (confirmed on iron stain) is present in hepatocytes and duct epithelium.

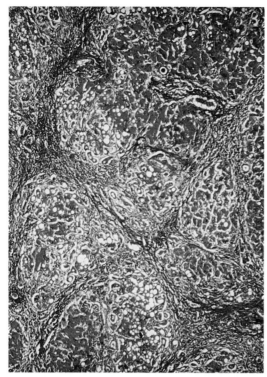

Figure 2-220 Nonalcoholic Steatohepatitis (Trichrome) This is from a wedge biopsy taken at the time of gastric bypass surgery for morbid obesity. The nodules are small, poorly defined, with considerable sinusoidal collagen deposition and variable fatty change.

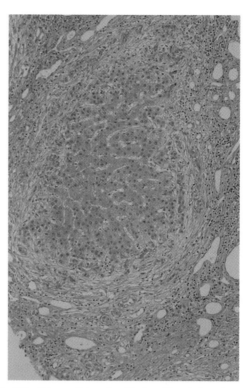

Figure 2-222 Primary Sclerosing Cholangitis As in primary biliary cirrhosis, the nodules exhibit a parallel array of lamellar fibrosis at the border of the nodules and fibrous bands (biliary type). No interlobular bile ducts are present.

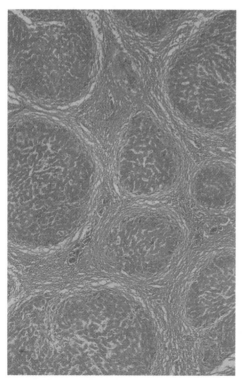

Figure 2-221 Primary Biliary Cirrhosis The regenerative nodules are small. Note parallel bands of fibrous tissue at the border of the nodules, characteristic of biliary type. Closer inspection in this example would reveal absence of interlobular bile ducts.

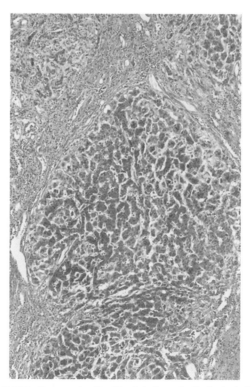

Figure 2-223 Progressive Familiar Intrahepatic Cholestasis (Byler's Syndrome) A micronodular (biliary) cirrhosis is present, with depletion of interlobular bile ducts.

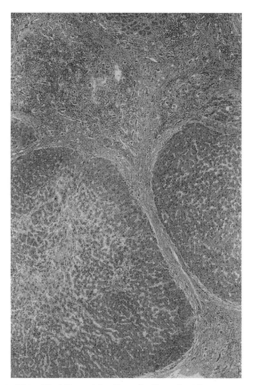

Figure 2–224 Viral Hepatitis, Chronic, Type B The regenerative nodules are well defined. In this photomicrograph, macronodules are seen; however, in other areas both macronodules and micronodules are present.

Portal Fibrosis *Without* Progression to Cirrhosis

Certain chronic liver diseases characteristically exhibit some degree of portal fibrosis that does *not* progress to cirrhosis with time (second part of Table 2–28). The value of listing these disorders separately is that if a liver disease such as idiopathic portal hypertension is clinically suspected, but a well-established cirrhosis is seen on biopsy, then that disease can be eliminated in the differential diagnosis.

Figures 2–226 through 2–228 demonstrate examples of liver disease in which portal fibrosis does *not* progress to cirrhosis.

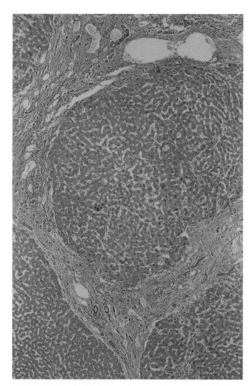

Figure 2–225 Wilson's Disease The regenerative nodules are well defined. The degree of inflammatory activity in this particular case is minimal.

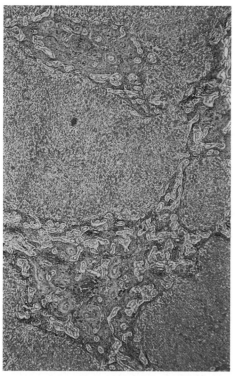

Figure 2–226 Congenital Hepatic Fibrosis (Trichrome) Although bridging fibrosis is seen, no regenerative nodules are present. Note the numerous dilated ducts within the fibrous regions.

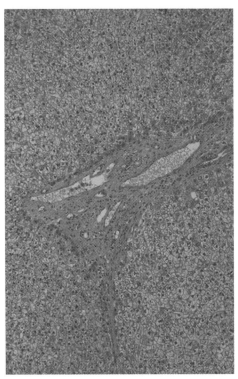

Figure 2–227   Idiopathic Portal Hypertension   The fibrotic portal tract exhibits a slightly dilated portal vein, with smaller portal venous radicles (suggestive of portal hypertension). No bridging fibrosis or cirrhosis was present at the time of portacaval shunt.

Sinusoids

Fibrosis

Sinusoidal collagen deposition may be present either as delicate fibrous strands that may or may not have a zonal distribution, or as striking and often diffuse interstitial bands involving virtually all the sinusoids in all zones. In some instances the strands may be quite thin and difficult to visualize on hematoxylin-eosin stain alone, but can best be seen on trichrome stain. In instances in which the sinusoidal collagen deposition is prominent (e.g., acute sclerosing hyaline necrosis), signs of portal hypertension such as ascites and esophageal varices may be present in a noncirrhotic liver. Associated sclerosis of the terminal hepatic venules may also be seen in some liver diseases, which are also listed in Table 2–37, Vessels (Excluding Sinusoids): Thrombosis and Occlusion. The liver disorders listed in Table 2–29 are divided into the degree of sinusoidal collagen most often present.

Figures 2–229 through 2–238 demonstrate sinusoidal collagen deposition in various diseases.

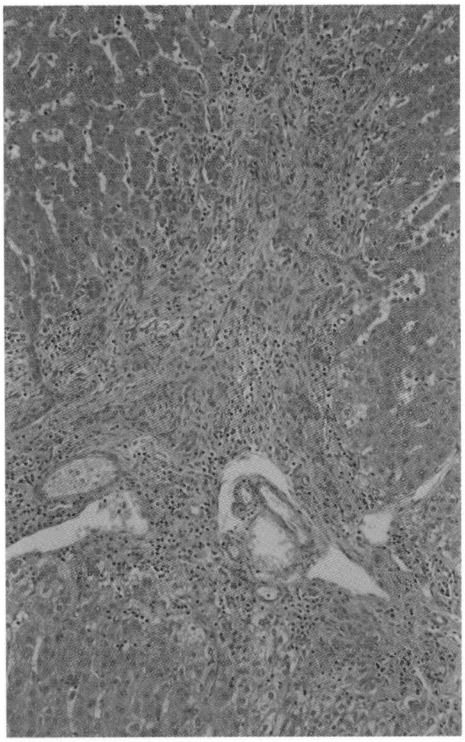

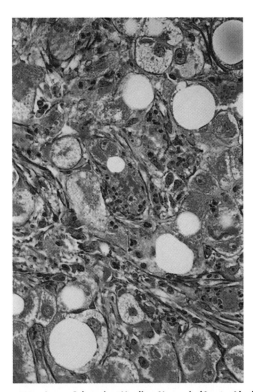

Figure 2–229   Acute Sclerosing Hyaline Necrosis (Acute Alcoholic Hepatitis) (Trichrome)   Extensive perivenular intrasinusoidal collagen deposition is seen. The liver cell in the center of the field shows the presence of Mallory bodies (staining red) with surrounding neutrophils (satellitosis).

Figure 2–228   Paucity of Ducts, Syndromatic (Alagille's Syndrome)   The fibrotic portal tract exhibits increased numbers of cholangioles; however, no interlobular bile ducts are seen. There is no bridging fibrosis or cirrhosis.

TABLE 2–29

Sinusoids: Fibrosis

Acute fatty liver, alcoholic etiology	+
Acute sclerosing hyaline necrosis (acute alcoholic hepatitis)	++
Alcoholic cirrhosis (active drinker)	++
Alcoholic foamy degeneration	+
Allograft, chronic (ductopenic) rejection	+
Allograft, fibrosing cholestatic hepatitis	++
Budd-Chiari syndrome, chronic	+
Cholangiocarcinoma	++*
Cholesterol ester storage disease	+
Crohn's disease	+
Cystic fibrosis	+
Down syndrome	++
Erythropoietic protoporphyria	+
Focal nodular hyperplasia	++†
Gangliosidosis, GM$_2$	+
Gaucher's disease	+
Heart failure, right-sided	+
Hepatocellular carcinoma, fibrolamellar type	++*
Hepatocellular carcinoma, trabecular, acinar, ductular type	+/++*
Hereditary fructose intolerance	++
Hyperalimentation, adult	+
Hyperalimentation, infants	+/++
Hypothyroidism	+
Idiopathic portal hypertension	+
Indian childhood cirrhosis	++
Leishmaniasis (chronic)	++
Lymphoma, non-Hodgkin's (B cell, high grade)	+
Mannosidosis	+
Mucopolysaccharidoses	++
Myeloproliferative disorders	+
Myoclonus epilepsy	+
Neonatal hepatitis	+
Niemann-Pick disease	+
Nonalcoholic steatohepatitis	+/++
Paucity of intrahepatic ducts, nonsyndromatic	++
Perivenular fibrosis, alcoholic etiology	+/++
Progressive perivenular alcoholic fibrosis	+/++
Schistosomiasis	+
Sickle cell anemia	+/++
Syphilis, congenital	++
Tyrosinemia	+
Veno-occlusive disease, chronic	+
Viral hepatitis, chronic, type C	+
Wilson's disease	+
Wolman's disease	+
Zellweger's syndrome	+

* Relates to the degree of collagen seen between tumor cells.

† Relates to the fibrous radiating band seen in the center of the tumor; away from this band, sinusoidal collagen is absent.

+ = Focal with or without zonal distribution; ++ = prominent and often diffuse.

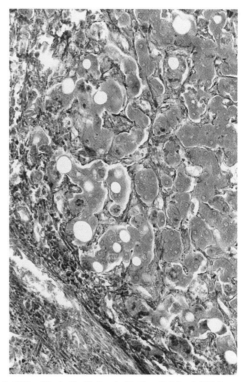

Figure 2–230 Alcoholic Cirrhosis (Active Drinker) (Trichrome) Prominent periseptal intrasinusoidal collagen is seen on high power in this cirrhotic liver.

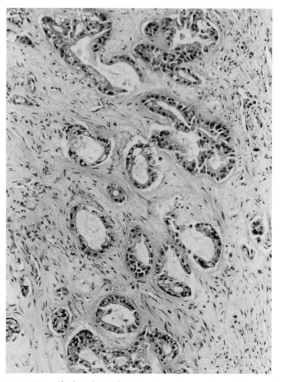

Figure 2–231 Cholangiocarcinoma Prominent sclerosis is seen between the neoplastic glands.

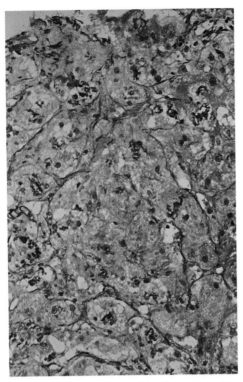

Figure 2–232   Drug-induced Sinusoidal Collagen Deposition (Amiodarone) (Trichrome)   Interstitial sinusoidal collagen deposition is seen. In addition, some of the hepatocytes contain Mallory bodies (staining blue).

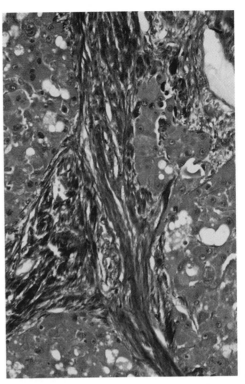

Figure 2–234   Hepatocellular Carcinoma, Fibrolamellar Type   Prominent bands of collagen laid down in a parallel (fibrolamellar) fashion are seen between the tumor cells.

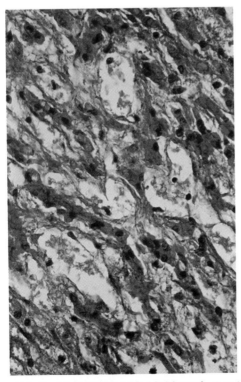

Figure 2–233   Heat Failure, Right-sided (Trichrome)   Prominent sinusoidal collagen is seen in these dilated sinusoids, also associated with variable liver cell atrophy.

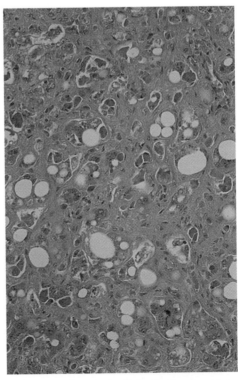

Figure 2–235   Hyperalimentation (Infant)   Prominent interstitial fibrosis is seen within the sinusoids. Cholestasis and fatty change are also present.

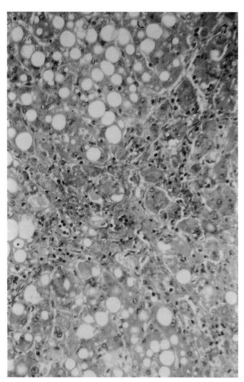

Figure 2–236 Nonalcoholic Steatohepatitis (Trichrome) The sinusoidal collagen has a perivenular and midzonal accentuation. Sclerosis of the terminal hepatic venule is also present.

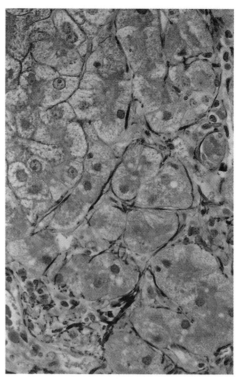

Figure 2–238 Viral Hepatitis, Chronic, Type C (Trichrome) The sinusoidal collagen is thin. Although a periportal accentuation is often seen, at times the collagen fibers may be randomly distributed.

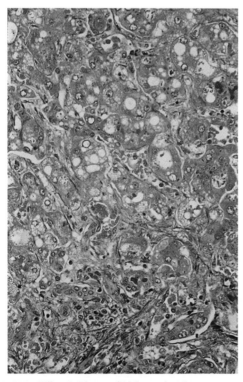

Figure 2–237 Wilson's Disease (Trichrome) Thin intrasinusoidal collagen bands are seen with no distinct zonal distribution pattern.

Sinusoids

Dilatation, Congestion, and Hemorrhage

The most common causes of sinusoidal *dilatation and congestion* relate to impaired hepatic venous outflow. In these instances, the histologic changes are most prominent in the perivenular zone and midzone (zones 3 and 2), although in severe instances the changes can be diffuse (Table 2–30). Generally, dilatation and congestion involve all lobules throughout the liver, although focal hepatic involvement is characteristic adjacent to mass lesions. When the congestion is severe, in conjunction with prominent vascular compromise (poor intrahepatic blood flow), perivenular liver cell dropout (ischemic necrosis) may occur, with resultant *hemorrhage*. Congestion and hemorrhage can also be seen focally without a distinct zonal distribution as a response to localized liver cell necrosis (e.g., adenovirus infection).

Figures 2–239 to 2–243 demonstrate examples of sinusoidal dilatation and congestion as well as hemorrhage.

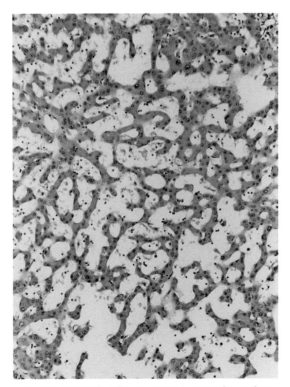

Figure 2–239   Sinusoids Adjacent to Space-occupying Lesions
This is a photomicrograph of the liver immediately adjacent to a hydatid cyst. The sinusoids show marked dilatation with atrophic liver cell cords due to impairment of hepatic venous outflow from compression by the cyst.

TABLE 2–30

Sinusoids: Dilatation, Congestion, and Hemorrhage

	Dilatation, Congestion	Hemorrhage
Acute fatty liver of pregnancy		+
Adenovirus infection		+
Adjacent to space-occupying lesions	+	
Allograft, acute graft failure		+
Allograft, harvesting (preservation) injury (severe)	+	+
Allograft, hyperacute (humeral) rejection		+
Amyloidosis*	+	
Angiosarcoma	+	
Aspergillosis		+
Borreliosis		+
Budd-Chiari, acute	+	+
Budd-Chiari, chronic	+	
Drugs/toxins (refer to Table 4–12)		
Heart failure, right-sided, acute	+	+
Heart failure, right-sided, chronic	+	
Hemolysis, elevation of liver enzymes, low platelet (HELLP) syndrome		+
Hereditary hemorrhagic telangiectasia	+	
Herpes simplex virus infection		+
Hypereosinophilic syndrome	+	
Hyperthyroidism	+	
Leukemia	+	
Light chain disease	+	
Lymphoma, Hodgkin's	+	
Malaria	+	
Myeloproliferative disorders	+	
Peliosis hepatis	+	
Pneumocystis carinii infection	+	
Rheumatoid arthritis	+	+
Sickle cell anemia	+	
Spontaneous rupture in pregnancy		+
Systemic lupus erythematosus	+	+
Toxemia of pregnancy	+	+
Veno-occlusive disease, acute	+	+
Veno-occlusive disease, chronic*	+	

*Although sinusoidal dilatation is present, congestion is uncommon.

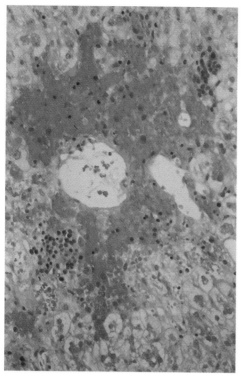

Figure 2–240 Allograft, Harvesting (Preservation) Injury The perivenular zone shows acute hemorrhage, without sinusoidal dilatation.

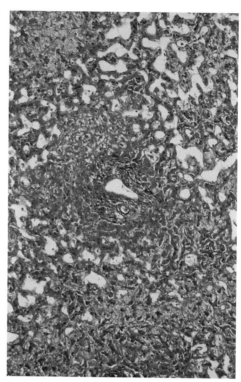

Figure 2–242 Heart Failure, Right-sided, Chronic (Trichrome) Prominent sinusoidal dilatation is seen involving the perivenular zones. Note that the perivenular zones connect with one another, with a centrally located normal-sized portal tract (reverse lobulation).

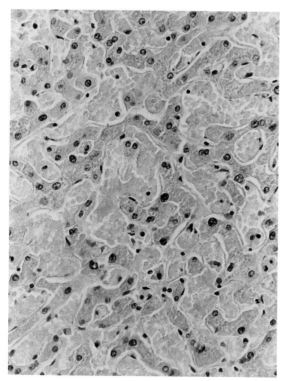

Figure 2–241 Heart Failure, Right-sided, Acute The sinusoids show marked dilatation and congestion, with slight atrophy of the adjacent liver cell plates.

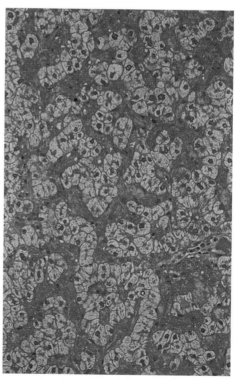

Figure 2–243 Sickle Cell Anemia The sinusoids are dilated and congested, and filled with sludged (sickled) red blood cells.

Sinusoids
Peliotic Lesions

Peliosis is a cystic space filled with red blood cells and is distributed randomly within the parenchyma (Table 2–31). It is formed either secondary to intrinsic weakness of the reticulin fibers or by focal liver cell dropout. These lesions initially do not have an endothelial lining, but endothelialization may in time occur. The lesion is usually microscopic, although in some instances (e.g., associated with AIDS) it can reach up to 2 cm in diameter and may be visualized on imaging. In rare instances, small capillaries may arise within the vascular spaces.

Figures 2–244 to 2–247 show peliotic lesions in various diseases.

TABLE 2–31
Sinusoids: Peliotic Lesions

Adenoma, liver cell
Angiosarcoma
Bacillary angiomatosis
Drugs/toxins (refer to Table 4–11)
Glycogen storage disease, type Ia
Hepatocellular carcinoma, fibrolamellar type
Hepatocellular carcinoma, trabecular, acinar, ductular type
Human immunodeficiency virus infection
Leukemia, hairy cell
Light chain disease
Lymphoma, Hodgkin's and non-Hodgkin's (B cell, high
  grade)
Marasmus
Peliosis hepatis
Systemic lupus erythematosus
Waldenströms macroglobulinemia

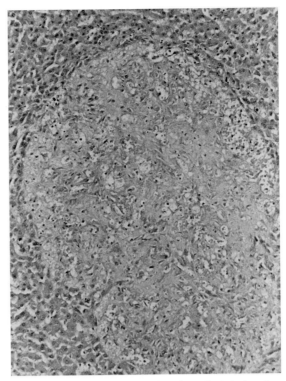

Figure 2–244   Bacillary Angiomatosis   This peliotic lesion shows numerous increased vascular channels on this hematoxylin-eosin stain. Gram-negative bacilli representing the rickettsial organism *Bartonella (Rochalimaea)* species were also identified by Warthin-Starry stain.

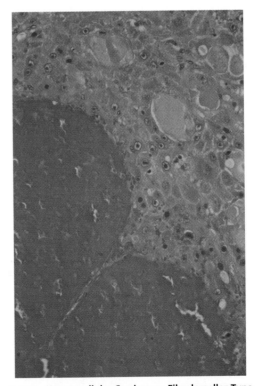

Figure 2–245   Hepatocellular Carcinoma, Fibrolamellar Type
Eosinophilic tumor cells are present, one of which contains a large cytoplasmic inclusion ("pale body"). Two peliotic lesions are also present.

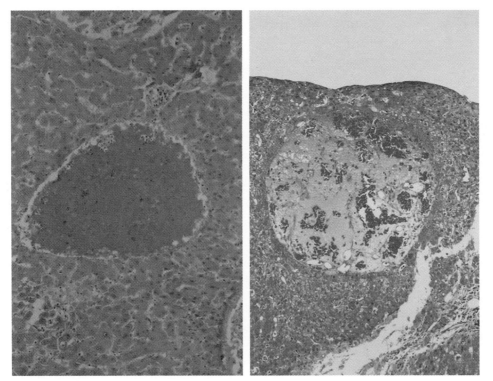

Figures 2–246, 2–247   Peliosis Hepatitis   (Fig. 2–246, *left*) The peliotic lesion is present within the parenchyma. (Fig. 2–247, *right*) In a patient with AIDS, the peliotic lesion on trichrome stain contains numerous small vascular channels.

Sinusoids

Red Blood Cell Extravasation

(Red Blood Cell–Trabecular Lesion)

The *red blood cell–trabecular lesion* represents red blood cell extravasation initially beneath the Kupffer and endothelial cells into the space of Disse, eventually replacing liver cells that have become atrophic or have dropped out due to ischemic injury (Table 2–32). It is often associated with acute hepatic venous outflow obstruction, but may also be seen in instances of poor arterial blood flow in the *absence* of hypotension. It also may be seen within the first few days to weeks after liver transplantation, in which liver cell dropout in the absence of hypotension may occur due to preservation injury. This lesion is seen most frequently within the perivenular zone (zone 3), although in severe cases zone 2 may also be involved.

Figures 2–248 to 2–250 demonstrate sinusoidal red blood cell extravasation in various diseases.

TABLE 2–32

Sinusoids: Red Blood Cell Extravasation

Adjacent to space-occupying lesions
Allograft, acute (cellular) rejection (severe)*
Allograft, acute graft failure
Allograft, harvesting (preservation) injury
Allograft, ischemia secondary to hepatic artery thrombosis
Budd-Chiari syndrome, acute
Drugs/toxins (refer to Table 4–13)
Heart failure, left-sided without hypotension
Myeloproliferative disorders
Veno-occlusive disease, acute

*Although acute rejection does not directly cause perivenular dropout, in severe rejection inflammation and occlusion of the hepatic arterioles may occur with secondary ischemia.

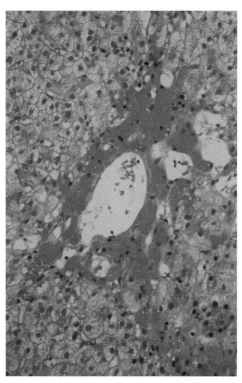

Figure 2–248 Allograft, Harvesting (Preservation) Injury The perivenular zone shows red blood cell extravasation into the hepatic cords with concomitant liver cell dropout.

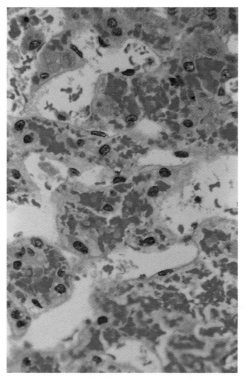

Figure 2–249 Budd-Chiari Syndrome, Acute Red blood cell extravasation into the hepatic cords can be seen. In this case it was due to hepatic venous outflow obstruction by a liver cell carcinoma occluding a large intrahepatic vein.

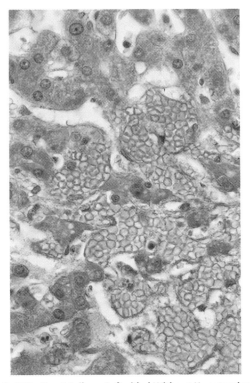

Figure 2–250 Heart Failure, Left-sided Without Hypotension (Trichrome) The liver cell cords within the perivenular zone (zone 3) show dropout of hepatocytes and their replacement by red blood cells. Note that the adjacent sinusoids are open and empty.

Sinusoids
Circulating Cells

Increased circulating cells within the sinusoids are usually associated with a high peripheral white blood cell count (Table 2–33). In many instances, variable degrees of lobular inflammation and necrosis (e.g., Epstein-Barr virus infection) may also be seen, usually associated with a portal inflammatory infiltrate.

Figures 2–251 to 2–254 show sinusoidal circulatory cells in various diseases.

TABLE 2–33
Sinusoids: Circulating Cells

Lymphocytes

Allograft, acute (cellular) rejection (severe)	Leukemia, chronic lymphocytic
Allograft, post transplant lymphoproliferative disease	Lyme disease
	Lymphoma, non-Hodgkin's
Borreliosis	Malaria
Cytomegalovirus infection	Nonspecific reactive hepatitis
Epstein-Barr virus infection	Rheumatoid arthritis
	Salmonellosis
Leishmaniasis	Viral hepatitis, acute, type C*
	Viral hepatitis, chronic, type C*

Neutrophils

Acute sclerosing hyaline necrosis (acute alcoholic hepatitis)	Leukemia, chronic myelogenous
Bacterial sepsis	Lyme disease
Borreliosis	Surgical hepatitis

*Although acute and chronic viral hepatitis in general may be associated with some degree of lymphocytosis, this feature is more often present in hepatitis C virus infection.

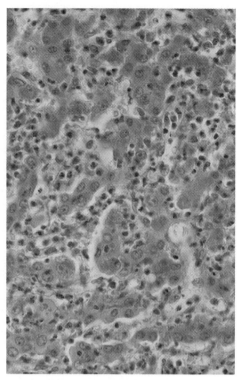

Figure 2–251 Acute Sclerosing Hyaline Necrosis (Acute Alcoholic Hepatitis) Neutrophils are often associated with Mallory body deposition in this disorder; however, leukocytosis is also a common feature, and at times can be marked. The white blood cell count on this patient at time of biopsy was 60,000.

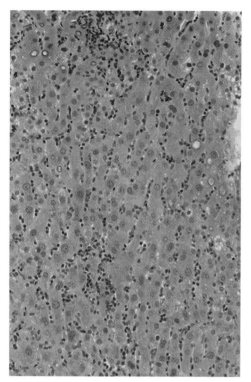

Figure 2–253 Epstein-Barr Virus Infection Prominent numbers of circulating lymphocytes are seen having a characteristic "beading" back-to-back appearance within the sinusoids.

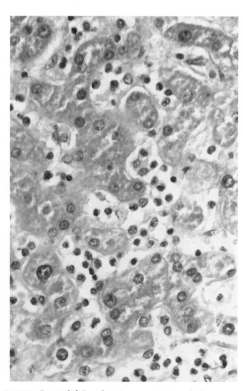

Figure 2–252 Bacterial Sepsis Increase in circulating neutrophils can be seen, associated with peripheral leukocytosis.

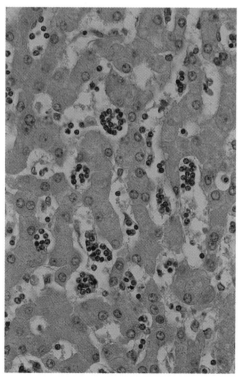

Figure 2–254 Leukemia, Chronic Lymphocytic Circulating leukemic cells are common within the sinusoids, the number seen in direct proportion to the white blood cell count.

Sinusoids

Extramedullary Hematopoiesis

Although extramedullary hematopoiesis (EMH) within the liver is most commonly seen in biopsies from neonates, it is also seen in various hematologic (e.g., myeloproliferative) disorders and certain neoplasms, such as hepatoblastoma (Table 2–34). In addition, EMH is also associated with various malignancies metastatic to the bone. It must be kept in mind that identification of a *single* megakaryocyte with no evidence of myeloid or erythroid precursors may rarely be encountered in an otherwise "normal" liver in which there is no clinical evidence of hematopoietic abnormalities or metastatic disease.

Figures 2–255 to 2–258 demonstrate EMH in various diseases.

TABLE 2–34

Sinusoids: Extramedullary Hematopoiesis

Adenoma, liver cell
Allograft, acute (cellular) rejection
Alpha$_1$-antitrypsin deficiency
Angiosarcoma
Down syndrome
Extrahepatic biliary atresia
Galactosemia
Hepatoblastoma
Hepatocellular carcinoma, trabecular, acinar, ductular type
Infantile hemangioendothelioma
Leukemia
Malignant neoplasms metastatic to bone*
Mesenchymal hamartoma
Myeloproliferative disorders
Neonatal hepatitis
Nodular regenerative hyperplasia
Paucity of intrahepatic ducts, nonsyndromatic and syndromatic
Sickle cell anemia
Tyrosinemia

*Not covered in Chapter 3, Liver Diseases: Pathology and Clinical Considerations.

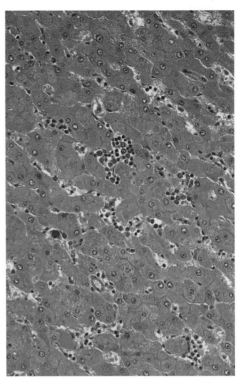

Figure 2–255 Adenoma, Liver Cell This benign hepatic neoplasm may rarely exhibit red and white cell precursors and megakaryocytes.

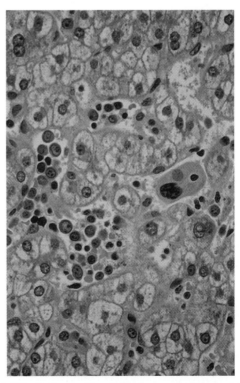

Figure 2–256 Leukemia, Chronic Myelogenous Extramedullary hematopoiesis is seen and is located within the sinusoids. All three cells lines are present in this field.

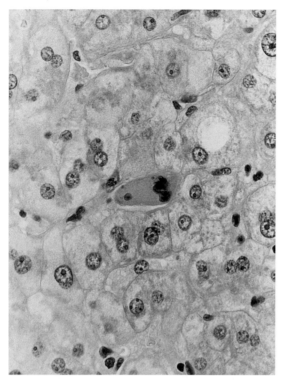

Figure 2–257 Myeloproliferative Disorders This field shows a megakaryocyte and normoblast within the sinusoid in a patient with myelofibrosis.

Syncytial Giant Cells

Syncytial giant cells (giant cell transformation) represent multinucleated hepatocytes. These cells are enlarged and have anywhere from 4 to over 50 nuclei, with an eosinophilic to slightly granular and sometimes hydropic cytoplasm (Table 2–35). These cells are most commonly seen in the neonate in a variety of liver diseases, and may involve all zones or tend to have a perivenular (zone 3) accentuation. In the adult this feature is less common; when present, the giant cells tend to be smaller and have fewer nuclei than those seen in the neonate. Syncytial giant cells most commonly occur due to inhibition of mitotic activity from viruses or drugs, and are seen in various inherited disorders. They may occur due to dissolution of cell membranes, and should not be confused with multinucleated giant cells (fusion of activated macrophages [*epithelioid cells*]) seen in granulomas.

Figures 2–259 through 2–264 demonstrate syncytial giant cells in various diseases.

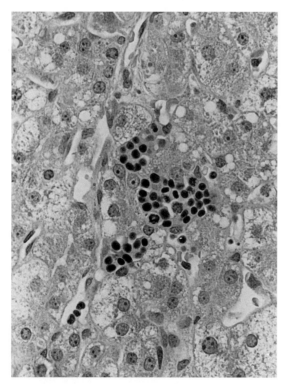

Figure 2–258 Paucity of Intrahepatic Ducts Clusters of normoblasts are seen within the lobule. This feature is not characteristic of the liver disease, but rather a manifestation of the patient's age (in this case an infant).

TABLE 2–35

Syncytial Giant Cells

Adenovirus infection
Alpha$_1$-antitrypsin deficiency
Autoimmune hepatitis
Cystic fibrosis
Cytomegalovirus infection
Epstein-Barr virus infection
Extrahepatic biliary atresia
Galactosemia
Hemochromatosis, neonatal variant
Hepatocellular carcinoma, trabecular type (poorly differentiated)
Hereditary fructose intolerance
Herpes simplex virus infection
Hyperalimentation, infants
Indian childhood cirrhosis
Neonatal hepatitis
Niemann-Pick disease
Paucity of intrahepatic ducts, syndromatic and nonsyndromatic
Progressive familial intrahepatic cholestasis
Recurrent cholestasis with lymphedema
Recurrent intrahepatic cholestasis of pregnancy
Rubella virus infection
Rubeola virus infection
Syphilis, congenital
Toxoplasmosis
Viral hepatitis, acute and chronic, type non A-G
Wilson's disease
Yellow fever

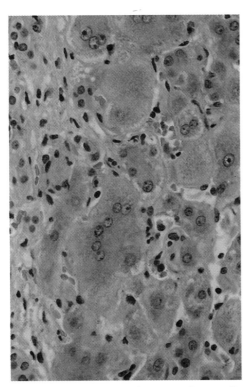

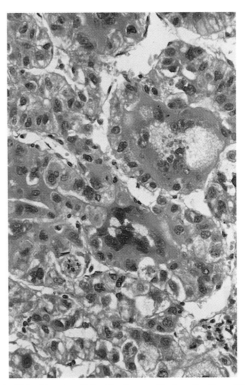

Figure 2-259 Autoimmune Hepatitis Syncytial giant cells can occasionally be seen in active stage disease, and are sometimes more prominent in the periportal zones.

Figure 2-261 Hepatocellular Carcinoma, Trabecular Type (Poorly Differentiated) This tumor may show syncytial giant cells in the less differentiated variants.

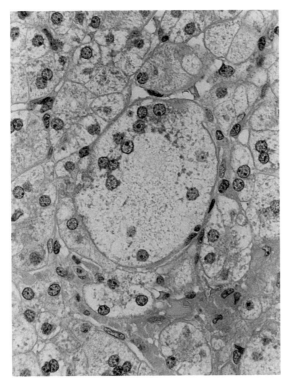

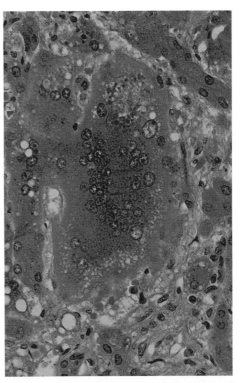

Figure 2-260 Extrahepatic Biliary Atresia A hydropic hepatocyte is seen having abundant somewhat clear cytoplasm and numerous nuclei. This feature is most prominent in the perivenular zone in this disorder.

Figure 2-262 Neonatal Hepatitis Multinucleated giant cells are a hallmark for this liver disease, and are usually seen diffusely throughout the lobule. In this example, the multinucleated cell is quite large, and also contains prominent hemosiderin pigment. Although increase in hemosiderin may be present in typical neonatal hepatitis, the differential diagnosis in this case would include neonatal variant of hemochromatosis, depending on the degree of iron on quantitation.

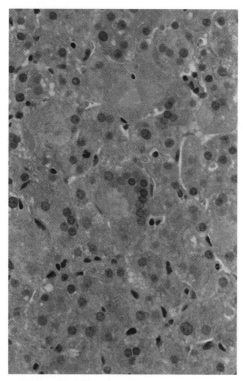

Figure 2–263 Paucity of Intrahepatic Ducts The giant cells may be seen anywhere in the lobule (in this case in zone 2), but are usually accentuated in the perivenular zone (zone 3).

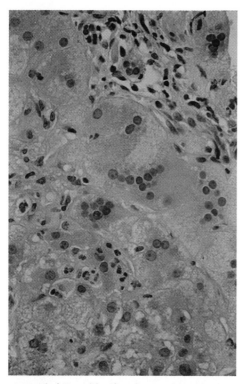

Figure 2–264 Viral Hepatitis, Chronic, Non A-G This liver disease is diagnosed on the basis of negative serologies for the other hepatotropic viruses, and exclusion of other viral etiologies (e.g., cytomegalovirus, adenovirus, exotic viruses). Multinucleated giant cells can occasionally be seen, and sometimes are present diffusely within the lobules.

Vessels (Excluding Sinusoids)
Inflammation

It is unusual to see inflammation of small arteries or arterioles in a biopsy specimen from a patient with systemic vasculitis, with the medium-sized vessels more characteristically involved. These changes are more frequently seen when the biopsy has been taken toward the hilum, where larger vessels are then available for evaluation. In some instances, when the vasculitis is severe and associated with partial or total occlusion of the lumen, the smaller arteries and arterioles as well as the interlobular bile ducts may undergo ischemic changes and become depleted (e.g., vascular rejection in an allograft). Secondary changes within the lobule may be seen due to hypoxemia and resultant ischemic necrosis. The inflammatory cells involving the arteries and arterioles are often mixed, including eosinophils, lymphocytes, and often neutrophils, sometimes associated with fibrin deposition. Depending on the etiology of the vasculitis, immunoperoxidase stain may demonstrate immunoglobulins (e.g., IgM, C1q deposits in hyperacute [humoral] allograft rejection). Inflammation of portal, terminal hepatic, and sublobular veins is usually mononuclear, with eosinophils less common; in instances of abdominal sepsis, however, neutrophils are usually present and may be prominent.

Figures 2–265 through 2–272 demonstrate nonsinusoidal vessel inflammation in various diseases.

TABLE 2–36

Vessels (Excluding Sinusoids): Inflammation

Arteries/Arterioles

Allograft, acute (cellular) rejection	Polyarteritis nodosa
	Rheumatoid arthritis
Allograft, hyperacute (humoral) rejection	Syphilis, secondary and tertiary
Allograft, vascular rejection	Systemic lupus erythematosus
Drugs/toxins (refer to Table 4–14)	Toxemia of pregnancy
Kawasaki disease	Toxic shock syndrome

Portal, Terminal Hepatic, and Sublobular Veins

Acute sclerosing hyaline necrosis (acute alcoholic hepatitis)	Perivenular fibrosis, alcoholic etiology
Allograft, acute (cellular) rejection	Progressive perivenular alcoholic fibrosis
Allograft, hyperacute (humoral) rejection	Pylephlebitis
	Recurrent pyogenic cholangiohepatitis
Crohn's disease	Salmonellosis
Epstein-Barr virus infection	Sarcoidosis
Graft-versus-host disease	Schistosomiasis
Inflammatory pseudotumor	Syphilis, secondary and tertiary
Lymphoma, non-Hodgkin's	
Nonalcoholic steatohepatitis	Toxic shock syndrome

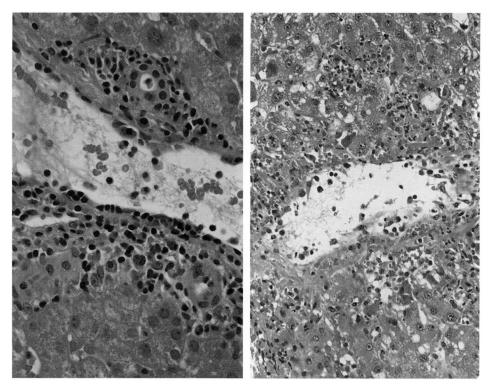

Figures 2–265, 2–266   Allograft, Acute (Cellular) Rejection   (Fig. 2–265, *left*) A portal vein shows lymphocytes hugging up against the damaged endothelium (endothelialitis). (Fig. 2–266, *right*) A terminal hepatic venule shows attachment of lymphocytes to the endothelium with endothelial damage. In severe rejection, perivenular sinusoidal lymphocytes are also present associated with variable liver cell dropout, as seen in this photomicrograph.

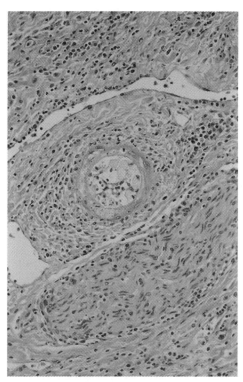

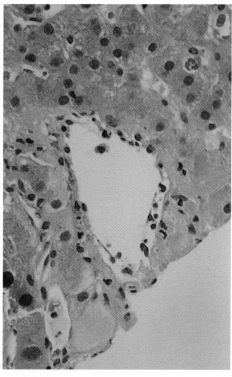

Figure 2–267   Allograft, Vascular Rejection   The small hepatic artery shows almost total occlusion by deposition of numerous foamy histiocytes.

Figure 2–268   Bacterial Sepsis   This terminal hepatic venule shows a mononuclear infiltrate hugging up against the endothelium. Although in bacterial sepsis the inflammation is usually neutrophilic, in some instances lymphocytes may predominate, as in this case of probable salmonellosis.

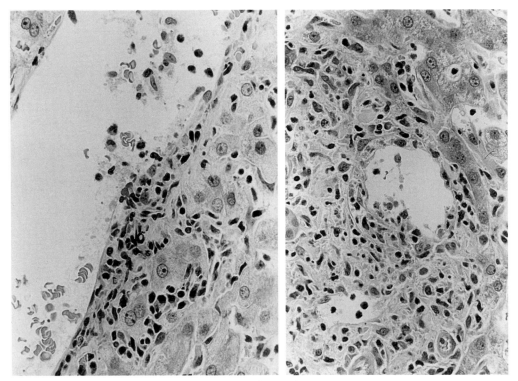

Figures 2–269, 2–270   Epstein-Barr Virus Infection   (Fig. 2–269, *left*) The terminal hepatic vein demonstrates lymphocytes focally abutting up against and infiltrating beneath the endothelium (endothelialitis). (Fig. 2–270, *right*) The portal tract in the same biopsy also shows inflammatory cells focally disrupting the portal vein.

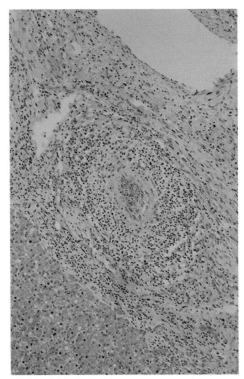

Figure 2–271   Polyarteritis Nodosa   A mixed inflammatory infiltrate consisting of lymphocytes, eosinophils, and occasional neutrophils is seen involving this hepatic artery; the smaller arterioles are seldomly histologically involved.

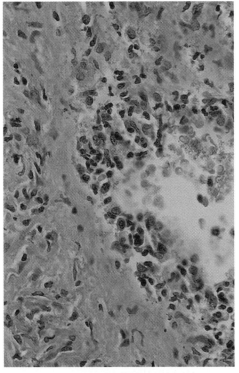

Figure 2–272   Syphilis, Secondary and Tertiary   Endarteritis, which may in some instances obliterate the lumen, is present. This photomicrograph shows a mononuclear infiltrate involving a sublobular vein.

Vessels (Excluding Sinusoids)

Thrombosis and Occlusion

This section includes disorders in which the vascular occlusion is *acute* and secondary to thrombosis (e.g., acute Budd-Chiari syndrome), or *chronic* in which significant perivenular fibrosis and even total luminal sclerosis may be present (e.g., chronic right-sided heart failure) (Table 2–37). Secondary hepatic injury in the acute phase consists of perivenular and sometimes midzonal sinusoidal congestion, acute hemorrhage, and liver cell ischemia. In addition, red blood cells may be seen within the space of Disse (refer to Table 2–32, Sinusoids: Red Blood Cell Extravasation). In *chronic* hepatic venous outflow obstruction, eventual bridging fibrosis between terminal hepatic veins may occur, leading to a "cardiac" cirrhosis (reverse lobulation, with sparing of centrally located portal tracts). *Veno-occlusive* change refers to sclerosis of the small terminal hepatic venules, with relative sparing of the larger outflow vessels.

Figures 2–273 to 2–279 demonstrates nonsinusoidal vessel thrombosis and occlusion in various diseases.

TABLE 2–37

Vessels (Excluding Sinusoids): Thrombosis and Occlusion

Thrombosis/Fibrous Obliteration (Terminal Hepatic and Sublobular Veins)

Acute sclerosing hyaline necrosis (acute alcoholic hepatitis)	Hypothyroidism
	Idiopathic portal hypertension
Alcoholic cirrhosis	Infantile hemangioendothelioma
Aspergillosis	
Budd-Chiari syndrome, acute and chronic	Inflammatory pseudotumor
	Myeloproliferative disorders
Cavernous hemangioma	Nodular regenerative hyperplasia
Congenital hepatic fibrosis	
Drugs/toxins (refer to Table 4–13)	Perivenular fibrosis, alcoholic etiology
Epithelioid hemangioendothelioma	Polyarteritis nodosa
	Progressive perivenular alcoholic fibrosis
Focal nodular hyperplasia	
Heart failure, right-sided, chronic	Pylephlebitis
	Schistosomiasis
Hepatoblastoma	Sickle cell anemia
Hepatocellular carcinoma, fibrolamellar type	Syphilis, secondary
	Toxemia of pregnancy
Hepatocelular carcinoma, trabecular, acinar, ductular type	

Veno-occlusive Changes (Terminal Hepatic Veins)

Acute sclerosing hyaline necrosis (acute alcoholic hepatitis)	Graft-versus-host disease
	Nonalcoholic steatohepatitis
Alcoholic cirrhosis	Perivenular fibrosis, alcoholic etiology
Allograft, chronic (ductopenic) rejection	Progressive perivenular alcoholic fibrosis
Drugs/toxins (refer to Table 4–13)	Veno-occlusive disease, acute and chronic

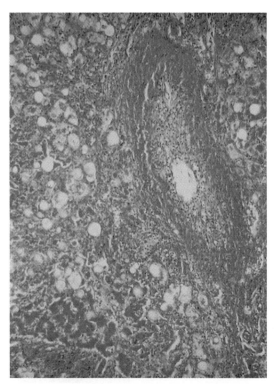

Figure 2–273   Alcoholic Cirrhosis   This low-power photomicrograph shows a sublobular vein with intraluminal fibrosis and almost total occlusion. The adjacent hepatocytes are hydropic and contain variable macrovesicular fat.

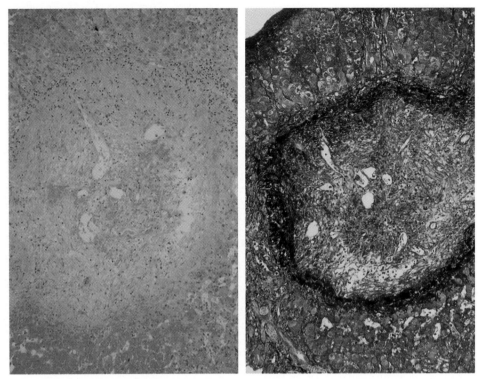

Figures 2–274, 2–275 Budd-Chiari Syndrome, Acute (Fig. 2–274, *left*) The sublobular vein is totally occluded by thrombosis. (Fig. 2–275, *right*) Trichrome stain of the same biopsy easily demonstrates the vein wall (dark blue), with new collagen deposition and early recanalization within the lumen.

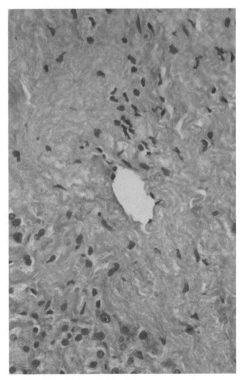

Figure 2–276 Hypothyroidism Concentric luminal thickening involving a terminal hepatic venule is present.

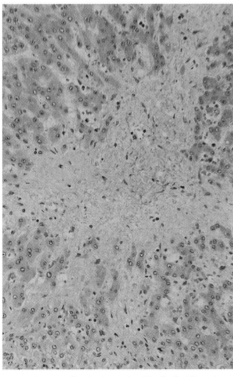

Figure 2–277 Progressive Perivenular Alcoholic Fibrosis The terminal hepatic venule shows total occlusion, with adjacent perivenular sinusoidal collagen deposition.

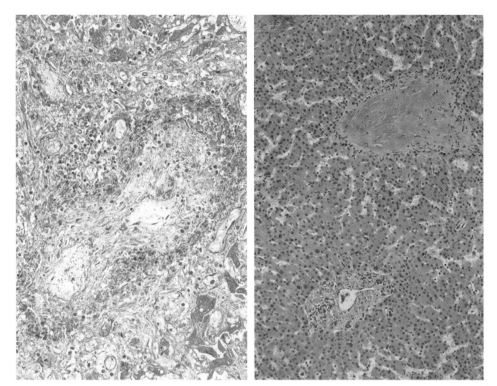

Figures 2–278, 2–279   Veno-occlusive Disease   (Fig. 2–278, *left*) In the acute phase, subintimal edema associated with perivenular and intraluminal sinusoidal collagen is seen on trichrome stain and is often associated with fibrin deposition. (Fig. 2–279, *right*) In the chronic phase, total luminal sclerosis is present.

Liver Diseases: Pathology and Clinical Considerations

TABLE 3-1

Abetalipoproteinemia[13-15]

Histology

- Variable macrovesicular fatty change is present, with a tendency to microvesicular fat deposition consequent to therapy.
- Portal fibrosis may progress to micronodular cirrhosis.
- Mallory bodies may be seen in the more advanced stages of disease.

Clinical/Laboratory Parameters

- Patients with this autosomal codominant disorder develop acanthocytosis, fat malabsorption, pigmentary retinal degeneration, spinocerebellar degeneration, and hepatomegaly.
- Extremely low serum cholesterol and triglyceride levels are present.
- Supplemental vitamins A and E and a low-fat diet are modes of treatment.
- It is uncertain whether the liver disease is directly part of the disorder or related to therapy.

TABLE 3-2

Actinomycosis (Actinomyces israelii)[16-18]

Histology

- Microabscesses are present that may coalesce.
- A surrounding fibrinoid reaction may be seen at the periphery of the abscesses, resembling granuloma formation.
- Organisms may be seen within the neutrophils and appear as radiating gram-positive bacilli.

Clinical/Laboratory Parameters

- This branched, gram-positive, filamentous, 1-μm-wide beaded organism is considered a prokaryotic bacterium and forms entire granules in tissue that range in size from 30 to 3000 μm in diameter.
- The organisms gain access through breaks in skin or mucosa and cause chronic suppuration with draining sinuses and fistulae.
- Portal seeding contributes to the development of hepatic disease, which is characterized by hyperbilirubinemia, elevated alkaline phosphatase activity, and mild increase in serum transaminase.
- Hypoalbuminia is common in severe disease.

TABLE 3-3

Acute Fatty Liver, Alcoholic Etiology[19-21]

Histology

- Marked predominantly macrovesicular fatty change is present involving virtually all hepatocytes.
- Variable sinusoidal collagen deposition may be seen but is generally mild.
- Megamitochondria may be present.
- Cholestasis is often seen and may be prominent.
- Portal tracts show a mild mononuclear inflammatory infiltrate.

Clinical/Laboratory Parameters

- These patients generally have a significant history of alcoholism and usually present with vague right upper quadrant abdominal pain.
- Jaundice may be present, with pruritus in some patients.
- The liver is enlarged and may be tender; ascites is absent.
- Laboratory tests show a normal white blood cell count, normal or mild impairment in serum albumin and prothrombin activity, slight abnormality in the serum transaminases, and moderately elevated serum bilirubin in those with cholestasis.
- The clinical course is benign with resolution of abnormalities after abstinence.

TABLE 3-4
Acute Fatty Liver of Pregnancy[22-30]

Histology

- Microvesicular fatty change is present in the perivenular and midzonal regions; in severe cases, the fatty change may be diffuse, with mild lobular inflammation.
- Cholestasis is seen in the perivenular zone.
- Mild macrovesicular fat may also be seen.
- Megamitochondria have been described.
- Intrasinusoidal fibrin deposition has been reported, occasionally associated with acute hemorrhage when concomitant disseminated intravascular coagulation (DIC) is present.
- Mild portal lymphocytic infiltration with occasional eosinophils and plasma cells are present.

Clinical/Laboratory Parameters

- Patients usually present in the third trimester of pregnancy with acute onset of mild to moderate hyperbilirubinemia, mild increase in serum transaminases, leukocytosis, and progression to liver failure characterized by hypoglycemia, encephalopathy, prolongation of prothrombin time, and sometimes DIC.
- Termination of pregnancy favors improvement and recovery and also allows survival of the fetus.
- In the rare case, deterioration in condition has been noted following delivery necessitating liver transplantation.

TABLE 3-5
Acute Sclerosing Hyaline Necrosis (Acute Alcoholic Heptatitis)[31-38]

Histology

- Marked perivenular fibrosis, often with obliteration of the terminal hepatic venules (veno-occlusive changes), is associated with striking intrasinusoidal (pericellular) collagen deposition accentuated in the perivenular zone, but often seen extending into the midzonal regions.
- Some degree of periportal sinusoidal collagen deposition is also present.
- Hydropic ballooning change of perivenular liver cells is seen.
- Mallory body deposition is present predominantly in perivenular liver cells, but may be diffuse in severe cases, often associated with neutrophilic infiltration surrounding *(satellitosis)* and infiltrating into liver cells containing the Mallory bodies.
- Megamitochondria may be seen.
- Variable degrees of macrovesicular and microvesicular fatty change are present.
- Sinusoidal leukocytosis may be seen.
- Portal tracts exhibit a moderate inflammatory infiltrate consisting of lymphocytes and neutrophils.
- A mild lymphocytic infiltrate may be seen involving some of the terminal hepatic venules and sublobular veins *(endophlebitis)*.
- Cholestasis is present, and is located predominantly in the perivenular zone.
- A variant of severe disease sometimes seen in autopsy specimens consists of marked enlargement of hepatocytes with lysis of liver cell membranes, usually associated with prominent Mallory body deposition *(lytic necrosis)*.

Clinical/Laboratory Parameters

- Clinically referred to as *acute alcoholic hepatitis,* the classic presentation consists of right upper quadrant abdominal tenderness, hepatomegaly, fever, and leukocytosis sometimes as high as 100,000/mm^3 with marked left shift, without evidence of sepsis.
- A systolic bruit over the liver is present due to increased hepatic arterial inflow.
- Depending on disease severity, liver test abnormalities demonstrate mild to marked hyperbilirubinemia, hypoalbuminemia, and marked prolongation of the prothrombin time.
- Serum transaminases are usually low with alanine aminotransferase (ALT) levels in the low normal range to only minimally raised, and aspartate aminotransferase (AST) levels elevated 2 to 3 times normal.
- Patients frequently demonstrate the stigmata of chronic liver disease with spider angiomas, palmar erythema, parotid enlargement, Dupuytren's contracture, and muscle wasting.
- Patients usually develop ascites, are clinically fragile, and may progress to renal insufficiency *(hepatorenal syndrome)* with encephalopathy in severe cases.
- The clinical course may be complicated by variceal bleeding and spontaneous bacterial peritonitis.
- Overall mortality is approximately 20% but increases to 80% after the hepatorenal syndrome develops.
- Corticosteroid treatment in a subset of patients with severe disease and without renal failure has been beneficial.

TABLE 3-6
Adenoma, Bile Duct[39-42]

Histology

- These lesions are usually solitary and subcapsular, nonencapsulated, white and firm, and less than 2 cm in diameter.
- Cytologically benign tubular ducts lined by a single layer of cuboidal cells are seen.
- A fibrous stroma is present, and can be hyalinized or cellular, with variable lymphocytes present at the border of the tumor.
- Normal portal tracts are often identified trapped within the tumor.
- Microcalcifications have been described.

Clinical/Laboratory Parameters

- These uncommon tumors of biliary epithelium are usually asymptomatic and are found incidentally on radiologic scans, at laparotomy, or at autopsy.
- Liver tests are usually normal.
- There is no evidence of malignant transformation.

TABLE 3-7
Adenoma, Liver Cell[41,43-52]

Histology

- The lesions are usually solitary, but may be multiple (2–6), are rarely pedunculated, and range in size from a few cm to 30 cm in diameter; they are well demarcated and seldom encapsulated.
- In some instances, multiple (>10) lesions can be seen *(multiple hepatocellular adenomatosis)*.
- The lesions are usually yellow to tan, soft to friable, with occasional foci of acute hemorrhage.
- Peliotic lesions may be seen, more commonly in those lesions induced by androgen usage.
- Microscopically the tumor consists entirely of cytologically benign liver cells forming cords no greater than 2 cells thick, lined by endothelial cells.
- Thin-walled vascular structures may be numerous, with scattered arterioles occasionally seen; larger feeding vessels may be identified at the margin of tumor and nontumor liver.
- The cytoplasm is usually uniformly pale eosinophilic to clear (abundant glycogen), and may contain macrovesicular fat, lipochrome (rare), bile, epithelioid granulomas, Mallory bodies, or extramedullary hematopoiesis.
- Dysplasia of tumor cells may be present but is uncommon; in these cases, malignant transformation to hepatocellular carcinoma has been reported.
- Increase in copper-binding protein has been described.
- Calcifications may be present but are uncommon.

Clinical/Laboratory Parameters

- These uncommon benign tumors are most often seen in young women on oral contraceptives.
- The tumors are also associated with use of androgens (17-alpha alkylated compounds for the treatment of Fanconi's anemia), and with other conditions such as glycogen storage disease type 1a, galactosemia, tyrosinemia, and diabetes mellitus.
- Although patients may present with abdominal pain or fullness, often they are asymptomatic.
- Liver tests are usually normal, with only mild elevations of serum transaminases and alkaline phosphatase activity in a minority of patients.
- Serum alpha-fetoprotein is normal.
- Computed tomography (CT) scan shows a well-circumscribed, usually single mass, most often located in the right lobe, and often subcapsular.
- There is no uptake of technetium on the technetium sulfur colloid scan (cold mass).
- Complications include rupture in women who continue to take oral contraceptives.
- Malignant transformation to well-differentiated hepatocellular carcinoma has been reported, although there is no evidence of these malignant tumors metastasizing.
- Therapy includes discontinuation of oral contraceptives, which may result in shrinkage of the tumor in a minority of cases; surgical removal is often indicated due to the possibility of malignant transformation.
- The prognosis is excellent when surgical removal is complete.

TABLE 3–8

Adenomatous Hyperplasia (Macroregenerative Nodules)[53–55]

Histology

- The nodules measure approximately 2 to 3 cm in diameter (range 1–15 cm), and most often occur in cirrhotic livers or after extensive liver cell injury.
- These nodules often bulge on cut section, and may compress the adjacent liver.
- The cytologically benign hepatocytes are often hydropic and may contain fat.
- Variable degrees of cytologic atypia can also be seen, ranging from dysplasia, acinus formation, and Mallory bodies (*borderline* lesions) to outright malignant transformation *(hepatocellular carcinoma)*.

Clinical/Laboratory Parameters

- A large well-circumscribed distinct nodule is seen in the setting of acute severe liver injury, such as submassive hepatic necrosis or in some patients with advanced cirrhosis.
- Discovery is incidental on scanning modalities.
- This lesion has no specific symptoms, signs, or laboratory test abnormalities except for those of the underlying liver disease.
- Because of the nodules' malignant potential, histologic evaluation is favored when considering surgical removal.

TABLE 3–9

Adenovirus Infection[56–59]

Histology

- In immunocompromised patients, the features are similar to herpes simplex virus infection (refer to Table 3–106), with extensive coagulative-type necrosis but little inflammation; these features may sometimes occur mainly in the perivenular zones.
- Intranuclear inclusions are prominent in viable liver cells.

Clinical/Laboratory Parameters

- Adenovirus is a DNA virus related to upper and lower respiratory tract infections, lymphadenopathy, and conjunctivitis, and may also cause gastrointestinal infections and hepatitis.
- The more severe infections occur in immunocompromised patients and are associated with markedly elevated serum transaminases.
- Mild elevations of serum transaminases may be noted with normal bilirubin in the setting of a respiratory tract infection in the immunocompetent patient.

TABLE 3–10

Adjacent to Space-occupying Lesions[60,61]

Histology

- The portal tracts exhibit variable edema and a mixed inflammatory infiltrate consisting chiefly of lymphocytes with occasional neutrophils.
- In some cases the neutrophils may surround and invade proliferating cholangioles and interlobular bile ducts; in these instances, cholestasis may be seen in the perivenular zone.
- Sinusoidal dilatation and congestion in the perivenular and midzonal regions is seen with adjacent liver cell atrophy; in addition, red blood cells may extravasate into the space of Disse when severe hepatic venous outflow obstruction is present.

Clinical/Laboratory Parameters

- Focal lesions which include primary and metastatic neoplasms and abscesses may produce obstruction to hepatic venous outflow.
- Obstruction to the biliary tract may also occur, especially in lesions located toward the hilum of the liver, and induce signs and symptoms of bile duct obstruction.
- Serum transaminases are only mildly abnormal, although hyperbilirubinemia and elevated alkaline phosphatase activity may be pronounced if bile flow is impeded.

TABLE 3-11
Adult Polycystic Disease[62-65]

Histology

- The liver is enlarged and diffusely cystic, the cysts ranging from less than 1 mm to greater than 12 cm in diameter.
- Occasionally only one lobe (usually the left) is involved.
- Diffuse ectasia of intra- and extrahepatic ducts may be seen.
- The cysts contain clear colorless or light yellow fluid, and are lined by columnar or cuboidal cells, the larger cysts lined by flattened cells.
- Cysts may collapse, the smaller ones resembling corpora atretica of the ovary.
- Von Meyenberg complexes may be seen.
- Infected cysts contain neutrophils, forming microabscesses.
- Calcifications may be seen.

Clinical/Laboratory Parameters

- An autosomal dominant disease, cysts may be incidentally found; however, hepatomegaly and renal masses may be clues to the diagnosis.
- Abdominal pain is common when there is massive hepatic enlargement.
- Liver function is well preserved even in extensive cystic disease, although portal hypertension may develop.
- Systemic hypertension, progressive renal insufficiency, and intracranial hemorrhage from aneurysms in the circle of Willis are complicating problems.

TABLE 3-12
Alcoholic Cirrhosis[21,31,37,67,74-77]

Histology

- Bridging portal and perivenular fibrosis eventually leads to a micronodular cirrhosis (nodules ≤3 mm in diameter).
- In the active alcoholic, variable macrovesicular fatty change, sinusoidal collagen deposition, and Mallory body formation are usually seen.
- The *active* alcoholic may show striking diffuse sinusoidal collagen deposition throughout the nodules *(diffuse interstitial fibrosis);* little to no regenerative activity is seen within the nodules.
- In the *inactive* alcoholic, regenerative nodules are well defined and bulging, and larger (>3 mm in diameter) than seen in the active alcoholic; with time the fibrous bands become thin, with an intact cord-sinusoid pattern visualized within the regenerative nodules.
- Sclerosis of terminal hepatic venules is present within the bridging fibrous bands.
- Hemosiderin deposition may be seen involving occasional periportal hepatocytes.
- Hepatocellular carcinoma is a known complication, occurring in from 4 to 10% of patients; however, many of these patients may also have chronic hepatitis C virus (HCV) infection, itself a risk factor for hepatocellular carcinoma.

Clinical/Laboratory Parameters

- Cirrhosis develops following a long history of alcoholism, with usually greater than 80 grams of daily alcohol intake over a range of from 15 to 20 years (time sequence is variable).
- Patients may present for the first time with hepatic decompensation, demonstrating marked generalized muscle wasting, ascites, peripheral edema, esophageal varices, and encephalopathy.
- In patients with recent binge drinking, associated decompensation evidenced by hyperbilirubinemia, marked hypoalbuminemia, and prolonged prothrombin time may be present.
- These patients are at risk of developing sepsis with the primary source in the urinary or respiratory tracts, or ascites may develop.
- Mortality is affected by the hepatic reserve, which is the ability of these patients to tolerate serious, life-threatening complications provided the disease is recognized early and treatment is instituted.
- The risk of developing hepatocellular carcinoma is increased in patients with cirrhosis, especially in those patients who abstain from alcohol and who do not succumb to the complications and severity of the liver disease.
- Liver transplantation should be considered only in patients who remain decompensated after a minimum of 6 months of abstinence and rehabilitation.

TABLE 3-13

Alcoholic Fatty Liver[31,32,37,66-70]

Histology

- Macrovesicular fat is seen, first laid down in the perivenular zone, with eventual involvement throughout the lobules.
- The fat may disappear within 2 to 4 weeks after cessation of alcohol intake, but it may persist for a longer time within portal macrophages.
- Sinusoidal collagen deposition is not present.
- The portal tracts do not exhibit fibrosis or inflammation.
- *Lipogranulomas* can be occasionally seen, most frequently in the perivenular zone, and consist of coalescent fat droplets with collections of lymphocytes, histiocytes, occasional eosinophils, and rarely multinucleated giant cells.
- The lipogranulomas are secondary to rupture of liver cells containing fat, with secondary inflammatory response to the extracellular fat.

Clinical/Laboratory Parameters

- Patients with a history of alcoholism may present with vague abdominal pain and are noted to have firm hepatomegaly on physical examination.
- Characteristic laboratory findings include mild to moderate increase in serum transaminases, mild increase in alkaline phosphatase activity, and normal serum bilirubin, albumin, and prothrombin time.
- On a complete blood count, an elevated mean corpuscular volume may provide a clue to alcoholism.
- Resolution of symptoms and hepatomegaly, with improvement of the liver tests, occurs with abstinence.

TABLE 3-14

Alcoholic Foamy Degeneration[31,71-73]

Histology

- Striking microvesicular foamy fatty change of predominantly perivenular hepatocytes is present, with some extension into the midzonal regions, usually associated with variable macrovesicular fatty change as well.
- Cholestasis in the perivenular zone is often seen, sometimes with a mild chronic inflammatory infiltrate.
- The portal tracts exhibit a mild lymphocytic infiltration with occasional neutrophils.
- Variable periportal intrasinusoidal collagen deposition is seen; perivenular collagen, when present, is mild.
- *Megamitochondria* (discrete, round, eosinophilic cytoplasmic inclusions) are often present within hepatocytes.
- Mallory body deposition with lobular neutrophilic infiltration is not characteristic of this disease, and when present is patchy and mild.

Clinical/Laboratory Parameters

- Patients present with right upper quadrant abdominal discomfort or pain in the setting of chronic alcoholism.
- Physical examination demonstrates spider angiomas, hepatomegaly, sometimes massive, and associated abdominal tenderness.
- Laboratory tests show an elevated serum bilirubin, and moderate to marked elevation of serum transaminases with ALT higher than AST in about 50% of cases; the aminotransferases may reach values up to 700 IU/L in the early stage, with modest decrease in serum albumin and prolongation of the prothrombin time.
- The clinical course is usually benign with resolution of the process with abstinence; in some patients, progression to severe dysfunction and liver failure have been noted.

TABLE 3-15

Allograft, Acute (Cellular) Rejection[78-88]

Histology

- The following triad of histologic changes may be seen to variable degrees, depending on the severity of the rejection, and is graded as mild, moderate, or severe. Note that at least two of the three listed parameters are necessary for a diagnosis of acute rejection.
  1. *Mixed portal inflammatory infiltrate:*
     - Activated lymphocytes, eosinophils, occasional plasma cells, and neutrophils are present.
     - The inflammatory cells are usually confined to the portal tracts; however, in severe rejection, spillover of these cells into the adjacent peri-portal regions is usually seen.
  2. *Venous endothelial inflammation (endothelialitis):*
     - Lymphocytes and immunocytes attach to the luminal surface of portal and terminal hepatic venules, involving part or all of the vascular luminal lining.
     - Subendothelial infiltration is often seen; in severe rejection, the inflammatory cells also involve the perivenular sinusoids and may be associated with perivenular ischemic necrosis of hepatocytes.
     - Arterioles may be involved in severe cases.
  3. *Nonsuppurative cholangitis, destructive or non-destructive:*
     - Interlobular bile ducts are surrounded and invaded by lymphocytes, immunocytes, and neutrophils.
     - Biliary epithelium shows variable cytoplasmic vacuolization and nuclear pyknosis.
- Cholestasis and mild mononuclear inflammatory infiltration may be present within the lobules.
- When perivenular necrosis and collapse are present in severe cases, red blood cells may be seen infiltrating into the hepatic cords.
- A semiquantitative grading system using the Rejection Activity Index (RAI)[80] on biopsy is useful to monitor response to therapy.

Clinical/Laboratory Parameters

- Since liver transplant does not require human leukocyte antigen (HLA) matching between donor and recipient, the possibility of multiple mismatches of class I and II major histocompatibility complex (MHC) antigens occurs, increasing the alloreactivity against donor cells.
- As a result, alloreactions against the processed alloantigens occur with specific targets against biliary epithelium and endothelial cells.
- Acute cellular rejection occurs from 5 to 30 days post transplant in 70% of patients receiving liver allografts; however, both earlier and later presentations may arise in patients on less than therapeutic immunosuppressive doses.
- In mild rejection, clinical signs and symptoms may be absent; however, in moderate to severe rejection, tender hepatomegaly and fever may be associated with swelling and graft tenderness.
- Rises in serum transaminases and alkaline phosphatase activity occur to variable degrees, sometimes associated with hyperbilirubinemia.
- Infections with cytomegalovirus or hepatitis viruses could present in similar fashion; however, these infections usually do not occur prior to 4 weeks post transplant.
- Response to a corticosteroid bolus dose and recyle is usually effective in resolving this process.

TABLE 3-16

Allograft, Acute Graft Failure[78,79,89]

Histology

- Extensive coagulative (ischemic) necrosis is present within the perivenular and midzonal regions; in severe cases, the entire lobule may be affected.
- Neutrophils may be seen adjacent to the areas of ischemic necrosis.
- Cholestasis and variable acute hemorrhage are usually present.
- Red blood cells may be present within hepatic cords, taking the place of ischemic hepatocytes.
- There is no histologic evidence of vascular inflammation or occlusion (refer to Table 3–20, Allograft, Hyperacute [Humoral] Rejection).

Clinical/Laboratory Parameters

- Also referred to as *primary nonfunction* (PNF), this complication occurs in 5 to 10% of cases during the first week post transplant.
- Although the exact mechanism is not certain, a number of factors have been postulated:
  1. Ischemic injury in the donor liver prior to harvesting
  2. Poor technique during procurement
  3. Poor flushing or reperfusion injury during preservation
  4. Prolonged cold or warm ischemic time
  5. Significant steatosis in the donor liver
- When PNF occurs intraoperatively, there is massive fibrinolysis, lactic acidosis, and no bile production, leading to renal failure, ascites, and anasarca.
- PNF can occur postoperatively and may be difficult to distinguish from accelerated or hyperacute rejection, resembling fulminant hepatic failure with all the attendant features.
- Spontaneous recovery does not occur and retransplantation is necessary.

TABLE 3-17

Allograft, Chronic (Ductopenic) Rejection (Vanishing Bile Duct Syndrome)[78,79,81,82,84,90–92]

Histology

- Duct loss involves 50% or greater of the portal tracts (when <50% the term *indeterminate* or *impending [evolving] chronic rejection* is used).
- The ducts that are present often show cytologic atypia.
- Portal tracts exhibit only a mild lymphocytic infiltrate; when duct loss is complete, portal inflammation may be absent.
- With time, depletion of hepatic arterioles may also occur.
- Severe canalicular bile stasis, most prominent in the perivenular zone, is present, but it may be diffuse with mild inflammatory infiltrates.
- Variable ballooning of liver cells may occur with perivenular necrosis in severe cases.
- Sclerosis involving terminal hepatic venules may also be seen, with variable degrees of adjacent sinusoidal collagen deposition.
- Occasionally bridging fibrosis leading to biliary cirrhosis may be present.
- Chronic rejection often (but not always) is associated with vascular rejection (refer to Table 3–23, Allograft, Vascular Rejection).

Clinical/Laboratory Parameters

- Chronic rejection is an irreversible process leading to unrelenting loss of bile ducts; it occurs from 60 days to years post transplant in from 2 to 17% of patients in different series, and is the commonest cause of late graft failure.
- This disorder most frequently occurs after (1) an unresolved episode of acute rejection; (2) multiple acute rejection episodes; or (3) indolently after many months to years.
- Patients may have no specific clinical symptoms; however, persistent elevations in alkaline phosphatase activity with hyperbilirubinemia occur.
- Biliary sludging, biliary strictures, and hepatic infarcts may also be late findings.
- The diagnosis can only be suspected clinically; biopsy is necessary for confirmation.
- Retransplantation is the only effective treatment.

TABLE 3-18

Allograft, Fibrosing Cholestatic Hepatitis[78,79,93,94]

Histology

- Ballooning degeneration of liver cells is seen, with dropout and variable degrees of lobular collapse.
- Periportal sinusoidal collagen deposition is present.
- Cholestasis is marked with variable chronic inflammatory infiltration.
- Only a mild portal lymphocytic infiltrate is present.
- Prominence of hepatitis B surface antigen (HBsAg) and hepatitis B core antigen (HBcAg) by immunoperoxidase stains in recurrent hepatitis B virus (HBV) infection is present.

Clinical/Laboratory Parameters

- Some patients with HBV or HCV who receive a liver transplant develop progressive hepatic failure, sometimes rapid (range, 3–6 months) due to recurrence of HBV or HCV in the graft in the immunosuppressed state; hepatic failure is characterized by hyperbilirubinemia, increased alkaline phosphatase activity, and moderate elevations in serum transaminases (200–600 IU/L).
- Measurement of viral titers demonstrates marked increased levels.
- Graft loss is frequent; disease recurrence is common, and is usually more accelerated after retransplantation.

TABLE 3-19

Allograft, Harvesting (Preservation) Injury (Functional Cholestasis)[78,79,95,96]

Histology

- Cholestasis associated with marked ballooning of liver cells in the perivenular and midzonal regions or diffusely throughout the lobules is present.
- In the more severe cases, perivenular dropout of hepatocytes may be present, associated with perivenular congestion, hemorrhage, and at times red blood cells within the hepatic cords, taking the place of damaged liver cells.
- Cholangiolar proliferation and ectasia may also be seen when the cholestasis is pronounced.

Clinical/Laboratory Parameters

- A common feature following liver transplantation, preservation injury usually occurs during the first few weeks post transplant.
- Although the exact mechanism is not fully understood, suggested causes relate to ischemia during harvesting and transport.
- Patients present with mildly elevated serum bilirubin or alkaline phosphatase activity; occasionally the serum bilirubin levels exceed 10 mg/dl, with bile duct obstruction and acute rejection included in the differential diagnoses.
- Recovery is the rule and no long-term sequelae have been observed.

TABLE 3-20

Allograft, Hyperacute (Humoral) Rejection[78,79,81]

Histology

- Ischemic coagulative and hemorrhagic necrosis is present, most prominent in the perivenular zone but often involving the entire lobule.
- Numerous neutrophils may also be seen in the sinusoids adjacent to ischemic hepatocytes.
- Cholestasis is often present.
- Necrotizing endothelial damage and denudation occurs predominantly involving medium-sized (>120 μm in diameter) arteries with neutrophilic infiltration, fibrin thrombi, and partial vascular occlusion; fibrin thrombi may also be seen within portal and outflow vessels.
- Immunoglobulin (Ig) M, IgG, C1q, C3, C4, and fibrinogen deposits in arteries, veins, and portal capillaries may be identified on immunoperoxidase stains.

Clinical/Laboratory Parameters

- Hyperacute allograft rejection is an infrequent event following liver transplantation and occurs immediately or within the first week post transplant.
- The disorder is antibody mediated; the antibodies are either preformed or represent antidonor antibodies (e.g., anti–major histocompatibility complex, anti-ABO) that develop after transplantation.
- A complex cascade of events is initiated including complement activation, endothelial cell expression of adhesion molecules for neutrophil binding, activation of coagulation, and production of vasoactive peptides, all of which contribute to vascular disruption, severe liver cell ischemia, and eventual hepatic failure.
- Patients are encephalopathic and deeply jaundiced and may develop ascites; marked increases in serum transaminases and prolongation of the prothrombin time are present.
- Death occurs if retransplantation is not performed.

TABLE 3–21

Allograft, Ischemia Secondary to Hepatic Artery Thrombosis[78,79,97]

Histology

- Marked lobular coagulative necrosis is present.
- Red blood cells may be present within hepatic cords, taking the place of ischemic hepatocytes.
- Interlobular bile ducts may exhibit severe cytologic atypia, with duct ectasia, necrosis, acute inflammatory infiltration, microabscesses within portal tracts, and duct strictures *(ischemic cholangitis),* with eventual ductopenia.
- Bile lakes may form adjacent to damaged ducts.

Clinical/Laboratory Parameters

- In the *early* postoperative period, thrombosis of the hepatic artery can present with acute liver failure, bile leaks, intrahepatic biloma, and/or intermittent bacteremia.
- The development of biliary strictures seen on cholangiography should also raise the issue of ischemia from artery thrombosis.
- Retransplantation is usually required in the acute setting to avoid the risk of serious infections while on immunosuppression; however, some patients, particularly children, may stabilize and tolerate hepatic artery thrombosis without the need for retransplantation.
- *Late* artery thrombosis may develop many years post transplant as a result of vascular stenosis or intimal hyperplasia; hepatic artery blood flow may be sustained by collateralization of vessels.
- The presence of bacteremia or abscess formation several years following liver transplant should raise the possibility of ischemia from hepatic artery occlusion.

TABLE 3–22

Allograft, Post Transplant Lymphoproliferative Disease[78,79,83,98–101]

Histology

- Mononuclear infiltrates are seen within the portal tracts; these cells are polymorphous with prominence of cleaved and noncleaved lymphocytes, and variable numbers of plasma cells and immunoblasts *(polyclonal disease).*
- Sheets of these cells may occur forming distinct mass lesions.
- Progression to a monomorphic (monoclonal) infiltrate can also occur (refer to Table 3–140, Lymphoma, Non-Hodgkin's).
- The lymphocytic infiltrates are usually B-cell type.
- Epstein-Barr virus infection is most often present and predates the occurrence of these infiltrates; it is demonstrated by nuclear staining of lymphoid cells via in situ hybridization (Epstein-Barr virus-encoded RNA [EBER-1] probe).

Clinical/Laboratory Parameters

- Lymphoproliferative disorders are seen in about 2% of liver transplant recipients.
- Overimmunosuppression and Epstein-Barr virus infection are implicated in the etiology.
- Presentation ranges from a mild mononucleosis-like syndrome to malignant lymphoma.
- Patients present with fever, lymphadenopathy, visceral masses, intestinal ulceration, or obstruction.
- Diagnosis is made by biopsy.
- Treatment is directed to markedly reducing or discontinuing immunosuppression, with initiation of antiviral therapy; polyclonal infiltrates then usually regress, but the prognosis is poor if the infiltrates are monoclonal.

TABLE 3–23

Allograft, Vascular Rejection[78,79,92,102]

Histology

- Foam cell arteriopathy (or arteritis when inflammation is also present) involves medium-sized to large hepatic arteries, the foam cells primarily involving the intima with variable and in some instances pronounced intimal thickening and luminal narrowing.
- Over time, replacement of foam cells by myofibroblasts *(fibromyointimal proliferation)* is also seen.
- This vascular lesion is often (but not always) associated with duct loss (refer to Table 3–17, Allograft, Chronic [Ductopenic] Rejection [Vanishing Bile Duct Syndrome]).

Clinical/Laboratory Parameters

- The clinical signs, symptoms, and laboratory data are similar to those seen in chronic rejection (refer to Table 3–17, Allograft, Chronic [Ductopenic] Rejection [Vanishing Bile Duct Syndrome]).

TABLE 3–24

Alpers' Disease[103–105]

Histology

- Microvesicular fatty change is present, and often extensive.
- Portal and periportal lymphocytic infiltration is present.
- Variable degrees of lobular mononuclear inflammatory infiltration may be seen.
- Bridging or panacinar hepatic necrosis with collapse may occur.
- Cirrhosis may develop with prominent fibrous scarring.

Clinical/Laboratory Parameters

- This autosomal recessive disease is a disorder of the mitochondria due to a deficiency of cytochrome C oxidase complex IV, which predominantly affects muscle and brain, and presents with progressive neuronal degeneration in young children.
- Death may occur with liver failure in the more severe cases.

TABLE 3–25

Alpha₁-Antichymotrypsin Deficiency[106,107]

Histology

- Portal lymphocytic infiltration with piecemeal necrosis leading to cirrhosis is present.
- Granular alpha₁ inclusions are seen in periportal and periseptal liver cells.

Clinical/Laboratory Parameters

- This autosomal dominant disorder is associated with both liver and lung disease.
- Associated low levels of alpha₁-antichymotrypsin are present.

TABLE 3-26

Alpha₁-Antitrypsin Deficiency[108-114]

Histology

- Multiple periodic acid–Schiff-positive after diastase digestion (diPAS) intracytoplasmic eosinophilic globules 1 to 20 μm in diameter are present predominantly in periportal liver cells, but may extend to the midzonal region.
- These globules may also involve bile duct epithelium.
- There may be slight variation in the number of inclusions seen from one lobule to the next; in cirrhosis, these inclusions may show marked variation, with some nodules showing absence of inclusions.
- In the neonate, neonatal hepatitis (refer to Table 3–155) may occur, although giant cell transformation is minimal.
- The globules may be difficult to see in neonates less than 12 weeks of age.
- Macrovesicular fatty change may be present, predominantly in periportal hepatocytes.
- Extramedullary hematopoiesis is often seen in neonates.
- Glycogen nuclei of hepatocytes may rarely be seen in adults.
- Portal tracts may exhibit lymphocytic infiltration, rarely with piecemeal necrosis; focal necrosis may be seen within the lobule.
- Mallory bodies may be seen in periportal liver cells, but are uncommon.
- This disorder may be associated with atypical duct proliferation leading to a paucity of ducts and eventual biliary cirrhosis with ductopenia in children.
- Increase in copper and copper-binding protein is present in periseptal liver cells when cirrhosis is present.
- Both macronodular and micronodular cirrhosis occurs in adults.

Clinical/Laboratory Parameters

- One of the most common genetic diseases of infants and children, this disorder occurs at a frequency of 1 per 6000 to 8000.
- The disease can present in the neonatal period and in the adult (4th to 6th decade), and may lead to cirrhosis and liver failure.
- Structural variants are classified according to a protease inhibitor (Pi) phenotype system based on electrophoretic mobility or isoelectric focusing of plasma. More than 75 allelic variants have been reported.
- The commonest variant associated with liver disease and emphysema is PiZZ (the Z allele has a single amino acid substitution [lysine[342 position] for glucose]).
- The heterozygote variants (e.g., PiMZ) overall are more common but are much less frequently associated with liver disease.
- Hyperbilirubinemia and elevated alkaline phosphatase activity are noted in the neonatal period and can mimic biliary tract disease; serum transaminases are only modestly elevated.
- Low serum levels of alpha₁-antitrypsin are present, although the levels are often misleading, as this protein may increase during various inflammatory conditions even in PiZZ individuals.
- In advanced cases, ascites and esophageal varices may occur; hepatocellular carcinoma has been reported.
- Although the mechanism of liver injury is not known, the accumulation of alpha₁-antitrypsin globules within the endoplasmic reticulum and inability to degrade this protein may be a cause of direct toxicity.

TABLE 3-27
Amebiasis *(Entamoeba histolytica)* [115-120]

Histology

- A grossly demonstrable cyst is present that usually involves the right lobe but may be multifocal.
- The fully developed cyst *(abscess)* has ragged non-encapsulated margins, and contains liquidy amorphous eosinophilic contents that are brown-red and "anchovy paste–like," surrounded by a fibrous wall.
- The earliest lesion may demonstrate trophozoites (10–60 μm in diameter, round to oval organisms that contain round nuclei, and central karyosomes (which are positive on periodic acid–Schiff [PAS] and Gridley stains) in sinusoids associated with coagulative necrosis initially in the midzone, with associated neutrophilic infiltration, edema, and granulation tissue formation.
- As the lesion enlarges, viable organisms can be seen at the edge of the lesion, while in the center there is abundant hemorrhagic granular necrotic debris.
- Lymphocytes and plasma cells may also be present at the outer border of the cyst wall, which may eventually become dense and fibrotic.
- The organisms often contain phagocytized red blood cells.
- If the organisms are viable, they are often surrounded by a clear space ("halo").
- Parasites may also be seen outside the cyst in sinusoids and areas of focal necrosis.
- Variable macrovesicular fatty change may be present.

Clinical/Laboratory Parameters

- This microaerophilic protozoa, acquired by contamination of food and drink, is passed in the feces of asymptomatic persons, causing intestinal infection by trophozoites released in the colon with subsequent invasion of the mucosa.
- The liver is invaded by trophozoites, which enter the portal circulation, traverse the sinusoids, and form an abscess.
- During the intestinal infection, fever, diarrhea, or dysentery can occur.
- The development of a hepatic abscess is associated with fever, right upper quadrant pain and tenderness, hepatomegaly, and minimal derangement of alkaline phosphatase activity and transaminases.
- Serum bilirubin and prothrombin time are usually normal but hypoalbuminemia, mild anemia, and leukocytosis are frequent.
- Elevated right hemidiaphragm on chest X-ray and detection of abscess on ultrasound and CT scan provide clues.
- The marked increase in amebic titers on serologic tests (rising on serial samples) using enzyme immunoassays or indirect hemagglutination inhibition is highly suggestive of the diagnosis.
- Therapeutic trial with chloroquine or metronidazole (the latter used provided anaerobic abscess is not included in the differential diagnosis) is also helpful.
- Mortality is increased in untreated patients in whom abscesses rupture into the pericardium (left lobe abscess) or peritoneum.

TABLE 3-28

Amyloidosis[121-129]

Histology

- The liver is usually enlarged, pale, rubbery, and sometimes waxy.
- Eosinophilic acellular deposits *(amyloid)* are present and demonstrated by positive staining with Congo red (apple green under polarized light), PAS, Sirius red, thioflavin-T (fluorescence), and immunoperoxidase stains (light chains, amyloid-associated protein, pentagonal [P] component).
- Amyloid is extracellular and seen within portal connective tissue, media of hepatic arteries and arterioles, and portal and sublobular vein walls.
- Sinusoidal deposits are present within the space of Disse, the deposits widening the sinusoids and pushing Kupffer cells toward the center of the sinusoids, with adjacent liver cell atrophy.
- The *globular* form consists of discrete, round to slightly irregular acellular bodies 5 to 50 μm in diameter having a concentric laminated pattern, often with intense central staining. These globules are seen within the sinusoids, portal tracts, and walls of portal and sublobular veins (but not within small arteries or arterioles).
- A mixed type of globular and more typical amyloid may also be present.
- Amyloid may also be seen beneath the lining epithelium of large intrahepatic bile ducts and in peribiliary glands.
- Variation in zonal involvement of the lobules is often present, with the perivenular zone less often affected.
- Portal lymphocytic infiltration is seen but is generally mild.
- Cholestasis may occur in 5% of cases.
- Microcalcifications have been described.

Clinical/Laboratory Parameters

- Amyloid is an amorphous extracellular protein characterized by rigid, nonbranching linear aggregates 7.5 to 10 nm in diameter that exhibit cross beta-pleated sheets on X-ray diffraction.
- The deposits are usually systemic, although localized involvement (e.g., heart, certain endocrine tumors such as medullary carcinoma of the thyroid) may also occur.
- Systemic amyloidosis is associated with chronic inflammatory conditions 5 to 11% of the time, while 6 to 15% of patients with multiple myeloma develop amyloidosis.
- The liver is one of the major sites of amyloid deposition, which occurs in 17 to 98% of systemic amyloidosis; isolated hepatic involvement is rare.
- Two amyloid proteins have been identified: AL (anti–light chains) seen in primary amyloidosis, and AA (amyloid-associated protein) seen in secondary amyloidosis.
- AL depositis are seen in patients with multiple myeloma, while AA deposits are seen in long-term chronic inflammatory conditions (e.g., rheumatoid arthritis).
- Other less common amyloid proteins identified are SSA (localized cardiac), CAA (cerebral) and AF (familial).
- Patients may present with hepatosplenomegaly, nephrotic syndrome, intestinal pseudo-obstruction or cardiac failure in varying degrees of severity.
- Liver tests are mildly abnormal with mild to moderate increase in serum alkaline phosphatase activity, normal bilirubin, and normal or mild increase in serum transaminases.
- Hypoalbuminemia may be marked and related to urinary protein loss.
- Diagnosis is made by biopsy of the subcutaneous fat, rectal mucosa, or liver.

TABLE 3-29

Angiomyolipoma[130-134]

Histology

- These lesions may be small incidental findings, or large (up to 20 cm in diameter).
- The tumor is composed of a mixture of benign vascular spaces, smooth muscle, fat, and hematopoietic elements.

Clinical/Laboratory Parameters

- These tumors are usually incidental findings, and may be seen in association with renal angiomyolipomas.
- Removal is not indicated when the diagnosis is established by needle biopsy.

TABLE 3-30

Angiosarcoma (Malignant Hemangioendothelioma)[41,130,135-138]

Histology

- Ill-defined, spongy, hemorrhagic to firm tumor masses may be focal or diffusely involve the liver.
- Large cavernous spaces lined by elongated, pleomorphic, multilayered endothelial cells that may form luminal projections are present.
- A solid growth pattern can be seen, with formation of small vessels lined by malignant endothelial cells.
- Proliferation of spindle cells forming small capillaries admixed with red blood cells may be seen, and occurs more frequently in immunocompromised patients (e.g., in Kaposi's sarcoma).
- Focal acute hemorrhage may be seen, with formation of pelioid-type lesions.
- Extramedullary hematopoiesis and erythrophagocytosis may be seen in the adjacent nontumor liver.
- Noncirrhotic portal fibrosis may be present in the adjacent nontumor liver.
- When induced by Thorotrast (thorium dioxide), this granular green-brown pigment is seen in the adjacent nontumor portal macrophages and Kupffer cells.
- A helpful immunoperoxidase marker for diagnosis is factor VIII-related antigen, which stains the malignant endothelial cells.

Clinical/Laboratory Parameters

- This very rare neoplasm occurs most often in men between 50 and 60 years of age.
- Exposure to vinyl chloride, arsenic, Thorotrast, and other drugs (e.g., diethylstilbestrol, phenelzine) have been implicated in the etiology.
- There is no relationship to chronic viral hepatitis, and the serum alpha-fetoprotein is not elevated.
- Patients may present with hepatomegaly ($>50\%$), ascites (25%), jaundice (25%), thrombocytopenia (25%), or rupture ($<15\%$) with hemoperitoneum.
- The clinical features may resemble decompensated chronic liver disease or hemorrhage from hepatocellular carcinoma.
- Hypodense lesions with vascular enhancement on CT scan, or filling defects with tumor blush or puddling, are useful findings on angiographic studies.
- Biopsy of the lesion for diagnosis is preferably performed under direct vision, such as laparoscopy or minilaparotomy, as this approach is not usually associated with bleeding.
- Metastases to the spleen and lung may occur.
- The prognosis is poor with a low likelihood of survival (mean, 6 months) after diagnosis.

TABLE 3-31

Ascariasis (Ascaris lumbricoides)[139-141]

Histology

- An eosinophilic and neutrophilic granulomatous reaction to small larvae and eggs is present.
- Acute cholangitis with numerous eosinophils and abscess formation may occur as a complication of the worm migrating within the biliary tree.
- Intrahepatic biliary calculi in large ducts may be seen as a response to trapped dead worms, with secondary duct damage and adenomatous proliferation of biliary epithelium.

Clinical/Laboratory Parameters

- This intestinal helminthic infestation occurs by ingesting infected cysts, which are digested in the small intestine, releasing larvae that enter the portal circulation and lymphatics, eventually reaching the lungs through the thoracic duct where an eosinophilic reaction develops.
- The larvae migrate through the tracheobronchial tree to be swallowed into the esophageal lumen and ultimately end up in the small intestine as mature roundworms.
- Reactions to the larvae in the liver can occur during the migratory process; however, the major clinical impact develops when these adult helminths migrate up the biliary tract, whereby patients present with fever, biliary colic, cholangitis (jaundice, leukocytosis, and increases in serum alkaline phosphatase activity, transaminases, and bilirubin), and bile duct obstruction.
- In unrecognized and untreated cases, abscesses and *pylephlebitis* (refer to Table 3-176) can occur.

TABLE 3–32

Aspergillosis *(Aspergillus flavus* and *A. fumigatus)*[142,143]

Histology

- Hyphae (3–6 μm septate branching) can be demonstrated within vessels, sometimes leading to thrombosis and infarction.
- Hemorrhagic necrosis may be seen within the lobules.

Clinical/Laboratory Parameters

- The liver is involved in disseminated aspergillus infections when patients are severely immunosuppressed (e.g., high-dose corticosteroid therapy for autoimmune disease, chemotherapy, and organ transplantation).
- Patients may become seriously ill, with fever unresponsive to antibiotics, pulmonary infiltrates, elevated alkaline phosphatase activity, and hyperbilirubinemia.
- The diagnosis is made by isolation of this fungus on cultures and biopsies.

TABLE 3–33

Autoimmune Hepatitis[144–152]

Histology

- Portal tracts exhibit a moderate to marked infiltrate of lymphocytes and numerous plasma cells, with piecemeal necrosis common and often striking.
- Portal neutrophils can occasionally be seen, the neutrophils not oriented to duct structures.
- The lobule exhibits focal necrosis and hepatocytolysis diffusely throughout all zones.
- In the *active* stage, perivenular liver cell necrosis and dropout may occur accompanied by marked, diffuse lobular necroinflammatory changes; collapse can also be seen in the periportal zones, with bridging necrosis between portal tracts.
- Nonsuppurative destructive interlobular duct lesions may be present, with lymphocytes surrounding and attacking duct epithelium accompanied by marked cytologic duct atypia; ductopenia may occur in some cases *(autoimmune cholangiopathy)*.
- Cholestasis is present, and may be prominent in the active stage, associated with variable syncytial giant cell transformation of hepatocytes.
- Variable degrees of portal fibrosis are present; in nontreated cases, a macronodular or micronodular cirrhosis may eventually occur; in autoimmune cholangiopathy, biliary cirrhosis may be seen.
- The degree of portal and lobular activity markedly diminishes after steroid therapy is initiated.

Clinical/Laboratory Parameters

- This liver disease occurs in persons with a genetic predisposition; 90% are women and 75% are positive for HLA-B8, -DR3, or -DR4.
- A chronic fluctuating course is common, and cirrhosis is present in 60% of patients at first presentation.
- Patients present with hyperbilirubinemia, moderate and less commonly marked increase in serum transaminases, mild decrease in serum albumin, marked hyperglobulinemia, and prolongation of the prothrombin time.
- Most patients have autoimmune serologic markers (antinuclear antibody, smooth muscle antibody), and some may also have other markers (e.g., anti–liver-kidney microsomal antibody [anti-LKM], VDRL, antithyroid antibody).
- Extrahepatic manifestations include arthralgia, glomerulonephritis, hemolytic anemia, hypothyroidism, and diabetes mellitus.
- Corticosteroid therapy results in dramatic improvement in liver abnormalities and can be used as a diagnostic test.
- A small group of patients present with an acute and rapidly progressive course and do not usually respond to corticosteroids, perhaps as a consequence of advanced disease.
- *Autoimmune cholangiopathy* is a recently introduced entity for a subset of patients with clinical features that overlap with primary biliary cirrhosis (refer to Table 3–172), but the antimitochondrial antibody is negative; the antinuclear and smooth muscle antibodies, however, are positive, and corticosteroid response is similar to typical autoimmune hepatitis.

TABLE 3–34

Babesiosis (*Babesia* species)[143–153]

Histology

- Focal coagulative necrosis is present within the lobules with little inflammatory infiltrate.
- Hypertrophic Kupffer cells containing parasites that look similar to malaria but without pigment are also seen.

Clinical/Laboratory Parameters

- Transmitted by the bite of *Ixodes* ticks, infection occurs usually during the summer months; patients with prior splenectomy are at increased risk.
- Clinical signs and symptoms relate to proliferation of the organism in red blood cells with eventual rupture of these erthyrocytes.
- Patients present with fever, myalgia, sweats and headache. Mild hepatosplenomegaly and elevations of serum transaminases, alkaline phosphatase, and bilirubin may be noted.
- The infection by *B. microti* is mild and self-limited; however, infection by *B. divergens* results in fever, jaundice, anemia, renal failure, hemoglobinuria, marked leukocytosis, elevation of serum transaminases and bilirubin, and has a high mortality.
- The immunofluorescent antibody titer of $\geq 1:64$ with demonstration by light microscopy of the organism in erythrocytes is diagnostic.

TABLE 3–35

Bacillary Angiomatosis (*Bartonella [Rochalimaea]* species)[154–156]

Histology

- Peliotic-type fibrovascular proliferation is present within the lobules associated with rare lymphocytic and neutrophilic infiltration.
- These lesions may have a myxoid stroma that contains clumps of granular material representing bacilli (visualized by Warthin-Starry reaction).

Clinical/Laboratory Parameters

- The causative rickettsial organism may be seen in patients with AIDS presenting with cutaneous and visceral organ involvement, and in relapsing fever with bacteremia, endocarditis, trench fever, and bacillary peliosis hepatis.
- Infections can occur from cat scratch and tick bites.
- Skin lesions occur in 50% of cases with erythematous papules, nodules, and hyperpigmented plaques.
- Other manifestations include arthritis, myositis, and mucosal or deep subcutaneous nodules that resemble angiomas.
- Hepatosplenomegaly can occur without skin changes.
- Elevation in serum alkaline phosphatase and mild increase in serum transaminases and bilirubin may be noted.
- The peliotic lesions seen on liver biopsy resolve with antibiotic therapy.

TABLE 3-36

Bacterial Sepsis[143,157,158]

Histology

- Portal tracts show edema with a mixed acute and chronic inflammatory infiltrate.
- The neutrophils within the portal tracts may be scattered, without orientation to vessels or ducts; however, depending on the mode of infection, bile duct and cholangiolar proliferation with acute cholangitis may be seen (spread via the biliary tree).
- Cholestasis is present, sometimes associated with inspissated bile within dilated canaliculi and periportal cholangioles.
- Variable degrees of mostly macrovesicular but also microvesicular fatty change are present.
- Focal necrosis is seen within the lobules associated with neutrophilic exudation.
- Leukocytosis may frequently be seen within the sinusoids.
- In severe cases, microabscesses may be present; in instances of confluent necrosis, enlarged *pyogenic abscesses* may form.
- Organisms in some cases may be demonstrable on Gram stain.
- Necrotizing granulomas have been described (most commonly associated with staphylococcal infection).

Clinical/Laboratory Parameters

- Patients with bacterial sepsis may present with jaundice and abnormal liver tests when the focus of infection is not localized to the liver or biliary tract.
- The mechanism is not clear but is considered to be related to bacterial toxins.
- The typical patient has features of sepsis with fever, has leukocytosis with left shift (band forms), and may have evidence of an abdominal or pelvic collection (e.g., appendicular or diverticular abscess).
- Serum bilirubin may be as high as 20 mg/dl, alkaline phosphatase is moderately or markedly elevated (in cases of abscess formation), and modest increases in serum transaminases are present.
- Treatment of sepsis results in amelioration of the hepatic abnormalities.

TABLE 3-37

Benign Postoperative Intrahepatic Cholestasis[159-161]

Histology

- Cholestasis is seen in the perivenular zones with minimal to absent lobular inflammation.
- Erythrophagocytosis and variable degrees of hemosiderin deposition within Kupffer cells may be seen.
- The portal tracts exhibit little if any inflammation.

Clinical/Laboratory Parameters

- This entity is characterized by the development of jaundice following surgery, with serum bilirubin levels rising to 10 to 15 mg/dl and not accompanied by pruritus or hepatic synthetic dysfunction.
- Serum transaminases may be mildly abnormal; serum alkaline phosphatase may be normal or moderately elevated.
- In the postoperative setting, intra-abdominal abscess, biliary tract obstruction, and drug-induced cholestasis need exclusion.
- The liver tests improve within 2 weeks.
- The cause of cholestasis is multifactorial; no specific mechanism has been identified.

TABLE 3-38

Benign Recurrent Intrahepatic Cholestasis[162-164]

Histology

- Cholestasis is seen in the perivenular zone, in some instances accompanied by a mild mononuclear inflammatory infiltrate.
- Portal lymphocyte infiltration is present and mild, without duct abnormalities.

Clinical/Laboratory Parameters

- In this poorly understood disease, patients present with recurrent episodes of pruritus, often severe and intractable, with jaundice, increase in alkaline phosphatase activity, and bilirubin ranging from 10 to 20 mg/dl.
- Hepatic synthetic function is normal although prothrombin time may be prolonged because of vitamin K deficiency.
- Fasting bile acids are markedly elevated.
- Liver tests return to normal between episodes.

TABLE 3–39

Biliary Hamartoma (von Meyenberg Complex)[41,165]

Histology

- These lesions may be single but are sometimes multiple, and measure less than 0.5 cm in diameter.
- Small irregular and ectatic ducts embedded within a fibrous stroma are present.
- The ducts may contain a proteinaceous material or bile.
- This lesion is often seen in association with fibrocystic diseases (e.g., congenital hepatic fibrosis [refer to Table 3–57], solitary nonparasitic cyst [refer to Table 3–190], adult polycystic disease [refer to Table 3–11], and Caroli's disease [refer to Table 3–47]).

Clinical/Laboratory Parameters

- The lesions are usually incidental findings at laparotomy or autopsy.
- No specific clinical features are present due to the hamartoma itself, except for those related to coexisting hepatic disorders.
- These lesions have no prognostic significance.

TABLE 3–40

Blastomycosis, North American (Blastomyces dermatitidis)[143]

Histology

- Microabscesses and epithelioid granuloma can develop within the parenchyma.
- Within the granuloma 6- to 15-μm budding yeast forms with thick refractile cell walls are seen.

Clinical/Laboratory Parameters

- This fungus present in the soil is acquired by inhalation of conidia with eventual localization within the lungs.
- Chronic pulmonary infection may be noted, with involvement of skin, bones, genitourinary tract, and liver in disseminated disease.
- An increased incidence in patients with AIDS is recognized.
- Enzyme immunoassays are not sensitive for diagnosis; detection of the organism in tissue samples is preferred.

TABLE 3–41

Borreliosis (Relapsing Fever, Borrelia species)[143,166]

Histology

- Focal necrosis with hemorrhage is seen in the perivenular and midzonal regions.
- Increase in sinusoidal lymphocytes and neutrophils is present.
- Kupffer cell hypertrophy with erythrophagocytosis is often seen.
- Organisms (spirochetes 10–20 μm demonstrated by the Warthin-Starry reaction) are present free within the sinusoids.

Clinical/Laboratory Parameters

- This infection is caused by spirochetes of the genus Borrelia, a gram-negative organism transmitted by lice and ticks, with sporadic occurrences.
- During acute infection, which is characterized by fever, headache, sore throat, and myalgia, spirochetes are isolated from blood culture; in the nonfebrile phase, organisms may be found in the liver, spleen, bone marrow, and central nervous system.
- In severe infections, miliary abscesses are found in the spleen, with perisplenitis.
- Infection may also involve the lungs, myocardium, and kidneys; rarely DIC develops.
- In tickborne and louseborne diseases respectively, hepatomegaly (17% and 65%), splenomegaly (37% and 72%), and jaundice (7% and 38%) are observed.
- Serologic tests are somewhat helpful in chronic disease, with presence of agglutinins to Proteus OX-K antigen (interpret cautiously in scrub typhus endemic areas).

TABLE 3–42

Boutonneuse Fever (*Rickettsia conorii*)[167–169]

Histology

- Focal necrosis and lymphocytic infiltration within the lobules are seen.
- Granulomas may also be identified.
- Immunoperoxidase stain demonstrates rickettsial antigen in endothelial cells lining the sinusoids.

Clinical/Laboratory Parameters

- This disease, also termed Mediterranean spotted fever, is caused by *Rickettsii conorii* and is usually seen in Tunisia and other countries bordering the Mediterranean and Black seas.
- It is transmitted by tick bite, causing a raised maculopapular eschar.
- Local lymphadenopathy and fever are frequent.
- Hepatomegaly and mildly abnormal serum aminotransferases may occur.
- Diagnosis is confirmed by complement fixation test.

TABLE 3–43

Brucellosis (*Brucella* species)[170–176]

Histology

- Portal lymphocytic hyperplasia is seen with occasional scattered neutrophils.
- Well to poorly formed granulomas composed of lymphocytes, plump histiocytes, and rare epithelioid cells are seen; rarely fibrinoid necrosis and giant cells may be present.
- Larger granulomas with central necrosis have been described.
- Prominent Kupffer cell hyperplasia and hypertrophy are seen, associated with variable focal necrosis and mononuclear inflammatory infiltration.
- In latter stages, granulomas may undergo healing with fibrosis and calcification.
- Microabscess formation may occur in severe cases.

Clinical/Laboratory Parameters

- This infection is caused by *Brucella* species, a gram-negative coccobacillus acquired by contact with infected farm animals and drinking unpasteurized milk.
- Four species are capable of infection in humans: *Brucella abortus, B. suis, B. melitensis* (most severe infection) and *B. canis* (rare).
- The *acute* infection occurs after an incubation period of 5 to 14 days, presenting with fever, chills, and lymphadenopathy; hepatosplenomegaly may also occur less commonly, with abscess formation described but infrequent.
- Mild to moderate elevations in serum alkaline phosphatase activity and mild increase in transaminases are commonly seen; hyperbilirubinemia is rare and only present in severe disease.
- In the *chronic* form, fever is relapsing, and lymphadenopathy and hepatosplenomegaly are common.
- Diagnosis is confirmed by serologic tests and positive culture of blood, bone marrow, or lymph nodes.

TABLE 3-44

Budd-Chiari Syndrome[177-185]

Histology

Acute

- Sinusoidal dilatation, congestion, and acute hemorrhage in the perivenular zone are present.
- Variable ischemic necrosis of perivenular hepatocytes is seen.
- Extravasation of red blood cells into the space of Disse is present, the red cells eventually occurring within the hepatic cords and replacing the necrotic liver cells.
- The sublocular and hepatic veins may undergo thrombus formation, often with recanalization.
- Variable macrovesicular and microvesicular fatty change is present.

Chronic

- As the disease progresses, variable atrophy of viable liver cells in the perivenular and midzonal areas occurs, associated with sinusoidal dilatation, collagen deposition, and variable occlusion of the terminal hepatic venules.
- Bridging fibrosis of terminal hepatic venules leads to a *cardiac cirrhosis* (reverse lobulation with portal tract sparing).
- Eventually bridging fibrosis occurs between terminal hepatic venules and portal tracts, leading to a micronodular cirrhosis.
- If transjugular biopsies are performed, a thin fibrous web forming a valve-like membrane overlying the entrance of the hepatic vein into the inferior vena cava may be identified, often with calcifications.

Clinical/Laboratory Parameters

- In this syndrome, thrombotic occlusion of the major hepatic veins occurs from a variety of hypercoagulable disorders such as oral contraceptive use, factor V Leiden mutation, paroxysmal nocturnal hemoglobinuria, deficiency of protein C and S, myeloproliferative disorders, lupus anticoagulant, and tumor invasion; some instances are idiopathic.
- Membranous obstruction of the large hepatic veins immediately superior to their entrance into the inferior vena cava is also a cause most frequently seen in South Africa, Japan, and India; hepatocellular carcinoma has been shown to be associated with up to 50% of all cases of membranous obstruction in South Africa.
- In the *acute* form, patients present with tender hepatomegaly, ascites, modest elevations in serum transaminases, and mild increase in serum bilirubin; progression to liver failure necessitates liver transplantation.
- In the *chronic* form, the presentation is indistinguishable from decompensated cirrhosis of other etiologies.
- The drainage of the caudate lobe is often spared, resulting in marked caudate enlargement (visualized on technetium-99m sulfur colloid and CT scans) secondary to compensatory hyperplasia.

TABLE 3-45

Candidiasis (Candida albicans)[186-189]

Histology

- Microabscesses can occur within the lobules, with occasional granulomatous reaction.
- Pseudohyphae and budding yeast forms are usually visible and are easily confirmed on PAS stain.

Clinical/Laboratory Parameters

- Hepatic candidiasis is a well-recognized infection in patients receiving chemotherapy for malignancy, immunosuppressive therapy for autoimmune disease, or following organ transplantation.
- Patients present with fever, moderate to marked increases in alkaline phosphatase activity, variable increases in serum bilirubin, and modest increases in serum transaminases.
- The primary source may be an infected intravenous catheter, and its removal with administration of antifungal medications results in improvement; however, in patients with marked immunosuppression or chemotherapy-induced marrow failure, prognosis is poor.

TABLE 3–46

Capillariasis (Capillaria hepatica) [143,190,191]

Histology

- A granulomatous response to adult worms and eggs occurs within the lobules, the granulomas containing prominent numbers of eosinophils.

Clinical/Laboratory Parameters

- This nematode is found in the small intestine; humans are infected by ingesting larvae that reside in muscles of freshwater fish.
- Patients present with abdominal pain, diarrhea, and protein-losing enteropathy.
- Liver involvement is rare and may be due to ectopic localization.

TABLE 3–47

Caroli's Disease [192–196]

Histology

- This disorder generally involves the entire liver but may be segmental or lobar.
- Round to oval cysts form that are 1 to 4.5 cm in diameter.
- The cystic structures are lined by cuboidal epithelium that may be ulcerated or hyperplastic.
- Bile duct proliferation and ectasia with microcyst formation are present and may be prominent.
- Inspissated bile and calculi may be seen within dilated duct lumen.
- Duct dysplasia leading to adenocarcinoma may occur.
- Secondary changes of bile duct obstruction may be present, including periductal fibrosis, acute cholangitis, cholestasis, and abscess formation in nontreated cases.

Clinical/Laboratory Parameters

- This disorder usually is diagnosed between the ages of 5 and 20 years, but it also may be seen in the older population.
- Cystic dilatation of intrahepatic bile ducts is present and is contiguous with unaffected bile ducts.
- Microcystic disease of the kidneys (*medullary sponge kidney*) may be associated.
- Patients present typically with recurrent cholangitis and have a predisposition to develop pigmented stones.
- Saccular dilatation of ducts is also seen with complications of abscess formation; the clinical course is often punctuated by multiple surgeries to remove stones or drain abscesses.
- Hepatosplenomegaly may be noted; alkaline phosphatase activity is moderately elevated.
- Portal hypertension, which may occur due to associated congenital hepatic fibrosis (refer to Table 3–57), usually develops with progression of the disease.

TABLE 3–48

Cat-Scratch Disease (Afipia felis) [143,197–200]

Histology

- Microabscesses with granulomatous borders may be seen.
- On Warthin-Starry reaction extracellular clumps of bacillary organisms may be seen at the edge of the abscesses.

Clinical/Laboratory Parameters

- Caused by a gram-negative bacillus, the vast majority of cases occur by contact with cats, often by way of cat scratch or bite.
- Skin lesions and regional lymphadenopathy are the commonest manifestation in the human immunodeficiency virus (HIV)–negative population, with children developing the infection more often than adults.
- Rarely, encephalopathy, lytic bone necrosis, and pneumonitis may develop.
- Hepatic involvement is seen most often with systemic infection in the immunocompromised patient.

TABLE 3–49

Cavernous Hemangioma[130,201–205]

Histology

- The lesion is usually solitary and less than 5 cm in diameter (may be up to 20 cm in diameter [*giant type*]), is well demarcated, flat, red-blue, and often subcapsular.
- Large cavernous vascular spaces are seen lined by flattened endothelial cells, and the empty spaces may become filled with red blood cells.
- Variable degrees of fibrous thickening are seen between the vascular spaces, these fibrous bands often containing scanty lymphocytes.
- Central fibrous scarring may occur, and may calcify.
- Thrombosis of the vascular lumen may occur, with resultant ischemic necrosis.

Clinical/Laboratory Parameters

- Cavernous hemangiomas are the most common mass lesion in the liver, and are seen in approximately 1% of the total adult population.
- Patients are rarely symptomatic unless the lesion is large.
- Liver tests are normal.
- On ultrasound these lesions appear hyperechoic, and are hypodense on CT scan with peripheral enhancement on contrast studies.
- Gradual increase in uptake of red blood cell–labeled technetium in a blood pool scan is characteristic in large, nonthrombosed lesions.
- Increased signal on T2-weighted MR scans is also typical.
- Management is conservative and surgery is recommended only for very large lesions that encroach on the hepatic hilum.

TABLE 3–50

Cholangiocarcinoma[41,194,206–213]

Histology

- The tumor is gray-white and firm, most commonly seen at the periphery of the liver; however, approximately 15% arise from the bifurcation of the main hepatic ducts at the hilum *(Klatskin tumor)*.
- Microscopically the most common type is a well-differentiated adenocarcinoma forming tubules with abundant fibrous stroma.
- The tumor cells form glands lined by small cuboidal cells having round to oval nuclei with small nucleoli and scanty to moderate cytoplasm.
- Variable histologic subtypes occur, including signet-ring, acinar, papillary, mucin-producing, adenosquamous, and mucoepidermoid differentiation; microcalcifications may be seen.
- Bile may be seen at the edge of the tumor adjacent to trapped hepatocytes; however, the tumor itself does not secrete bile.
- The tumor cells merge into the adjacent hepatic parenchyma via the sinusoids, not cords.
- The hilar lesions may exhibit perineural invasion.
- When induced by Thorotrast (thorium dioxide), this granular green-brown pigment is seen in the adjacent nontumor portal macrophages and Kupffer cells.
- Helpful immunoperoxidase markers for diagnosis are the following: broad-spectrum cytokeratins, carcinoembryonic antigen, and epithelial membrane antigen (EMA) (which all help to differentiate cholangiocarcinoma from hepatocellular carcinoma but not from metastatic adenocarcinoma).

Clinical/Laboratory Parameters

- Cholangiocarcinoma represents approximately 8 to 12% of all hepatic primary malignancies in the adult, and is seen most often in middle-aged men.
- Predisposing conditions include primary sclerosing cholangitis with or without inflammatory bowel disease, biliary cystic diseases (e.g., choledochal cyst), hepatolithiasis, recurrent pyogenic cholangiohepatitis, biliary parasitic infestations, and toxins such as Thorotrast.
- Jaundice is frequent in hilar lesions when the major ducts are involved, resulting in significant biliary obstruction associated with pruritus, elevations in serum bilirubin, marked increases in alkaline phosphatase activity, and mild increases in serum transaminases with preserved hepatic synthetic function.
- Prothrombin time may be prolonged because of vitamin K deficiency related to bile duct obstruction, confirmed by correction with vitamin K replacement.
- Lesions located peripherally within the liver are identified by incidental ultrasound and CT scans, or for investigation of abdominal masses, which indicates advanced disease.
- Definitive diagnosis of intraductal hilar lesions is made by endoscopic retrograde cholangiopancreatography, with brushings and biopsies of suspicious lesions.
- The presence of perineural involvement is associated with a risk of recurrence after surgery.
- Liver transplantation is not recommended because of the high incidence of recurrence in the graft.

TABLE 3-51

Choledochal Cyst[214-216]

Histology

- The extrahepatic biliary cysts vary in size, but may be large and contain 5 to 10 L of bile.
- The wall is fibrotic and thickened, and may exhibit variable lymphocytic infiltration.
- The inner wall may contain inspissated bile.
- Generally there is no epithelial lining, but islets of cylindrical or columnar epithelium, intestinal metaplasia with goblet and Paneth cells, and neuroendocrine differentiation may be present.
- Malignant transformation to adenocarcinoma or to anaplastic or squamous cell carcinoma may be seen overall in about 3% of cases, but is age related (0.7% in the first decade, 6.8% in the second decade, 14.3% thereafter).
- Secondary changes of bile duct obstruction may be present, including bile duct proliferation and ectasia, periductal fibrosis, acute cholangitis, cholestasis, and abscess formation in nontreated cases.

Clinical/Laboratory Parameters

- The clinical presentation may occur at any age, with almost one fifth occurring during the first year of life.
- The disorder is three times more frequent in females.
- Other bile duct anomalies such as double gallbladder or double common bile duct may also be seen; intrahepatic duct dilatation (refer to Table 3-47, Caroli's Disease) may also be present.
- Infants present with clinical features simulating duct obstruction and have progressive disease, while older children and adults have a less severe course.
- Abdominal pain is a common symptom, with jaundice less frequent.
- Cholangiocarcinoma can develop in untreated patients along the cyst lumen or in residual cyst tissue if surgical resection is incomplete.

TABLE 3-52

Cholesterol Ester Storage Disease[217-220]

Histology

- Hypertrophic Kupffer cells and portal macrophages contain DiPAS-positive birefringent crystals on frozen section, confirmed by positive oil red O stain as neutral fat.
- Variable macrovesicular and microvesicular fatty change is present within hepatocytes.
- Although portal fibrosis and intrasinusoidal collagen deposition may be present, cirrhosis is quite uncommon.

Clinical/Laboratory Parameters

- This autosomal recessive disorder resembles *Wolman's disease* (refer to Table 3-227) but is generally milder.
- Low acid lipase levels are found in tissues, including leukocytes and cultured fibroblasts.
- Patients present in childhood with hepatomegaly and diarrhea, and they may have early onset of atherosclerosis.
- Only mildly abnormal serum aminotransferases are present; however, serum bile acids are elevated.

TABLE 3-53

Chronic Granulomatous Disease of Childhood[221-224]

Histology

- Granulomas are composed of epithelioid cells, lymphocytes, plasma cells, and occasional giant cells with peripheral palisading and centrally located eosinophilic necrotic material.
- Granulomas may coalesce, with more extensive necrosis and neutrophilic infiltrates, forming microabscesses.
- Portal lymphocytic and plasma cell infiltration is present.
- Mild to moderate macrovesicular fatty change may be present.
- Increase in lipochrome pigment is seen in hypertrophied Kupffer cells and portal macrophages.
- Cirrhosis has been reported, with large dense scar formation and associated "potato-like" nodules *(hepar lobatum)*.

Clinical/Laboratory Parameters

- A heterogeneous group of defects secondary to decreased neutrophilic production of oxidants, the white blood cells can phagocytize organisms but are not able to kill them; as a result, patients develop in the first year of life recurrent bacterial and fungal infections.
- Clinical findings include marked lymphadenopathy, pneumonia, dermatitis, splenomegaly, and hepatic and perihepatic abscesses.
- Liver tests are usually normal although hypoalbuminemia caused by chronic infections and elevated bilirubin due to sepsis may be noted.

TABLE 3-54
Ciliated Hepatic Foregut Cyst[225,226]

Histology

- Occurs as a solitary unilocular cyst (<4 cm) having four layers:
  - Pseudostratified ciliated columnar mucosa
  - Subepithelial collagen
  - Adjacent smooth muscle elements
  - Outermost fibrous capsule

Clinical/Laboratory Parameters

- This disorder is clinically asymptomatic and incidentally discovered by radiologic imaging.
- Infrequently, patients may present with vague abdominal pain.
- If large, the cysts may be palpable on abdominal examination.
- Liver tests are normal.
- The clinical course is benign, although rarely spontaneous rupture can occur.

TABLE 3-55
Clonorchiasis *(Clonorchis sinensis)*[143,227-230]

Histology

- This liver fluke is seen mainly within distal ducts, but with heavier parasite loads the proximal ducts and gallbladder may also be involved.
- The left lobe is more often affected than the right lobe.
- *Segmental* duct dilatation (up to 3–6 mm in diameter) with thickened walls and worms in the duct lumen are seen.
- The duct epithelial lining adjacent to the worms is hyperplastic *(adenomatous ductular hyperplasia),* often with goblet cell metaplasia, increased mucin production surrounding the ducts, and variable infiltration by eosinophils.
- Fibrosis around ducts is present with variable acute and chronic inflammatory infiltration.
- Cysts may form in severe cases secondary to marked duct dilatation, the cysts containing clear bile.
- Associated bile duct obstruction may produce cholestasis with lobular neutrophils and acute cholangitis.
- Cholangiocarcinoma is a known complication.

Clinical/Laboratory Parameters

- *Clonorchis sinensis* is a liver (bile duct) fluke, similar to *Opisthorchis viverrini* (opisthorchiasis[701-703]), which resides in the biliary tract of the definitive host (humans) and is a common infection in Asia.
- The adult worm (10–20 mm in length) lays eggs that travel down the bile ducts and are excreted in the feces into fresh water; the eggs are ingested by snails (intermediate host); miracidia hatch from the ingested eggs and develop into cercariae, which eventually break out of the snail and enter fresh water.
- Cercariae penetrate the scales of fish, encyst, develop into metacercariae, and are eaten by humans in raw or poorly cooked fish.
- The worm then develops and migrates into the main bile ducts, causing liver disease.
- During acute infection, fever, abdominal pain, and jaundice related to cholangitis develop; in some patients, abscesses or cholecystitis may be seen.
- In the late stages with recurrent cholangitis, cystic dilatation and biliary strictures may develop.

TABLE 3-56
Coccidioidomycosis *(Coccidioides immitis)*[143,174,231-233]

Histology

- Epithelioid granulomas are present, with prominent multinucleated giant cells containing spherules 20 to 200 μm in diameter, which are positive on methenamine silver stain. The spherules have 2-μm-thick walls and contain endospores (2–5 μm) or granular eosinophilic material.
- The granulomas may coalesce.
- The spherules may rupture, with endospores released adjacent to empty distorted spherules.
- Smaller immature spherules (10–20 μm) may also be seen.
- With resolution, granulomas may become fibrotic.

Clinical/Laboratory Parameters

- *Coccidioides immitis* is endemic in the southwestern United States, occurs within the soil, and is acquired by inhalation of spores.
- Disseminated infection occurs in both immunocompetent and immunosuppressed individuals; the patient presents with fever, meningitis, and skin lesions. Hepatomegaly suggests liver involvement.
- Liver tests may be normal or mildly abnormal with increases in serum alkaline phosphatase activity.
- Peritoneal involvement also occurs in the disseminated form, mimics tuberculous peritonitis, and can only be distinguished by culture and positive fungal stains.

TABLE 3-57

Congenital Hepatic Fibrosis[234-241]

Histology

- Biliary fibrosis with thick fibrous bands is present, and may occasionally encircle groups of liver cells, *without* formation of regenerative nodules.
- Prominent bile duct and cholangiolar proliferation and ectasia are present, with anastomosing structures often containing inspissated bile plugs.
- Although there is little portal inflammatory infiltrate, acute cholangitis may at times occur and be associated with cholestasis.
- There is a paucity of portal veins and portal venous radicles.
- Duct rupture may lead to microabscesses.
- Increase in copper-binding protein has been described.

Clinical/Laboratory Parameters

- With this recessive genetic disease, patients present in childhood or young adulthood with hepatomegaly and some degree of abdominal discomfort.
- Bleeding esophageal varices may be the first manifestation.
- Liver function is well preserved except for elevated alkaline phosphatase activity when the disorder is complicated by biliary tract infection.
- Associated renal changes such as polycystic kidneys or tubular defects are seen in 50% of patients.

TABLE 3-58

Crigler-Najjar Syndrome[242-244]

Histology

- Cholestasis may be seen in the perivenular zone.
- Portal and lobular inflammation are usually absent.

Clinical/Laboratory Parameters

- Crigler-Najjar syndrome is characterized by unconjugated hyperbilirubinemia since birth.
- Two subtypes are present:
  - In *type 1,* the defect is complete deficiency of the enzyme bilirubin uridine diphosphate (UDP) glucuronosyltransferase; infants present with marked elevations in serum bilirubin (exceeding 350 mmol/L) with kernicterus.
  - In *type 2,* the defect is partial deficiency of this enzyme, whereby the bilirubin levels are usually less elevated.
- Although phenobarbital reduces serum bilirubin levels, liver transplantation is the treatment of choice in type 1 disease.

TABLE 3-59

Crohn's Disease[61,245-247]

Histology

- 1+ to 2+ macrovesicular fatty change is present in the majority of cases.
- Portal lymphocytic infiltration is seen; piecemeal necrosis may also be present.
- Focal necrosis and lymphocytic infiltration are present within the lobules, but are generally mild.
- Epithelioid and inflammatory granulomas are present (5% of cases).
- Variable degree of sinusoidal collagen deposition may be present.
- Amyloidosis has been described.
- Macronodular cirrhosis may occur but is rare.
- Pyogenic abscesses, pylephlebitis, and hepatic venous outflow obstruction (Budd-Chiari syndrome) have been reported.

Clinical/Laboratory Parameters

- Liver dysfunction is seen in up to 10% of patients with either *ulcerative colitis* (refer to Table 3-203) or Crohn's disease.
- Patients may develop elevated alkaline phosphatase activity associated with granulomas.
- Intra-abdominal abscesses can occur and are often frequent.
- Liver abscesses are uncommon; when present, the prognosis is dim.
- Cholecystitis with gallstones is not infrequent and may in part be related to malabsorption of bile acids.

TABLE 3–60

Cryptococcosis *(Cryptococcus neoformans)*[143,248–250]

Histology

- Hypertrophic Kupffer cells and portal macrophages contain yeast forms 5 to 20 μm in diameter, which are encapsulated and budding, with thick walls having an empty rim (best visualized with mucicarmine and PAS stains).
- Epithelioid granulomas may also be present within the lobules.
- Rarely sclerosing cholangitis may be seen secondary to involvement of the extrahepatic biliary system.

Clinical/Laboratory Parameters

- Seen usually in the immunocompromised individual, this infection often occurs with encephalitis or pneumonitis.
- The alkaline phosphatase activity may be elevated when there is hepatic involvement.
- Diagnosis is confirmed on spinal fluid analysis with India ink wet mounts as well as organisms identification in tissues on biopsy.

TABLE 3–61

Cryptosporidiosis *(Cryptosporidium parvum)*[251–253]

Histology

- These small 1- to 2 μm organisms are seen adherent to the luminal surface of large- to medium-sized bile ducts.
- Rarely the organisms can be demonstrated involving smaller interlobular ducts.
- These smaller ducts may show periductal sclerosis; in some cases, ductopenia can occur (refer to Table 3–110, Human Immunodeficiency Virus–associated Cholangiopathy).

Clinical/Laboratory Parameters

- This small protozoan organism is found in the small intestine and has a predilection for infecting biliary epithelial cells.
- Approximately 20% of cases of HIV-associated cholangiopathy are detected to have cryptosporidium on biopsy.
- Patients may present with right upper quadrant pain, elevated alkaline phosphatase activity, and sometimes hyperbilirubinemia.
- Ultrasound may demonstrate dilated bile ducts.
- Endoscopic retrograde cholangiopancreatography has the advantage of permitting biopsies for diagnosis, with sphincterotomy to relieve symptoms.

TABLE 3–62

Cystadenoma With or Without Mesenchymal Stroma[41,254–256]

Histology

- The cysts are multilocular and range from 5 to 25 cm in diameter, with the contents clear and cloudy to mucinous.
- The inner surface of the cysts is smooth to trabeculated, and may show small sessile projections.
- Microscopically the cysts are lined by columnar, cuboidal to flattened, usually mucin-secreting, nonciliated duct epithelium that is single-layered, but may show papillary projections or infoldings.
- The underlying stroma may be acellular and hyalinized; *mesenchymal stroma* is composed of hypercellular spindle cells and is usually seen in the majority of cases but may be absent or present only focally.
- The outer layer of the cyst is composed of dense collagen containing large vessels, nerves, fat, and small glands, and is sharply demarcated from the adjacent liver.
- The septa may also contain foamy histiocytes, pigmented macrophages, cholesterol clefts, acute hemorrhage, and calcifications.
- Dysplasia of the lining cells may occur in up to 25% of cases; these cells are multilayered, sometimes exhibiting a solid growth (borderline lesions); capsular invasion may occur (malignant transformation to cystadenocarcinoma).

Clinical/Laboratory Parameters

- Cystadenomas are benign intrahepatic multiloculated cystic tumors that are subdivided as present with or without mesenchymal stroma.
- Lesions with mesenchymal stroma are seen exclusively in women, while there is a male predominance in lesions without a stromal component.
- An abdominal mass and pain develop in about half of patients.
- Elevations in serum alkaline phosphatase may be seen in lesions at the hepatic hilum, with associated increases in serum bilirubin and mild elevations in serum transaminases.
- On ultrasound and CT scans, cystic lesions with thickened walls are noted; in lesions with mesenchymal stroma, a complex mass with irregularities of the cyst wall is seen.
- Malignant transformation in lesions with mesenchymal stroma may occur.
- Surgical resection is indicated; however, marsupialization of large, nonresectable tumors may be an alternative treatment.

TABLE 3-63

Cystic Fibrosis[257-263]

Histology

- In the early stages there may be features resembling neonatal hepatitis (refer to Table 3–155), with portal and lobular inflammatory infiltrates and syncytial giant cell reaction.
- Macrovasicular fatty change is seen, first in the periportal zones, but often diffuse throughout the lobules. Some degree of microvesicular fat may also be present.
- Hemosiderin may be seen in periportal hepatocytes.
- Sinusoidal collagen deposition may also be present.
- Variable but often prominent cholangiolar proliferation and ectasia are present, sometimes with rupture and prominent neutrophilic response, the cholangioles often containing amorphous eosinophilic concretions or inspissated DiPAS-positive bile.
- Marked cholestasis with variable acute and chronic inflammatory infiltration is present, predominantly in the periportal zones.
- Paucity of bile ducts due to large duct damage may also be present.
- A mild focal increase in copper and copper-binding protein is present in periportal liver cells.
- Mucinous material is often seen in both extra- and intrahepatic bile ducts in a minority of cases.
- Biliary fibrosis is present, with eventual progression to focal biliary fibrosis in 25 to 30% of patients, or multilobular (multinodular) biliary cirrhosis in 5 to 10% of patients. The nodules are often quite large and potato-like (resembling hepar lobatum).
- Secondary changes of bile duct obstruction may be present, including periductal fibrosis, acute cholangitis, cholestasis, and abscess formation in non-treated cases.

Clinical/Laboratory Parameters

- Cystic fibrosis is an autosomal recessive disorder with an incidence of 1 in 2000 live births in the white population; the disorder is uncommon in the black population and in Asians.
- The liver and biliary tract exhibit common complications of this predominantly respiratory disease.
- In the neonatal period, jaundice, acholic stools, and meconium ileus are manifestations.
- Liver disease in children and young adults is usually asymptomatic, although manifestations of pulmonary involvement such as bronchiectasis and pneumonia are often present.
- Firm, sometimes nodular hepatomegaly and splenic enlargement may coincide with the development of portal hypertension.
- When supported by a positive family history, the sweat test is performed for diagnosis (a positive test yields values >60 mEq of chloride per liter).
- The clinical course is complicated by bleeding esophageal varices and, in severe cases, ascites, encephalopathy, and liver failure.
- In the absence of pulmonary infections and hypertension, liver transplantation should be considered.

TABLE 3-64

Cystinosis[264,265]

Histology

- Deposition of water-soluble hexagonal and cylindrical cystine crystals in hypertrophic Kupffer cells and portal macrophages are present; the crystals are brightly silver colored on birefringence under polarized light.
- Cystine crystals within the lobule are seen predominantly in the perivenular zone, and are best identified on frozen section or liver fixed in alcohol.

Clinical/Laboratory Parameters

- Cystinosis is a rare lysosomal disorder due to defective carrier-mediated transport of the amino acid cystine.
- Cystine crystals accumulate in the eye, reticuloendothelial system, kidneys, and other organ systems.
- Renal disease and failure, acidosis, hypophosphatemic rickets, corneal erosions, diabetes mellitus, and neurologic deterioration are complications.
- Massive hepatomegaly has been reported; however, most patients do not have significant liver disease.

TABLE 3-65

Cytomegalovirus Infection[100,266–272]

Histology

- Portal lymphocytic infiltration is present and often prominent, with occasional clusters of atypical lymphocytes present.
- Sinusoidal lymphocytosis is often seen.
- Focal necrosis is present and often granulomatous in type, rarely with epithelioid multinucleated giant cell formation.
- Some degree of predominantly macrovasicular but also microvasicular fatty change may be present.
- Occasionally lymphocytes may attack bile duct epithelium, with minimal duct atypia; however, in the neonate this type of biliary damage may lead to duct depletion with concomitant giant cell transformation of hepatocytes.
- Viral inclusions may be seen in duct epithelium, hepatocytes, or endothelial cells. In the immunocompromised patient, the inclusions are generally large, amphophilic, and intranuclear with a surrounding clear space ("owl's eye"), sometimes associated with numerous smaller cytoplasmic inclusions.
- These inclusions may be seen with or without an inflammatory reaction; when inflammation is seen, poorly formed granulomatous necrosis is present, or inclusions are surrounded by small clusters of neutrophils forming *microabscesses* (the latter most frequently noted after liver transplantation).
- Viral inclusions that involve duct epithelium may cause duct damage, sclerosing cholangitis, and eventual duct depletion in HIV-associated cholangiopathy (refer to Table 3–110).
- Note that viral inclusions may occasionally be seen in the neonate in immunocompetent patients.

Clinical/Laboratory Parameters

- This DNA virus is a member of the herpesvirus group and causes cytomegaly and large intranuclear inclusion bodies of infected cells.
- About 50 to 80% of adults are exposed to this virus; thus manifestations in the immunosuppressed state are mostly secondary to reactivation of the latent virus.
- In congenital infection, neonates present with hepatosplenomegaly, jaundice, and thrombocytopenia and may develop chorioretinitis and other signs of intrauterine infection.
- In the adult who is immunocompetent, the infection is self-limited, with serum transaminases seldom above 500 IU/L; serum bilirubin is rarely elevated except in severe, untreated or disseminated cases associated with renal failure.
- Only rare cases of fulminant hepatitis have been reported.
- Atypical lymphocytosis may be seen in the peripheral blood.
- In the immunocompromised patient, infection may be chronic and persistent.
- The risk of developing cytomegalovirus (CMV) infection in post transplant patients is highest in weeks 4 to 12 postoperatively and occurs more frequently in recipients of organs from CMV seropositive donors.
- The recognition of cytomegalic cells with inclusion bodies in the tissues is diagnostic.
- Positive viral cultures may not reflect active infection and disease.
- Detection of the viral antigen (PP65) or virus by polymerase chain reaction is helpful for quick diagnosis and treatment.

TABLE 3-66

Dengue Fever[143,273–275]

Histology

- Focal perivenular coalescent liver cell necrosis with dropout of hepatocytes but little inflammation is present.

Clinical/Laboratory Parameters

- This arbovirus (RNA virus) is transmitted by the *Aedes* mosquito, with infection endemic in tropical countries.
- The disease is characterized by fever, severe myalgias (breakbone fever), headache, malaise, and prostration.
- Liver tests are mildly abnormal, and fulminant liver failure has not been reported.

TABLE 3–67
Down Syndrome[276–279]

Histology

- Diffuse interstitial fibrosis may be present within all zones.
- Extramedullary hematopoiesis may be seen.
- The lobules may exhibit parenchymal hemosiderin.
- Ductopenia has been described.

Clinical/Laboratory Parameters

- The clinical features of Down syndrome (trisomy 21) include mental retardation, hypotonia, congenital heart disease, duodenal atresia, Hirschprung's disease, an increased propensity to infection, immunodeficiency, thyroid abnormalities, and increased incidence of leukemia and Alzheimer's disease.
- Patients may present with severe liver disease at or shortly after birth, with associated hyperbilirubinemia.

TABLE 3–68
Dubin-Johnson Syndrome[243,280–282]

Histology

- Grossly the liver is dark green to black.
- Coarsely granular, dark, melanin-like pigment is seen in perivenular liver cells with pericanalicular localization.
- The pigment may disappear after acute hepatitis of any cause, with eventual reaccumulation.
- Portal and lobular inflammation are usually not present.

Clinical/Laboratory Parameters

- The Dubin-Johnson syndrome is familial and characterized by chronic and intermittent jaundice and identified black pigment in the liver.
- Patients are asymptomatic except for occasional mild jaundice; some patients present with weakness, nausea, and vomiting.
- The serum conjugated bilirubin is elevated, rarely as high as 20 mg/dl (360 mmol/L).
- The sulfobromophthalein test is abnormal and characterized by normal plasma concentration at 45 minutes followed by a secondary rise in plasma levels 45 to 90 minutes after injection.
- There is no progression of the liver disease and the prognosis is excellent.

TABLE 3–69
Ebola Virus Infection[275,283,284]

Histology

- Coagulative-type necrosis without inflammation is present scattered within the lobules, with numerous acidophil bodies.
- The necrosis is usually patchy but in some cases may be confluent.

Clinical/Laboratory Parameters

- Outbreaks of infection by this RNA virus are associated with severe and often fatal hemorrhagic fever.
- Patients present with sudden onset of fever, malaise, nausea and vomiting, myalgias, maculopapular rashes, and conjunctivitis.
- Liver dysfunction develops during the second week of illness, although hyperbilirubinemia is uncommon.

TABLE 3–70
Enterobiasis (Enterobius [Oxyuris] vermicularis)[143,285,286]

Histology

- Up to 1 cm, round granulomatous nodules composed predominantly of acellular eosinophilic debris are present.
- The nodules contain a centrally located degenerating worm that sometimes is surrounded by eggs.
- A mixed inflammatory infiltrate including eosinophils is present at the periphery of the nodules.

Clinical/Laboratory Parameters

- The most cosmopolitan of all nematodes, this pinworm affects mainly children who present with perianal pruritus.
- The worm resides in the lumen of the cecum and colon, and may be linked to appendicitis.
- Ectopic localization of the worms has been noted in the peritoneal cavity, fallopian tubes, and rarely in the liver, forming mass lesions.

TABLE 3-71
Eosinophilic Gastroenteritis[287,288]

Histology

- Numerous eosinophils are present within portal tracts.
- Granulomas have also been described containing eosinophils.

Clinical/Laboratory Parameters

- This rare disease may present with recurrent abdominal pain, sometimes with associated steatorrhea.
- Intestinal perforation has been reported.
- Hepatic involvement is unusual.

TABLE 3-72
Epithelioid Hemangioendothelioma (Vasoablative Endotheliosarcoma)[41,130,289-294]

Histology

- Multiple firm fibrous masses are present.
- Histologically, the *dendritic* component consists of elongated stellate eosinophilic processes containing well-defined cytoplasmic vacuoles, usually within a myxoid or pseudocartilaginous stroma.
- The *epithelioid* component consists of rounded, relatively abundant eosinophilic cytoplasm, hyperchromatic nuclei, and prominent nucleoli, forming cords or tubular structures.
- Tumor growth within outflow vessels (terminal hepatic and sublobular veins) frequently occurs.
- Stromal fibrosis may be extensive, with the tumor cells at times appearing isolated.
- Microcalcifications may occur.
- A helpful immunoperoxidase marker for diagnosis is factor VIII–related antigen, which stains the malignant endothelial cells.

Clinical/Laboratory Parameters

- This neoplasm is a slow-growing variant of *angiosarcoma* (refer to Table 3-30) with an overall better prognosis.
- There is a slight predominance in middle-aged women.
- Hepatomegaly, right upper quadrant pain, and weight loss occur.
- Hyperbilirubinemia with jaundice is seen in up to 10% of patients.
- A slight increase in alkaline phosphatase activity is present, usually with normal serum bilirubin.
- The alpha-fetoprotein level is normal.
- Resection has allowed better survival in up to 30% of patients with 5-year follow-up; liver transplantation has been performed.

TABLE 3-73
Epstein-Barr Virus Infection[98,100,295-298]

Histology

- The histologic features are similar to cytomegalovirus infection (refer to Table 3-65) in immunocompetent patients except that atypical portal and sinusoidal lymphocytes are more prominent.
- Portal eosinophils and plasma cells in some instances may be increased.
- Endothelialitis may occasionally be demonstrated involving portal and terminal hepatic veins.
- Viral inclusions are rarely seen on routine staining except in severe fatal cases; however, positive staining for virus may be demonstrated in portal lymphocytes by in situ hybridization (Epstein-Barr virus-encoded RNA [EBER] probe).
- In liver transplant patients, infection may be associated with post transplant lymphoproliferative disease (PTLD; refer to Table 3-22); lymphoproliferative disease may also be seen in AIDS patients.

Clinical/Laboratory Parameters

- The Epstein-Barr virus is a DNA virus belonging to the herpesvirus group that causes a self-limited systemic infection usually of young adults.
- The acute infection is characterized by fever, pharyngitis, prominent lymphadenopathy, splenomegaly, malaise, anorexia, and hepatitis in more severe infections.
- Leukopenia, atypical lymphocytosis, thrombocytopenia, moderate to marked increases in serum alkaline phosphatase, mild to moderate increase in transaminases, and normal to mild increases in bilirubin occur in most cases of hepatitis.
- In the severe or the rare fulminant case, marked hyperbilirubinemia may also be seen.
- The diagnosis is made by observing atypical lymphocytosis in a patient with a positive heterophil antibody, and confirmed by high titers of EB viral capsid antigen IgM and IgG.
- The ability to test tissue for EBV by in situ hybridization (EBER probe) may improve the diagnosis of post transplant lymphoproliferative disease.

TABLE 3-74

Erythropoietic protoporphyria[299-304]

Histology

- Grossly the liver is black.
- Accumulation of dark brown pigment in liver cells, biliary canaliculi, interlobular bile ducts, Kupffer cells, and portal collagen is present, the pigment representing protoporphyrin crystals.
- Intense red autofluorescence of pigment on frozen sections is present.
- The pigment under polarized light has a maltese cross appearance.
- Portal lymphocytic infiltration may be present; in some instances in which chronic liver disease develops, piecemeal necrosis may be seen.
- Cholestasis with mononuclear inflammation may be present in those patients in whom chronic liver disease develops.
- Portal and intralobular fibrosis may progress to cirrhosis.

Clinical/Laboratory Parameters

- This disorder is a probable autosomal dominant inherited defect with variable penetrance of the ferrochelatase enzyme resulting in the accumulation of protoporphyrin IX in red blood cells, skin, and liver.
- Photosensitivity skin changes are usually minor, and anemia is generally mild and may be hemolytic.
- Liver disease is rare; when it is present, patients present with hepatosplenomegaly, ascites, hyperbilirubinemia, modest elevations of serum transaminases, and encephalopathy.
- Death from liver failure or variceal hemorrhage can be prevented by liver transplantation.

TABLE 3-75

Extrahepatic Biliary Atresia[305-315]

Histology

- Three types of extrahepatic biliary remnants are present:
  - Type 1: Absence of ducts.
  - Type 2: Small lumen (diameter <50 μm) containing neutrophils; cellular debris, bile, and epithelial necrosis are found in the lumen of ducts greater than 300 μm.
  - Type 3: Central lumen with incomplete lining, and ducts similar to type 2.
- Markedly dilated proliferating ducts and cholangioles with inspissated bile plugs may be seen.
- Giant cell transformation of perivenular hepatocytes occurs in 15% of cases.
- Perivenular cholestasis is usually present.
- Mallory bodies, bile lakes, and/or infarcts may be seen in the periportal zones.
- Extramedullary hematopoiesis may occur.
- Increase in copper and copper-binding protein may be present in the periportal liver cells.
- Portal lymphocytic and neutrophilic infiltration is seen.
- Biliary fibrosis eventually occurs in nontreated patients, leading to biliary cirrhosis with ductopenia.

Clinical/Laboratory Parameters

- Extrahepatic biliary atresia is responsible for up to 50% of all cases of cholestasis in the neonatal period; the overall incidence ranges from 1 per 8000 to 1 per 20,000 live births.
- The newborn presents with jaundice within 1 to 3 weeks after birth with failure to thrive, progressing to liver failure with portal hypertension, bleeding varices, and ascites in untreated patients.
- Hyperbilirubinemia, elevated alkaline phosphatase activity, hypoalbuminemia, and prolonged prothrombin time are common.
- Hepatosplenomegaly is usual.
- Relief of obstruction by hepatoportoenterostomy (Kasai procedure) in some patients prevents progression of the liver disease and delays the need for transplantation.

TABLE 3–76

Extrahepatic Biliary Obstruction, Early[316,317]

Histology

- Grossly the liver is enlarged and green, with dilatation of the large intrahepatic bile ducts, which may contain bile, or pus if ascending cholangitis is also present.
- Portal edema is present, and may be most prominent surrounding interlobular ducts.
- Periductal neutrophilic infiltration is present, with neutrophils surrounding and invading duct epithelium *(acute cholangitis)*.
- Prominent proliferation and ectasia of cholangioles is present, the cholangioles often containing bile plugs and surrounded by neutrophils *(acute cholangiolitis)*.
- Periductal fibrosis may be seen, but is minimal in the early stages.
- Cholestasis, both intrahepatic and intracanalicular, is most prominent in the perivenular zone, with or without acute and chronic lobular inflammatory infiltrate.
- Microabscesses may form within the portal tracts and parenchyma as a consequence of ascending cholangitis.
- Note: Neutrophilic clusters resembling microabscesses may be seen within the lobules and immediately beneath Glisson's capsule after laparotomy and are secondary to manipulation of the liver (surgical hepatitis; refer to Table 3–193); the adjacent liver cells are usually normal and *not* infiltrated by neutrophils.

Clinical/Laboratory Parameters

- Obstruction of the biliary tract occurs commonly from choledocholithiasis (stones within the common bile duct), and inflammatory or neoplastic diseases of the head of the pancreas.
- Less frequently, gallbladder carcinoma extending along the cystic duct to obstruct the common bile duct, cholangiocarcinoma of the extrahepatic bile ducts, and periampullary tumors need consideration.
- Lymphoma with extrinsic compression of the bile duct from enlarged hilar nodes; metastases from breast, pancreas, lung, and colon; and benign biliary strictures are also possibilities.
- In patients with choledocholithiasis, abdominal pain occurs in about 80% of cases and may be associated with jaundice, fever, pruritus, and leukocytosis (features of acute cholangitis).
- In obstruction by neoplasms, patients present with painless jaundice and pruritus.
- Laboratory tests confirm hyperbilirubinemia, marked elevation in serum alkaline phosphatase activity, modest elevations in serum transaminases (rarely can be as high as 2000 IU/L), and normal or mild decrease in serum albumin.
- A prolonged prothrombin time which completely corrects with vitamin K is useful corroborative evidence for biliary tract obstruction.
- The diagnosis is based on the presence of dilated bile ducts on ultrasound or CT scans.
- Endoscopic retrograde cholangiopancreatography is useful in determining the site of obstruction and provides an opportunity to relieve the obstruction until definitive therapy is offered.

TABLE 3-77

Extrahepatic Biliary Obstruction, Late (Months)[316,317]

Histology

- Prominent bile duct proliferation and ectasia are present, with periductal edema, acute cholangitis, and early periductal fibrosis.
- Portal inflammation is usually mixed, consisting of both lymphocytes and neutrophils.
- Portal fibrosis occurs, the fibrosis tending to be laid down in a parallel fashion in the periportal zones *(biliary fibrosis),* with eventual bridging of portal tracts but sparing of the terminal hepatic venules.
- Lobular cholestasis with mixed acute and chronic inflammatory infiltrates is more prominent, and may extend to the midzone and periportal zone, sometimes with bile plugs in dilated cholangioles. With persistent obstruction, microabscesses may occur.
- *Feathery degeneration* of hepatocytes (swollen, finely reticular pattern, containing intracellular bile) is seen; these foci may become confluent, leading to *lytic necrosis* and *bile infarct* formation (extracellular bile deposition associated with liver cell necrosis and histiocytic response).
- Interlobular ducts and cholangioles may be damaged, with bile leakage and bile accumulation *(bile lakes).*
- Both bile lakes and infarcts tend to be periportal, but may be seen anywhere within the lobule.
- Mallory bodies may rarely be seen in periportal hepatocytes.

Clinical/Laboratory Parameters

- If the biliary obstruction is not relieved, pruritus persists and serum bilirubin levels remain persistently elevated although fluctuations in the levels may provide a confusing picture.
- On physical examination, the liver may be enlarged and firm.
- In distal bile duct obstruction, a distended gallbladder may be palpable.
- Serum alkaline phosphatase activity also remains persistently elevated with mild to moderate increases in serum transaminases.
- Decrease in serum albumin may be noted but prothrombin time may be normal.
- The diagnostic tests and management are the same as for acute obstruction (refer to Table 3-76, Extrahepatic Biliary Obstruction, Early).
- Relief of obstruction leads to improvement and halts the progression of the liver disease.

TABLE 3-78

Extrahepatic Biliary Obstruction, Late (Years)[316-319]

Histology

- Bridging portal-portal and portal-terminal hepatic venular fibrosis occurs leading to a secondary *biliary* cirrhosis, the regenerative nodules exhibiting a jigsaw-type geographic pattern, associated with prominent lamellar fibrosis at the border of the septa and parenchyma.
- Periductal fibrosis and bile duct and cholangiolar proliferation are present, often with bile plugs within the cholangioles.
- Duct loss may be present but is not common, and may only focally involve the portal septa.
- Mild portal lymphocytic infiltration is present.
- Cholestasis may be seen, predominantly periseptal in location.
- Variable acute and chronic lobular inflammation may be present; with persistent obstruction, acute cholangitis with microabscess formation may occur.
- Mallory bodies may be seen in periseptal liver cells, but are infrequent (approximately 2% of cases).
- Increase in copper (rubeanic acid stain) and copper-binding protein (orcein stain) is present in periseptal hepatocytes.

Clinical/Laboratory Parameters

- The patient with long-standing biliary tract obstruction may present with isolated elevation in serum alkaline phosphatase activity, sometimes with associated hyperbilirubinemia, hypoalbuminemia, and prolongation of the prothrombin time.
- Decompensated liver disease with portal hypertension may develop with bleeding esophageal varices and ascites.
- On physical examination the liver may be enlarged; in extreme cases the liver may be small and not palpable.
- Splenomegaly may also be present.
- Relief of obstruction will not lead to reversal of the process at this stage of the disease.

TABLE 3–79
Fabry's Disease (Glycosphingolipidosis) [320–322]

Histology

- Kupffer cells, portal macrophages, and vascular endothelial cells are swollen and contain a finely granular, light tan pigment that is strongly DiPAS-positive.
- These cells also contain birefringent crystals on frozen section examination.

Clinical/Laboratory Parameters

- This X-linked disease caused by alpha-galactosidase deficiency results in the deposition of glycosphingolipids in the endothelium, heart, kidney, eyes (corneal and lenticular opacities), and skin (angiokeratosis).
- Cardiac, cerebral, and renal involvement is common.
- The hepatic vasculature is involved but there is no hepatosplenomegaly.

TABLE 3–80
Familial Hyperlipoproteinemia [323–325]

Histology

- Lipid-laden foamy Kupffer cells and portal macrophages are present.
- Crystalline megamitochondria may be seen (types IV and V).

Clinical/Laboratory Parameters

- Increased secretion and elevated serum levels of various lipoproteins are present, with five patterns recognized.
- Liver function is generally normal.

TABLE 3–81
Farber's Lipogranulomatosis (Ceramidase Deficiency) [326–328]

Histology

- Granulomas composed of lymphocytes, histiocytes, and PAS-positive foam cells develop.
- Associated granulomatous necrosis and reactive fibrosis occur in older lesions.

Clinical/Laboratory Parameters

- This genetically determined disorder of lipid metabolism is due to a deficiency of lysosomal acid ceramidase with accumulation of gangliosides within the lungs, heart, lymph nodes, and liver.
- The disease is characterized by subcutaneous nodules, painful deformed joints, hoarseness from laryngeal involvement, and corneal opacities.
- In the neonatal type, hepatosplenomegaly is common.
- Death occurs in the more severely affected within a few years, with no therapy available.

TABLE 3–82

Fascioliasis (Fasciola hepatica)[143,230,329–331]

Histology

- Yellow surface nodules are present ranging from 5 to 20 mm in diameter.
- A track containing the organisms with surrounding eosinophils and variable tissue necrosis is present, eventually leading to subcapsular scar formation.
- Segmental duct dilatation with a centrally located worm is present, associated with duct erosion and prominent reactive adenomatous duct hyperplasia.
- Large necrotic granulomas can develop around trapped eggs.
- Acute cholangitis may also occur, with eosinophils prominent.
- Portal fibrosis occurs without progression to cirrhosis.

Clinical/Laboratory Parameters

- The life cycle of this trematode is similar to that of *Clonorchis sinensis* (refer to Table 3–55, Clonorchiasis) except that the cercaria released from the snail (intermediate host) attaches to aquatic plants (like watercress), with infection of humans occurring by drinking contaminated water or ingesting these plants.
- The metacercariae released in the duodenum migrate to the biliary ducts and produce inflammation and obstruction of the biliary radicles, presenting as biliary colic, hepatomegaly with acute cholangitis, formation of strictures and pigmented stones, and abscesses.
- During attacks of acute cholangitis, the presence of eosinophilia should raise this diagnostic possibility in endemic areas.
- Diagnosis is made by demonstrating the characteristic biliary tract abnormalities on scanning modalities or at cholangiography.

TABLE 3–83

Fibrinogen Storage Disease (Afibrinogenemia and Hypo[dys]fibrinogenemia)[332–335]

Histology

- Round to oval, globular, eosinophilic cytoplasmic inclusions representing fibrinogen are present in hepatocytes; these inclusions are sometimes vacuolated, strongly phosphotungstic acid–hematoxylin (PTAH)-positive, and weakly PAS-positive to PAS-negative.
- Perivenular intracytoplasmic globular inclusions within liver cells are also seen representing C3 and C4 complement components.
- Cirrhosis has been described.

Clinical/Laboratory Parameters

- This is a rare autosomal recessive disease characterized by complete (afibrinogen) to reduced (hypofibrinogen) levels of fibrinogen.
- Dysfibrinogenemia can also occur, where there are functionally abnormal fibrinogen molecules caused by mutations that usually result in amino acid cleavage.
- Patients present with bleeding problems (e.g., epistaxis, menorrhagia, recurrent abortions, intracranial hemorrhage) and thromboembolic events.

TABLE 3–84

Focal Fatty Change[336–340]

Histology

- Single or multiple tumor-like masses distinctly visualized on imaging are entirely composed of liver cells with abundant macrovesicular fat, but without architectural disruption (the portal tract–terminal hepatic venule–portal tract relationship is maintained).

Clinical/Laboratory Parameters

- This lesion is usually seen in asymptomatic individuals and is detected incidentally by ultrasound or CT scan.
- No abnormalities of liver tests are present.
- Physical examination is usually normal although some patients may be overweight; however, the lesions may not disappear with weight loss.

TABLE 3-85

Focal Nodular Hyperplasia[41,44,47-49,341-345]

Histology

- The tumor is usually yellow-brown to white, solitary, well circumscribed, bulging on cut section and less than 5 cm in diameter; however, the lesions may occasionally be larger (up to 15 cm in diameter) and pedunculated or multiple.
- A characteristic central radiating stellate fibrous septa that subdivides the lesion into multiple segments is present.
- The radiating scars exhibit lymphocytic infiltration, numerous small vessels, and occasional arterioles.
- Proliferating ductules (metaplastic liver cells) with no distinct lumen having a serpentine growth pattern and located at the border of the fibrous septa and parenchyma are present.
- Larger vessels within the fibrous band may show irregular fibrointimal thickening.
- Adjacent cytologically benign hepatocytes are present forming cords no greater than two cells thick.
- Both endothelial and Kupffer cells are present lining the sinusoids.
- The hepatocytes within the tumor may contain glycogen, bile, macrovesicular fat, lipochrome, and rarely Mallory bodies; copper and copper-binding protein has also been reported.
- Rupture with hemorrhage can occur, but is not frequent.
- Calcifications may be present but are uncommon.

Clinical/Laboratory Parameters

- This lesion is not a true neoplasm, but rather a reactive hyperplastic process secondary to vascular insult, liver cell ischemia, and adjacent regenerating hepatocytes.
- Most patients are women, and present usually in the 3rd through 5th decades; however, the age ranges from 14 to 74 years.
- The lesion is usually found incidentally at surgery, with only one third of patients presenting with abdominal pain and a palpable mass.
- Liver tests including alpha-fetoprotein are normal.
- The uptake of technetium in the technetium-99m sulfur colloid scan helps to distinguish this lesion from hepatic adenomas.
- Angiography shows centrifugal blood flow, and hypervascularity with dense capillary blushing.
- Bleeding is extremely rare, and malignant transformation has not been reported.
- Resection is not necessary and management is conservative.

TABLE 3-86

Galactosemia[346-350]

Histology

- Histologic changes are seen in two stages:
  - By 10 days: Macrovesicular and microvesicular fatty change is present, with marked cholangiolar proliferation often containing bile plugs and surrounded by neutrophils.
  - At 2 to 6 weeks: Pseudoacinar changes surround dilated canaliculi, often containing bile or eosinophilic material.
- Extramedullary hematopoiesis and hemosiderosis of hepatocytes may be seen.
- Syncytial giant cell transformation of liver cells may be present.
- Fibrosis leads to micronodular cirrhosis by 3 to 6 months; macroregenerative nodules (1.0-2.9 cm in diameter) may also occur.
- Increase in copper-binding protein in hepatocytes has been described.

Clinical/Laboratory Parameters

- A deficiency of galactose-1-phosphate uridyltransferase results in the abnormal accumulation of galactose in the liver and lens.
- The disease severity varies from mild to fulminant with onset occurring at first ingestion of milk by the infant.
- Failure to thrive, anorexia, vomiting, diarrhea, hypoglycemia, hepatomegaly, cataracts, and jaundice are frequently present; ascites is seen in severe cases.
- Other abnormalities include hyperchloremic acidosis, albuminuria, aminoaciduria from renal tubular defects, hyperbilirubinemia, and hypoalbuminemia.
- Diagnosis is confirmed by galactosuria.

TABLE 3–87

Gangliosidosis,[351–354] GM$_1$: Infantile Form (Type I), Juvenile Form (Type II); GM$_2$: Tay-Sachs Disease, Sandhoff's Disease

Histology

- Lipid-laden finely vacuolated Kupffer cells and portal macrophages are present in GM$_1$, type I, while lipid-laden, foamy, pale-staining intensely diPAS-positive Kupffer cells and portal macrophages are seen in GM$_1$, type II.
- GM$_2$ shows no changes on hematoxylin-eosin stain on light microscopy, but Sandhoff's disease shows PAS-positive, Luxol–fast blue-positive granules in Kupffer cells, with periportal fibrosis also reported.
- Both GM$_1$ and GM$_2$ show characteristic cytoplasmic bodies on electron microscopy.

Clinical/Laboratory Parameters

- An autosomal recessive disease caused by deficiency of beta-galactosidase leads to the accumulation of galactosyl oligosaccharides and keratan sulfate degradation products in the brain and other organs.
- In the infantile form, hepatosplenomegaly is present in addition to involvement of the musculoskeletal and central nervous systems.
- In the juvenile and adult forms, hepatosplenomegaly is not present.

TABLE 3–88

Gaucher's Disease (Glucocerebrosidase Deficiency)[355–359]

Histology

- Kupffer cells and portal macrophages are large (up to 100 μm in diameter) and contain striated, wrinkled cytoplasm, best seen on Masson and PAS stains.
- The distribution of these cells is focal or zonal (zone 3 predominantly); in the cirrhotic liver these cells may be periseptal.
- Sinusoidal collagen deposition may be seen.
- Calcifications may be seen but are rare.
- Iron has been described in hypertrophic Kupffer cells.
- Fibrosis and micronodular cirrhosis may develop in some cases.

Clinical/Laboratory Parameters

- There is an accumulation of cerebrosides, specifically glucosylceramide, in the lysosomes of the reticuloendothelial cells due to a deficiency of glucocerebrosidase.
- The disease manifests in infancy with hepatosplenomegaly and progressive neurologic deterioration.
- In adults, massive hepatosplenomegaly, portal hypertension, thrombocytopenia, skeletal fractures, and coagulation disorders occur.
- Infusions of glucocerebrosidase has prevented progression and, in some cases, caused amelioration of the disease.

TABLE 3–89

Gilbert's Syndrome[243,360–362]

Histology

- Increase in lipochrome pigment is present in perivenular hepatocytes (inconstant finding).
- Portal and lobular inflammation are usually absent.

Clinical/Laboratory Parameters

- Gilbert's syndrome is characterized by mild indirect hyperbilirubinemia in the absence of bilirubinuria, with normal serum transaminases, and normal hepatic synthetic function, with no evidence of liver disease.
- The abnormality is caused by a 30% reduction of hepatic bilirubin UDP glucuronyltransferase activity.
- Fasting and nicotinic acid increase the indirect hyperbilirubinemia by different mechanisms.

TABLE 3-90
Glycogen Storage Diseases[51,52,363-370]

Histology

- Grossly the liver is enlarged and pale; depending on the subtype, the capsule ranges from smooth to nodular.
- Most cases show hydropic vacuolated liver cells, centrally located nuclei, and cytoplasm containing excess glycogen.
- Histologic changes characteristic of certain subtypes include:
  - I, II, VI: Prominent neutral fat.
  - IX, X: Thin fibrous septa without cirrhosis.
  - III, IV, VI: Fibrosis and cirrhosis.
  - Ia: Liver cell adenoma (multifocal), hepatocellular carcinoma, Mallory bodies, peliosis.
  - I, III, VI: Glycogenated nuclei.
  - IV: Eosinophilic cytoplasmic DiPAS-positive inclusions, predominantly in the periportal zone, representing amylopectin-like material.
- Note that types V and VII do *not* involve the liver.

Clinical/Laboratory Parameters

- Approximately 10 types are known, some of which are listed below:
  - I: Glucose-6-phosphatase deficiency, with stunted growth, recurrent infections, xanthomas, nephropathy.
  - II: Lysosomal alpha-1,4-glucosidase deficiency, with muscular hypotonia, renal failure, and death within the first year.
  - III: Amylo-1,6-glucosidase deficiency, with growth retardation, infections, and consequences of portal hypertension.
  - IV: Alpha-1,4-glucan-6-glycosyltransferase deficiency, with gastroenteritis, osteoporosis, failure to thrive, death from cirrhosis and cardiac failure.
  - VI: Hepatic phosphorylase deficiency, with growth retardation and consequences of portal hypertension.
  - VIII: Phosphorylase kinase deficiency, with hepatomegaly and progressive neurologic deterioration.
  - IX: Phosphorylase kinase deficiency, with hepatomegaly.
  - X: Cyclic adenosine monophosphate–dependent kinase deficiency with hepatomegaly.

TABLE 3-91
Graft-Versus-Host Disease[84,371-375]

Histology

- Prominent portal lymphocytic infiltration is present; although this inflammatory infiltrate is usually confined to the portal tracts, some degree of spillover of these inflammatory cells into the adjacent periportal zones may be seen.
- Nonsuppurative destructive cholangitis is present, the inflammatory cells chiefly lymphocytes, with variable cytologic atypia of duct epithelium.
- Eventual biliary fibrosis occurs with ductopenia.
- Endothelialitis may be seen involving portal and terminal hepatic veins.
- Cholestasis may be present with variable lobular chronic inflammatory infiltration.
- Veno-occlusive changes with fibrous obliteration of the terminal hepatic venules has been described.
- Occasionally bridging fibrosis leading to biliary cirrhosis may be present.

Clinical/Laboratory Parameters

- Graft-versus-host disease is usually seen in the setting of bone marrow transplantation (BMT), although other grafts may also initiate the process.
- Skin and intestinal involvement predominate, with the clinical manifestations staged as follows:
  - Stage I: Maculopapular rash involving less than 25% of the body, with a serum bilirubin level of 2 to 3 mg/dl.
  - Stage II: Rash involving 25 to 50% of body surface with a bilirubin level of 3 to 6 mg/dl.
  - Stage III: Generalized erythroderma, with a bilirubin level of 6 to 15 mg/dl.
  - Stage IV: Desquamation and bullae, with a bilirubin level greater than 15 mg/dl.
- Diarrhea of increasing severity is seen in all stages, and in severe cases may be due to protein-losing enteropathy.
- Patients may present with hepatomegaly, elevation in serum alkaline phosphatase activity, and serum transaminases elevated 5- to 10-fold.
- The disease course is variable, occurring usually in the second week following BMT and rarely after 6 months or a year.
- Death in unrecognized or severe disease occurs from sepsis and multiorgan failure; however, death from liver failure is uncommon.

TABLE 3-92

Group B Coxsackievirus Infection[376]

Histology

- A mixed portal and sinusoidal inflammatory infiltrate is present consisting of both mononuclear cells and neutrophils.
- Perivenular cholestasis and hydropic change of hepatocytes may be present.

Clinical/Laboratory Parameters

- A member of the enteroviruses, group B coxsackievirus may be associated with respiratory tract infection, myocarditis, pericarditis, aseptic meningitis, pleurodynia, and vesicular and papular rashes, and in epidemic situations can cause hepatitis.
- The mild to modest increase in serum transminases associated sometimes with hepatomegaly and with common manifestations of the disease suggests the diagnosis.
- Positive specific antibodies to coxsackie B virus are helpful in confirming the diagnosis.

TABLE 3-93

Heart Failure, Left-sided with Hypotension (Acute Circulatory Failure, Shock)[377–381]

Histology

- Coagulative (ischemic) liver cell necrosis is seen in the perivenular zone, with eventual dropout of hepatocytes and perivenular collapse; in more severe cases, the necrosis may extend into the midzonal regions.
- Neutrophils may be present at the border of liver cell necrosis and viable hepatocytes.
- Cholestasis may be present in severe cases.
- Both extracellular (sinusoidal) and intracytoplasmic eosinophilic hyaline globules up to 4 μm in diameter may be seen in the perivenular zone.
- Calcifications may occur within areas of necrosis.

Clinical/Laboratory Parameters

- Patients with circulatory failure due to an acute, low left-ventricular output state with severe hypotension (as in massive bleeding or during surgery [especially in older patients]) present with marked increases in serum transaminases (several thousands), prolongation of the prothrombin time, and mild increases in alkaline phophatase activity and serum bilirubin (1–3 mg/dl) with mild hypoalbuminemia.
- The rapidity of the improvement in liver tests is dependent on the left ventricular output state and extent of permanent left ventricular dysfunction.
- Improvement can be seen within 24 to 48 hours.
- Liver failure is seen only in patients with severe, persistent left ventricular failure.

TABLE 3-94

Heart Failure, Left-sided Without Hypotension[382,383]

Histology

- Red blood cells may be seen beneath the space of Disse and within the hepatic cords, replacing liver cells that had undergone ischemic necrosis (refer to Table 2–32, Sinusoids: Red Blood Cell Extravasation).
- The perivenular sinusoids are open *without* perivenular collapse (as opposed to left-sided failure with hypotension, in which collapse is often present).
- Cholestasis may be present in severe cases.

Clinical/Laboratory Parameters

- The cardiac findings predominate but nausea, dyspepsia, elevations in serum transaminases (100–300 IU/L), mild hyperbilirubinemia, hypoalbuminemia, and modest elevations in the serum alkaline phosphatase activity are present.
- Sometimes the liver test abnormalities may be more prominent and mimic acute viral hepatitis.
- Rapid improvement in liver tests occurs with successful treatment of the cardiac disorder.

TABLE 3–95

Heart Failure, Right-sided[377–380]

Histology

Acute

- Sinusoidal congestion and dilatation are present in the perivenular zone.
- Acute hemorrhage may also be seen associated with ischemic necrosis of perivenular hepatocytes in severe cases.
- Cholestasis may also be present in severe cases.
- Both extracellular (sinusoidal) and intracytoplasmic eosinophilic hyaline globules up to 4 μm in diameter may be seen in the perivenular zone.

Chronic

- Sinusoidal dilatation is present with adjacent liver cell atrophy, sinusoidal fibrosis, and variable occlusion of the terminal hepatic venules.
- Bridging fibrosis of terminal hepatic venules leads to a *cardiac cirrhosis* (reverse lobulation with portal tract sparing).
- Eventually bridging fibrosis occurs between terminal hepatic venules and portal tracts, leading to a micronodular cirrhosis.

Clinical/Laboratory Parameters

- The hepatic dysfunction in right-sided heart failure is overshadowed by the findings of elevated jugular venous pressure, a pulsatile and sometimes enlarged liver, peripheral edema, ascites in severe or chronic cases, and the findings on physical examination and echocardiography of cardiomegaly, pulmonary hypertension, and tricuspid regurgitation.
- Infrequently, constrictive pericarditis may be the cause of the ascites.
- In the *acute* presentation, elevations of serum bilirubin, mostly indirect; mild to moderate increases in serum transaminases and alkaline phosphatase activity; and hypoalbuminemia are noted.
- Analysis of ascites reveals high total protein and high serum : ascites albumin gradient.
- Liver test abnormalities resolve quickly if treatment of cardiac failure is effective.
- In the *chronic* stage, manifestations of portal hypertension may occur.

TABLE 3–96

Heat Stroke[384–387]

Histology

- Variable degrees of microvesicular fatty change may be seen.
- Coagulative-type (ischemic) necrosis of perivenular hepatocytes may often occur.
- Cholestasis may be present.
- Proliferation of cholangioles may be seen, with acute cholangitis less frequent.

Clinical/Laboratory Parameters

- Exertional heat stroke may be associated with marked elevations of the serum aminotransferases, sometimes with associated hyperbilirubinemia.
- Complications include shock, sepsis, and coagulopathy.
- The outcome is dependent on the degree of liver cell necrosis, with transplantation sometimes warranted.

TABLE 3–97

Hemochromatosis[388–396]

Histology

- Hemosiderin (golden-brown pigment) accumulates first in periportal hepatocytes, eventually diffusely involving all hepatocytes, the cytoplasmic pigment often accentuated surrounding the biliary canaliculi.
- Although occasionally Kupffer cells and portal macrophages may contain hemosiderin, this feature is not common, and when present it is usually secondary to superimposed necroinflammatory change from other causes (e.g., acute viral hepatitis).
- Hemosiderin in bile duct epithelium is frequent and usually prominent; hemosiderin may occasionally be seen within endothelial cells.
- Variable macrovesicular fatty change is seen, with occasional glycogenated nuclei in instances in which diabetes is also present (secondary to hemosiderin deposition within the pancreas).
- Eventual fibrosis leads to a micronodular cirrhosis.
- In cirrhosis, the center of the nodules may have less pigment than the periseptal regions when regenerative activity is prominent.
- There is a high incidence of hepatocellular carcinoma in cirrhotic livers (200 times the general population).

Clinical/Laboratory Parameters

- Hemochromatosis is an HLA-linked autosomal recessive disorder with increased iron absorption from the intestine resulting in excessive deposition of iron in the liver and multiple organ systems.
- The gene responsible for the disease is present on the short arm of chromosome 6, and its frequency is 1 in 300 to 400.
- The disorder presents clinically between 40 and 60 years of age in men; women develop the disease less commonly, and clinically present at an older age (in part secondary to menstruation, pregnancy, and lactation).
- Diabetes, chondrocalcinosis and degenerative arthritis, hypogonadism, and pigmented skin are complications.
- Patients may be asymptomatic or present with abnormal liver tests, hepatosplenomegaly, and bleeding esophageal varices.
- The diagnosis is made by elevated iron saturation ($>55\%$) and a hepatic iron index of greater than 1.9 (calculated from quantitative hepatic iron measurements in micromoles divided by the patient's age).
- Frequent phlebotomy is effective in removing body iron and ameliorating liver disease if diagnosed early.
- The risk of developing hepatocellular carcinoma is *not* decreased if phlebotomy is offered after cirrhosis is well established.

TABLE 3–98

Hemochromatosis, Neonatal Variant[397–400]

Histology

- Hemosiderin (golden-brown pigment) accumulates first in periportal hepatocytes, eventually diffusely involving all hepatocytes, the cytoplasmic pigment often accentuated surrounding the biliary canaliculi.
- Although occasionally Kupffer cells and portal macrophages may contain hemosiderin, this feature is not common, and when present it is usually secondary to superimposed necroinflammatory change from other causes (e.g., acute viral hepatitis).
- Hemosiderin in bile duct epithelium is frequent and usually prominent; hemosiderin may occasionally be seen within endothelial cells.
- Histologic features of neonatal hepatitis are also present, with syncytial giant cell transformation, variable fibrosis, and often extensive lobular collapse.

Clinical/Laboratory Parameters

- This perinatal recessively inherited disorder is uncommon, is usually rapidly fatal, and often occurs in siblings.
- The infants may be born prematurely, with complications of pregnancy including intrauterine growth retardation.
- Infants may present with ascites, jaundice, and bleeding abnormalities.
- Low serum transferrin levels, hyperbilirubinemia, and elevated alkaline phosphatase activity are usually present.
- The iron stores are similar to that seen in hemochromatosis (refer to Table 3–97).
- Chelation and antioxidant therapy may have some benefit.
- Liver transplantation may be considered.

TABLE 3-99

Hemolysis, Elevated Liver Enzymes, Low Platelet (HELLP) Syndrome[22,29,401-407]

Histology

- Periportal and/or focal lobular necrosis with fibrin deposition may occur (similar to that seen in toxemia).
- Intrahepatic and subcapsular hemorrhage with rupture may also occur.
- Portal lymphocytic infiltration, mild lobular inflammation, and macrovesicular fatty change are present.

Clinical/Laboratory Parameters

- The HELLP syndrome is seen in patients with pregnancy-induced hypertension and is characterized by hemolysis, moderate elevations in serum transminases, thrombocytopenia, and preservation of hepatic synthetic function.
- Recovery is the rule following termination of pregnancy.
- The etiology is not clear, although a microangiopathic process may be involved.

TABLE 3-100

Hemosiderosis (Secondary Iron Overload)[394,408-413]

Histology

- Hemosiderin deposition occurs in hepatocytes, but the amount of pigment is not as prominent as in primary hemochromatosis.
- When hemosiderin deposition is transfusion related or secondary to chronic hemolysis, prominent uptake within the reticuloendothelial system (Kupffer cells, portal macrophages) is present.
- Bile duct epithelium only rarely contains hemosiderin, and when present is only scanty.
- In instances in which there are numerous transfusions (e.g., patients with beta-thalassemia) the total amount of iron in the liver may be striking.
- In some instances, cirrhosis may occur when associated with prominent increase in dietary iron uptake *(Bantu siderosis)*, with the iron seen predominantly within Kupffer cells and portal macrophages.

Clinical/Laboratory Parameters

- Hemosiderosis develops in patients who receive frequent blood transfusions for chronic anemia caused by thalassemia major, sideroblastic anemia, hemolytic disorders such as sickle cell anemia, and with excessive oral iron therapy.
- Patients may present with elevated serum transaminases, elevations in serum iron, and increases in serum iron saturation and ferritin levels.
- Cirrhosis and portal hypertension leading to liver failure are not usually encountered in these patients.
- Since phlebotomy cannot be offered because of the underlying hematologic disorder, chelation therapy with desferrioxamine is recommended.

TABLE 3-101

Hepatoblastoma[41,414-424]

Histology

- Usually a single mass, the tumor may be quite large (up to 25 cm in greatest dimension, and weigh up to 1000 grams), and may be brown-green and cystic.
- Histologically two subgroups are present: *epithelial* (67% of cases) or *mixed epithelial–mesenchymal* (33% of cases).
- The *epithelial* component consists of three variants:
  1. *Fetal*
     - Polygonal small cells are present with round to oval nuclei, prominent single nucleoli, and granular to clear cytoplasm.
     - The cells are arranged into irregular cords and sinusoids, with bile canaliculi occasionally containing bile.
     - Extramedullary hematopoiesis is common.
  2. *Embryonal*
     - Small, round to elongated, and fusiform cells that have hyperchromatic nuclei and little cytoplasm are present, these cells arranged in rosettes, cords, and ribbons; the cells may have a clear cytoplasm or may contain glycogen or fat.
  3. *Anaplastic small cell*
     - Sheets of small, primitive, loosely cohesive cells are present.
- The *mesenchymal* component consists of immature mesenchymal elements composed of cellular spindle cells, and may contain osteoid, chondroid, collagen, microcalcifications, and undifferentiated cells, rarely cartilage, striated muscle, neural tissue (*teratoid* type), and melanin.
- Invasion into the hepatic and portal veins with thrombosis may occur.
- Increase in copper-binding protein has been described.
- Helpful immunoperoxidase markers for diagnosis are the following: alpha-fetoprotein, human chorionic gonadotropin, carcinoembryonic antigen, epithelial membrane antigen, alpha$_1$-antitrypsin, ferritin, S100, chromogranin A, neurone-specific enolase.

Clinical/Laboratory Parameters

- Hepatoblastoma is the most common hepatic neoplasm in children, responsible for approximately 40% of all tumors in pediatric patients up to 2 years of age.
- The onset ranges from time of birth to 48 months.
- Hepatomegaly, failure to thrive, intermittent vomiting, and diarrhea are common.
- Slightly abnormal serum transaminases and hyperbilirubinemia may be present in the minority of cases.
- Alpha-fetoprotein (AFP) is elevated in up to 90% of patients. It should be noted that the AFP is normally elevated at birth (10–14 μg/ml) but rapidly decreases to normal values (5–10 ng/ml) by 1 year of age; the AFP in neonates with hepatoblastoma is disproportionately high.
- Other associated conditions include osteopenia, hemihypertrophy, macroglossia, sexual precocity secondary to ectopic gonadotropin levels, and cardiac and renal malformations.
- The tumor shows calcifications on imaging in approximately 50% of cases.
- Angiography usually exhibits hypervascularity.
- Characteristic features are seen on magnetic resonance imaging (MRI) and can often distinguish between the different types of hepatic neoplasms seen in the pediatric age group.
- Surgical resection is indicated for smaller isolated tumors, for which survival is excellent after tumor removal.
- Transplantation can also be offered in some patients when the lesions are larger and there is no evidence of metastasis.

TABLE 3–102

Hepatocellular Carcinoma, Fibrolamellar Type[41,425–431]

Histology

- This neoplasm is usually solitary, well demarcated, often large, most often involves the left lobe, and characteristically arises in noncirrhotic livers.
- A lobular arrangement with central fibrous septa may be present.
- Histologically the tumor cells are large, polygonal, and eosinophilic, with round nuclei and prominent nucleoli.
- Abundant hypocellular fibrous stroma arranged in parallel fashion is present around nests, cords, and sheets of tumor cells.
- Endothelial lining cells can be visualized, but definite cords and sinusoids are usually not apparent.
- Cytoplasmic DiPAS-positive globules are often seen.
- Characteristic *pale bodies* (lightly eosinophilic cytoplasmic inclusions) are present in approximately one half of the cases.
- The tumor cells may contain bile, copper, and copper-binding protein; peliotic lesions may also be seen.
- Invasion into the hepatic and portal veins with thrombosis may occur, but not as frequently as in typical hepatocellular carcinoma.
- Mallory bodies, epithelioid granulomas, and calcifications have been described.
- *Mixed* forms of typical trabecular and fibrolamellar hepatocellular carcinoma may also be seen within the same mass lesion.

Clinical/Laboratory Parameters

- This tumor is uncommon in the middle-aged to elderly population, but is responsible for 14 to 40% of all hepatic neoplasms in patients under the age of 35.
- There is an equal sex distribution.
- There is no known association with viral hepatitis.
- Clinically patients present with abdominal pain, malaise, and hepatomegaly; an abdominal mass is often appreciated.
- Slight elevations of the serum transaminases and alkaline phosphatase activity are present.
- The alpha-fetoprotein is seldom elevated.
- A high serum unsaturated vitamin B_{12} binding capacity may be identified.
- Calcifications may be seen on imaging.
- The tumor is generally slow growing, with surgical resection often curative.
- Surgical resection of extrahepatic sites and tumor recurrence may be helpful in some patients.
- Liver transplantation including block resections of adjacent nodes (when positive) can be beneficial.

TABLE 3-103

Hepatocellular Carcinoma, Trabecular, Acinar, Ductular Type[41,52,414,417,419,430-442]

Histology

- This neoplasm may be soft, hemorrhagic, and bile stained and may form variably sized masses (solitary or multinodular, diffuse, rarely pedunculated or encapsulated), with direct involvement of the portal (34% of cases) and/or hepatic (22% of cases) veins.
- Microscopically the hepatic cords are greater than or equal to 3 cells thick, lined by endothelial cells, without fibrous stroma (when ≥ 10 cells thick, the cords are termed *macrotrabecular*).
- Ductular, acinar patterns may be seen secondary to marked dilatation of canaliculi, which may contain bile (5–10% of cases).
- Duct-like spaces secondary to central necrosis with eventual central clearing may also occur, the space then containing eosinophilic proteinaceous material (fibrin).
- Papillary-type projections may be seen.
- Solid growth patterns may be present; in addition, abundant fibrous stroma may at times be present.
- Less commonly, clear cells, spindle cells, and pleomorphic mononuclear and multinucleated giant cells may be present.
- Cytologic features include a polygonal, round to oval nucleus and prominent nucleolus, with an increase in the nuclear-cytoplasmic ratio.
- The cytoplasm of tumor cells may be finely granular eosinophilic to hydropic; bile canaliculi sometimes containing bile plugs may be seen, as may intracellular components such as fat, glycogen, Mallory bodies, DiPAS-positive cytoplasmic inclusions, "ground glass"–like cytoplasmic inclusions, and glycogen nuclei.
- Highly vascularized tumors may have a *pelioid*-type pattern.
- Tumor growth into nontumor liver is via the trabeculae, not sinusoids; invasion into the hepatic and portal veins with thrombosis is common.
- Cirrhosis is present in anywhere from 60 to 90% of cases.
- Extramedullary hematopoiesis and microcalcifications may also be seen.
- Helpful immunoperoxidase markers for diagnosis include alpha-fetoprotein, polyclonal carcinoembryonic antigen (bile canaliculi), cytokeratins (CAM 5.2), alpha$_1$-antitrypsin, ferritin, albumin, and chymotrypsin.

Clinical/Laboratory Parameters

- This tumor is the most common hepatic neoplasm in adults worldwide and accounts for almost three fourths of cases of solid hepatic tumors.
- The incidence is most frequent in sub-Saharan Africa and Southeast Asia.
- The tumor is seen most frequently in men in the 3rd through 5th decades.
- Predisposing conditions include chronic viral hepatitis (HBV and HCV), aflatoxin exposure, alcoholic cirrhosis, and hemochromatosis.
- These tumors may be detected incidentally during surveillance or may present with overt manifestations including massive hepatomegaly and evidence of metastases.
- Paraneoplastic syndromes such as erythrocytosis, hypercalcemia, and hypoglycemia can occur.
- Patients may also present with decompensation of the underlying liver disease with ascites, variceal hemorrhage, and liver failure.
- Liver test abnormalities suggest hepatic decompensation with hypoalbuminemia, hyperbilirubinemia, prolongation of the prothrombin time, and mild to modest elevations in alkaline phosphatase activity and serum transaminases.
- Serum AFP values greater than 400 ng/ml are seen in up to 85% of patients with hepatitis B–related liver disease and in 60% of patients with alcoholic cirrhosis; the AFP is also elevated in cirrhosis secondary to chronic HCV.
- These tumors can be detected by ultrasound or CT scan (double spiral); gallium uptake by the tumor is seen in about 85% of cases.
- Although hepatocellular carcinoma generally has a bleak prognosis, smaller localized lesions have surgery as an option; large tumor size (>5 cm), multiple tumor nodules, and invasion of the major portal veins are features of poor prognosis.

TABLE 3–104

Hereditary Fructose Intolerance[448–453]

Histology

- Changes of neonatal hepatitis (refer to Table 3–155) with giant cell transformation are present, with duct reduplication and ducts containing inspissated bile described.
- Predominantly macrovesicular with some degree of microvesicular fatty change is often seen.
- Sinusoidal and portal fibrosis may occur leading to cirrhosis.
- Increase in copper-binding protein has been described.

Clinical/Laboratory Parameters

- The clinical and biochemical abnormalities in this disease arise from a deficiency of fructose-1-phosphate aldolase, which catalyzes the conversion of fructose-1-phosphate to D-glyceraldehyde, with resultant accumulation of fructose-1-phosphate in the liver.
- Infants develop vomiting, anorexia, diarrhea, failure to thrive, and aversion to sweet foods.
- Hepatomegaly, modest elevations of serum transaminases, prolonged prothrombin time, and jaundice are present in untreated cases.
- Avoidance of fructose-containing foods ameliorates the disease, although once significant fibrosis is present, progression can be expected leading to liver failure.

TABLE 3–105

Hereditary Hemorrhagic Telangiectasis (Osler-Rendu-Weber Disease)[443–447]

Histology

- Biopsy demonstrates a honeycomb meshwork of dilated sinusoids or tortuous thick-walled veins and adjacent arteries within the lobules intermixed within a fibrous stroma.
- Numerous dilated vessels (veins, arteries, lymphatics) within a fibrous stroma may also be present.
- Variable degrees of portal fibrosis may be present.
- Cirrhosis may occur but is uncommon.

Clinical/Laboratory Parameters

- Mucocutaneous telangiectasias are typical with episodic bleeding starting at the second decade.
- Epistaxis is common.
- Portal hypertension may occur, but liver failure is rare.

TABLE 3–106

Herpes Simplex Virus Infection[454–459]

Histology

- Herpes simplex virus (HSV) infection is usually disseminated in immunocompromised patients with irregular, often confluent, coagulative-type necrosis without associated inflammatory exudate.
- Acute hemorrhage may be seen in necrotic areas.
- Two types of intranuclear inclusions are seen in hepatocytes located at the border of viable and necrotic regions:
  - Large eosinophilic inclusions with a peripheral halo *(Cowdry type A)*.
  - Basophilic inclusions taking up the entire nuclear volume, with a peripheral rim of chromatin *(Cowdry type B)*.
- Cells containing the viral inclusions may be multinucleated.
- In the neonate, giant cell transformation of hepatocytes is often seen.

Clinical/Laboratory Parameters

- About 80% of adults have previously been infected with this DNA virus, which can primarily clinically affect the neonate or reactivate in immunocompromised individuals.
- This primarily systemic infection (HSV type 1 in adults and HSV type 2 in neonates) is characterized by mucocutaneous vesiculation (which also recurs in reactivation), ulcerative gingivostomatitis, esophagitis, keratoconjunctivitis, encephalitis, hepatomegaly, and hepatitis.
- Serum transaminases are modestly elevated, hyperbilirubinemia is rare, and elevated alkaline phosphatase activity may be present.
- In immunosuppressed patients, particularly following transplantation, mucocutaneous lesions predominate with mild hepatic involvement.
- The diagnosis is usually made clinically in the immunosuppressed patient and can be confirmed by neutralizing and complement fixing antibodies.

TABLE 3-107

Herpes Zoster Virus Infection[460-461]

Histology

- Focal or confluent coagulative-type necrosis without inflammation is present (similar to that seen with herpes simplex infection).
- Variable numbers of intranuclear inclusions within hepatocytes are identified.

Clinical/Laboratory Parameters

- The predominant manifestations are the vesicular skin lesions associated with pain and neuralgia.
- Liver disease is restricted to those who are immunocompromised, in whom liver involvement may be severe.

TABLE 3-108

Histoplasmosis *(Histoplasma capsulatum)*[143,174,176,462-464]

Histology

- Epithelioid granulomas containing intracytoplasmic encapsulated yeast forms 2 to 5 μm in diameter with a retracted clear space *(halo)* are present within Kupffer cells and portal macrophages.
- Larger granulomas (1–3 mm in diameter) have been described having central necrosis; on resolution, fibrosis with scar occurs with microcalcification and ossification.

Clinical/Laboratory Parameters

- This organism, prevalent in the east central plains of the United States, is present in the soil in a mycelial state.
- Infection of humans occurs by inhalation of spores causing primarily a pulmonary infection.
- Hepatic involvement is seen in disseminated infection, which usually occurs in the immunosuppressed patient who presents with fever and hepatosplenomegaly.
- Elevated serum alkaline phosphatase activity and mild increases in serum transaminases and bilirubin may be seen.

TABLE 3-109

Homocystinuria (Cystathionine Beta-Synthase Deficiency)[465-468]

Histology

- Fatty change is present that is most accentuated in the perivenular zone.
- Mild to moderate portal fibrosis occurs without progression to cirrhosis.

Clinical/Laboratory Parameters

- This autosomal recessive disease is due to cystathionine beta-synthase deficiency leading to the accumulation of homocystine, methionine, and other related metabolites.
- Patients present with mental retardation, seizures, and involvement of the vascular and skeletal systems, eye (dislocation of the lens), liver, hair, and skin.
- Hepatomegaly is present and thromboembolic events are common.

TABLE 3–110

Human Immunodeficiency Virus–associated Cholangiopathy[143,478,479]

Histology

- Interlobular bile ducts show cytologic atypia, occasionally with plasma cells within the portal tracts.
- Cytomegalovirus inclusions may be seen on multiple levels involving duct epithelium, but they may also be identified in hepatocytes, Kupffer cells, and endothelial cells.
- Both cryptosporidiosis (refer to Table 3–61) and microsporidiosis (refer to Table 3–148) may also involve the larger intrahepatic duct segments.
- Both bile duct depletion and changes of sclerosing cholangitis can be seen.

Clinical/Laboratory Parameters

- This entity is seen in patients with AIDS, with a frequency as high as 15% in advanced disease.
- Patients may be asymptomatic or may present with abdominal pain and jaundice similar to sclerosing cholangitis.
- Elevation in serum alkaline phosphatase is always present; serum bilirubin and transaminases are usually normal or mildly elevated.
- Abdominal ultrasound demonstrates dilatation of the common bile duct; endoscopic retrograde cholangiopancreaticography demonstrates a papillitis in addition to the duct dilatation.
- *Cryptosporidium parvum* is the confirmed pathogen and is cytopathic to biliary epithelia by an apoptotic mechanism.

TABLE 3–111

Human Immunodeficiency Virus Infection[143,375,469–477]

Histology

- There is a paucity of inflammatory cells within the portal tracts.
- Kupffer cells may exhibit variable degrees of erythrophagocytosis.
- Mild macrovesicular and microvesicular fatty change within the lobules is often seen.
- Secondary superinfection often characterized by variable lobular inflammation with little portal reaction is common; note, however, that in superinfection with hepatotropic viruses, the portal inflammation is usually *not* depleted.
- Duct damage may occur, with or without a mononuclear inflammatory exudate, and may in some cases cause duct depletion (refer to Table 3–110, Human Immunodeficiency Virus–associated Cholangiopathy); serial sections may demonstrate cytomegalovirus inclusions in the damaged duct epithelium.
- Peliotic lesions have been described.

Clinical/Laboratory Parameters

- Human immunodeficiency virus types 1 and 2 (HIV-1 and HIV-2) belong to the lentivirus subfamily of retroviruses.
- On infection the reverse transcriptase catalyzes the synthesis of haploid double stranded DNA, which is inserted into the chromosomal DNA of the host cell.
- The major cell surface receptor for adsorption of both HIV-1 and HIV-2 is the CD4 differentiation antigen expressed on T helper lymphocytes, which results in eventual depletion of CD4 and immune deficiency.
- Primary infection of HIV is asymptomatic; however, 50 to 80% of patients may have symptoms if questioned.
- Symptomatic primary infection is characterized by fever, headache, malaise, myalgia, arthralgia, pharyngitis, meningitis, pneumonitis, and less frequently liver test abnormalities (mild increase in serum transaminases without elevation of serum bilirubin or alkaline phosphatase).
- Leukopenia and lymphopenia are frequently present.
- HIV-1 antibodies are present within several weeks.
- Serum p24 and proviral DNA by polymerase chain reaction is more sensitive in detecting primary infection.
- The absolute CD4 count is a predictor of diseae progression.

TABLE 3-112

Hydatid Disease *(Echinococcus granulosus* and *E. multilocularis)*[143,480-485]

Histology

- Spherical cysts up to 30 cm in diameter having a fibrous rim are present.
- The cysts are secondary to infection by *E. granulosus;* they are unilocular and characteristically contain many daughter cysts.
- The wall of these cysts is composed of three components:
  1. An outer layer of acellular, laminated, dense hyalinized membrane up to 1 mm thick, ivory-white, and friable.
  2. An inner germinal membrane.
  3. Underlying endogenous daughter cysts arising from the germinal membrane. These daughter cysts are thin walled and bulb-like *(brood capsules)* containing protoscolices (ovoid structures 100 μm in diameter with two circles of refractile hooklets and a sucker) attached to the membrane.
- Granulation tissue with eosinophils and plasma cells is present overlying the cyst.
- Degenerating cysts contain amorphous, often calcified granular sediment; calcification frequently occurs within the cyst wall itself.
- If a cyst ruptures, a granulomatous reaction occurs with numerous eosinophils, giant cells, and secondary acute cholangitis and sclerosing cholangitis.
- The alveolar (multilocular) cysts secondary to *E. multilocularis* are characterized by:
  - Daughter cysts forming outside the poorly formed cyst wall.
  - Absence of a germinal layer.
  - Laminated fragmented membranes with granulomatous infiltration by neutrophils and eosinophils, with calcifications.

Clinical/Laboratory Parameters

- The cestode (tapeworm) *Echinococcus granulosus* has worldwide distribution, and is common in sheep-rearing areas with the dog as the definitive host; *Echinococcus multilocularis* is seen in colder climates with a variety of carnivores (e.g., foxes, wolves) as the definitive hosts.
- The gravid proglottid when ingested releases the eggs, which hatch in the intestinal lumen and gain access to the portal circulation, eventually being trapped in the liver and less commonly in the spleen, lungs, central nervous system, and bone.
- The larvae then encyst, forming the characteristic hydatid cyst.
- The cysts gradually increase in size, causing pain and sometimes bleeding or infection.
- Cystic lesions are identified on ultrasound and CT scan, demonstrating a calcific rim.
- Aspiration of the hepatic cysts without prior therapy can release the scolices into the peritoneum, forming cystic masses over time.
- The diagnostic protoscolex with refractile hooklets can be seen under the microscope.
- The injection of hypertonic saline or formalin at surgery kills the scolices, but care must be taken to avoid peritoneal and biliary tract spillage.
- Liver tests are usually normal unless the biliary tract is obstructed.
- Serologic tests using enzyme immunoassays (e.g., enzyme-linked immunosorbent assay) have a sensitivity of greater than 90%.

TABLE 3–113

Hyperalimentation (Total Parenteral Nutrition)[486-491]

Histology

Infants

- Intracellular and intracanalicular cholestasis is present, predominantly in the perivenular zone, with mild chronic lobular inflammation.
- Rosettes of liver cells form around dilated canaliculi containing bile plugs.
- Bile may be seen within cholangioles and interlobular bile ducts.
- Fatty change is present but infrequent.
- Syncytial giant cell transformation of hepatocytes may be seen in the perivenular zone.
- Sinusoidal collagen deposition is present to variable degrees, but can be prominent in a minority of cases.
- Portal tracts exhibit mixed lymphocytic and neutrophilic infiltration.
- In prolonged hyperalimentation, cholangiolar proliferation may be present along with biliary fibrosis leading to biliary cirrhosis.

Adults

- Cholestasis is seen with no distinct zonal distribution and only mild associated chronic inflammatory infiltration.
- Macrovesicular fatty change (often periportal) is seen with or without chronic inflammatory infiltration.
- Mallory bodies have been described but are rare.
- Portal lymphocytic infiltration is present.
- Portal fibrosis may occur, with eventual micronodular cirrhosis in a minority of cases; sinusoidal collagen can occasionally be seen in these cases.
- An increase in copper and copper-binding protein is seen in periportal hepatocytes.
- Hemosiderin is also noted within Kupffer cells and periportal hepatocytes.

Clinical/Laboratory Parameters

- Liver abnormalities may develop in patients who receive total parenteral nutrition (TPN), and consist of elevated bilirubin levels as well as modest increases in serum transaminases and alkaline phosphatase activity.
- Hyperbilirubinemia occurs between 4 and 47 days after the onset of TPN.
- In the adult, liver test abnormalities begin approximately 1 week after TPN, with bilirubin rising to approximately 3 mg/dl.
- In neonates, hyperbilirubinemia may occur in up to 25% of cases; however, when TPN is prolonged (60–90 days), hyperbilirubinemia may develop in from 80 to 90% of patients.
- Gallstones and sludge are often present secondary to bile stasis within the gallbladder.
- Fatty change may be secondary to imbalance of fatty acid and lipoprotein synthesis.
- The pathogenesis in the neonate is multifactorial, and includes immaturity, associated sepsis, absence of oral feeding leading to inadequate gastric-duodenal stimulation, and relative amino acid and essential fatty acid deficiency.
- With cessation of TPN, cholestasis resolves, with liver tests returning to normal.
- In cases in which TPN cannot be discontinued, chronic liver disease including cirrhosis may develop.

TABLE 3–114

Hypereosinophilic Syndrome[492-495]

Histology

- Prominent numbers of eosinophils are present within portal tracts and sinusoids.
- Sinusoidal congestion may also be seen.
- Portal lymphocytic infiltration is seen, with variable portal fibrosis, and sometimes piecemeal necrosis; although bridging fibrosis has been reported, no true progression to well-established cirrhosis has been described.

Clinical/Laboratory Parameters

- This idiopathic disorder occurs predominantly in young to middle-aged men who have persistent eosinophilia of unknown cause (hypersensitivity reactions, parasitic infestation, and other causes of eosinophilia must be ruled out).
- Hepatomegaly with minimally abnormal liver tests occurs in approximately 30% of these patients.
- Complications include congestive heart failure, myocarditis, and various neurologic abnormalities.
- Overall the prognosis is poor, although chemotherapy may be promising in some cases.

TABLE 3-115
Hyperpyrexia[496]

Histology

- Microvesicular fatty change is seen.
- Coagulative-type necrosis of perivenular hepatocytes may be present.
- Cholestasis may occur, sometimes associated with acute cholangitis and cholangiolitis.

Clinical/Laboratory Parameters

- Patients develop marked increases in serum transaminases and bilirubin.
- Occasionally progression to death may occur with terminal hypotension and renal failure.

TABLE 3-116
Hyperthyroidism[497–501]

Histology

- Mild portal lymphocytic infiltration, macrovesicular fatty change, and mild necroinflammatory changes may be seen.
- Sinusoidal congestion with adjacent liver cell atrophy may be present.

Clinical/Laboratory Parameters

- Patients may present with clinical features of hyperthyroidism including a palpable thyroid gland, bruit, tremors, lid lag, and exopthalmos.
- Serum bilirubin is minimally elevated (3 mg/dl), and mild increases in serum transaminses (ALT higher than AST) are noted.
- In patients with associated cardiac disease, the liver test abnormalities may be markedly deranged.

TABLE 3-117
Hypothyroidism[500,502,503]

Histology

- Concentric thickening of the terminal hepatic venules may be seen, associated with perivenular fibrosis.

Clinical/Laboratory Parameters

- Liver tests are usually normal.
- In some patients with severe hypothyroidism, ascites may be present.

TABLE 3-118
Idiopathic Adulthood Ductopenia[504–507]

Histology

- Portal lymphocytic infiltration is seen, with variable nonsuppurative duct damage.
- Small ducts may exhibit periductal fibrosis, mimicking primary sclerosing cholangitis (refer to Table 3–173).
- Cholestasis may be seen associated with variable mononuclear inflammatory infiltration.
- Biliary fibrosis occurs with eventual biliary cirrhosis and ductopenia.
- Increase in copper and copper-binding protein are seen in periportal and periseptal hepatocytes as the disease progresses.

Clinical/Laboratory Parameters

- In this cholestatic disorder of uncertain etiology, patients present with pruritus and jaundice; elevations in serum bilirubin and alkaline phosphatase activity, and mild increases in serum transaminases are noted.
- Hepatic synthetic function is well preserved, although prothrombin time may be prolonged if cholestasis is long-standing.
- Bile ducts are not dilated and are normal at endoscopic retrograde cholangiopancreatography.
- Some patients improve spontaneously, but others progress to liver failure and may need transplantation.
- A careful drug history is essential to exclude drug-related vanishing bile duct syndrome.

TABLE 3-119

Idiopathic Granulomatous Hepatitis[61,174,176,508-513]

Histology

- This liver disease is loosely defined as an inflammatory condition histologically manifested by the presence of a circumscribed collection of inflammatory cells *(granulomas)* within portal tracts and lobules in which no specific etiologic diagnosis has been established.
- The granulomas are usually of *epithelioid* type (transformed activated macrophages, lymphocytes, and multinucleated giant cells).
- It is postulated that some of these cases may represent sarcoidosis (refer to Table 3-187) confined to the liver without pulmonary manifestations.

Clinical/Laboratory Parameters

- The initial report on this disorder included 12 patients who presented with prolonged fever, elevated alkaline phosphatase activity, and no evidence of infection.
- None of these patients had lymphadenopathy, hypercalcemia, or pulmonary disease (features seen in sarcoidosis).
- In some patients, hepatomegaly is noted and therapy with corticosteroids is beneficial.
- Fever recurs when steroid therapy is withdrawn, and temperature returns to normal when steroids are reintroduced.
- The long-term course is benign without progression to advanced liver disease.

TABLE 3-120

Idiopathic Portal Hypertension (Noncirrhotic Portal Fibrosis)[343,446,514-520]

Histology

- Portal fibrosis is present, with stellate periseptal collagen strands sometimes seen.
- Increased dilated portal venous radicles are present.
- Only minimal portal and lobular inflammation is present.
- There is a lack of orientation between portal tracts and terminal hepatic venules.
- Larger portal veins may show eccentric intimal thickening.
- Bridging fibrosis between portal tracts has been described; the fibrous bands are thin, without development of cirrhosis.

Clinical/Laboratory Parameters

- Also termed *noncirrhotic portal fibrosis,* this disease of uncertain etiology is seen most commonly in Japan and India but is not frequent in developed countries.
- Patients present with manifestations of portal hypertension such as bleeding esophageal varices and hypersplenism.
- The liver is usually normal in size but splenomegaly is common and sometimes striking.
- Liver function is normal, with leukopenia and thrombocytopenia related to the splenomegaly.
- Ultrasound and CT scans demonstrate portal hypertension with collateral circulation.

TABLE 3-121

Indian Childhood Cirrhosis[521-525]

Histology

- Diffuse interstitial fibrosis may be present.
- Mallory bodies are seen in the majority of hepatocytes in the advanced stage of disease.
- Focal necrosis and hepatocytolysis are present, the inflammatory cells chiefly consisting of lymphocytes and neutrophils.
- Mild fatty change is present in the early stages, but is unusual in the cirrhotic stage.
- Syncytial giant cell transformation of hepatocytes may be seen, but these cells are relatively small (2-3 nuclei per cell).
- An increase in copper and copper-binding protein is present in periseptal liver cells, but it may also occur diffusely.
- Micronodular cirrhosis develops, with poorly formed nodules exhibiting little regeneration.

Clinical/Laboratory Parameters

- First described in Indian male infants, this rare disorder is characterized by failure to thrive, hepatosplenomegaly, neurologic symptoms, and death from liver failure usually within 1 to 2 years after diagnosis.
- Copper toxicity resulting from the ingestion of milk boiled in copper vessels has been considered a possible cause of this disease.

TABLE 3-122

Infantile Hemangioendothelioma[130,531-534]

Histology

- This tumor is usually multinodular or diffuse, spongy, and red-brown with variable scarring.
- Two histologic subtypes are often seen within the same tumor:
  a. Type 1
    - Numerous intercommunicating vascular channels lined by a single layer of cytologically benign endothelial cells are present, with numerous small bile ductules scattered throughout.
    - Centrally located large cavernous spaces, sometimes with thrombosis and infarction, are seen.
    - Extramedullary hematopoiesis may be present.
  b. Type 2
    - Nuclear atypia is seen, with pleomorphism, multilayered endothelial cells, papillary projections, and intravascular budding of endothelial lining.
    - Solid growth patterns with mitoses may be present.
    - Note that although this type histologically resembles angiosarcoma, these lesions do not metastasize.

Clinical/Laboratory Parameters

- This tumor acounts for about 12% of childhood hepatic neoplasms, occurs more frequently in females, and affects other organs such as skin, lung, lymph nodes, and bone.
- The vast majority of the tumors are detected within 6 months of age.
- Hepatomegaly is common and congestive cardiac failure from large arteriovenous shunts may be present in up to 25% of cases.
- Cutaneous hemangiomas are often present.
- Thrombocytopenia due to sequestration of platelets within the vascular channels, hemoperitoneum from rupture, and jaundice have been reported.
- Surgical resection is indicated in small solitary lesions or in clusters of lesions confined to a single segment.
- Hepatic artery ligation and irradiation is considered for large unresectable tumors.
- Spontaneous involution may occur in limited disease in some patients.
- Malignant transformation with metastases has been described.

TABLE 3-123

Infantile Microcystic Disease[526-530]

Histology

- The cysts are quite small; grossly recognizable cysts are uncommon.
- Bile duct proliferation and ectasia are present, forming rings at the periphery of the portal tracts and lobules.
- Bile ducts branch and anastomose, with polypoid projections.
- Normal interlobular bile ducts are absent.
- Dilated duct channels may contain pink to orange material and/or pus, and may exhibit acute cholangitis.
- Portal fibrosis may be present without progression to cirrhosis.

Clinical/Laboratory Parameters

- Massive enlargement of the liver and kidneys may be present at birth.
- Respiratory difficulty, congestive cardiac and renal failure with acidosis, and failure to thrive leading to death in the first month may occur.
- Liver function is not impaired, but portal hypertension may develop.

TABLE 3-124

Inflammatory Pseudotumor (Myofibroblastic Tumor)[41,130,535-540]

Histology

- These lesions are solitary or multiple, and may measure up to 25 cm in diameter.
- A mixed inflammatory infiltrate is seen consisting chiefly of lymphocytes and plasma cells, with eosinophils and macrophages also present.
- A fibroconnective tissue framework is present with variable sclerosis.
- Trapped bile ducts may be seen within the tumor, as are trapped hepatocytes toward the periphery of the lesion.
- Obliterative endophlebitis and giant cell granulomas have been reported.

Clinical/Laboratory Parameters

- This mass clinically often resembles a healed abscess (pyogenic or amebic) or post traumatic hepatic injury.
- The lesion is much more commonly seen in young men.
- Patients may present with fever, usually intermittent, nausea, and diarrhea.
- Surgical resection is curative, although complications related to portal hypertension have been described when the lesion is located toward the hepatic hilum.

TABLE 3-125

Inspissated Bile Syndrome[316,541,542]

Histology

- Perivenular cholestasis is present with prominent bile plugs but little lobular inflammation.
- Portal tracts may exhibit a mild lymphocytic and neutrophilic infiltrate.
- Hemosiderin in Kupffer cells may be seen.

Clinical/Laboratory Parameters

- This syndrome presents as obstructive jaundice in infancy and occurs in the setting of ABO- and Rh-incompatible transfusions.
- Bile duct obstruction is due to inspissated concretions and bile.
- Removal of the obstruction and concretions by washing or mucolytic agents at surgery or endoscopy is helpful.
- In some patients spontaneous resolution may be seen.

TABLE 3-126

Kawasaki Disease[543-547]

Histology

- Acute cholangitis with bile duct damage may be seen.
- Vasculitis involving the main hepatic artery branches may be present.

Clinical/Laboratory Parameters

- Also termed *mucocutaneous lymph node syndrome,* the disorder is characterized by arteritis, with cardiac complications developing in 22% of patients.
- Hepatosplenomegaly may be present.
- Hydrops of the gallbladder may develop; patients present with biliary colic, elevated serum transaminases, and increased serum bilirubin.
- Acute cholangitis may develop clinically, and aneurysms of the hepatic artery have also been described.

TABLE 3–127

Kwashiorkor[548–551]

Histology

- Marked fatty change is present.
- The fat initially is microvesicular and is oriented in the perivenular zone.
- As the disease progresses, macrovesicular fat is seen involving all zones.
- With refeeding, the perivenular fat disappears first.
- Mallory bodies have been described.

Clinical/Laboratory Parameters

- This distinct syndrome in children, similar to marasmus (refer to Table 3–143), is primarily a deficiency of protein intake.
- Patients present with pallor, lethargy, edema, and hepatomegaly.
- Marked hypoalbuminemia, mild to moderate increases in serum transaminases, and normal prothrombin time are typical findings.
- Refeeding and restitution of protein in the diet is carried out slowly to prevent diarrhea and electrolyte abnormalities.

TABLE 3–128

Langerhans' Cell Histiocytosis[552–559]

Histology

- Poorly formed granulomas consisting of histiocytes, eosinophils, neutrophils, lymphocytes, and multinucleated giant cells are present in both the portal tracts and lobules.
- Both extra- and intrahepatic bile duct damage may occur, resembling primary sclerosis cholangitis, with periductal fibrosis and eventual intrahepatic duct loss.
- Variable portal fibrosis may be present; cirrhosis has been described.

Clinical/Laboratory Parameters

- This disorder, integrated from three previously known diseases (eosinophilic granuloma of bone, Hand-Schüller-Christian disease, and Letterer-Siwe disease), is estimated to occur in 1 in 200,000 children.
- Patients present with hepatosplenomegaly, edema, and ascites.
- Modest elevations of serum transaminases and bilirubin may be observed.
- Liver involvement is progressive and potentially life-threatening.

TABLE 3–129

Lassa Fever[275,283,560–563]

Histology

- Coagulative-type necrosis without inflammation is present within the lobules, with acidophil bodies common.
- The necrosis is usually patchy, although confluent necrosis can also be seen.
- Although no inclusions are seen on light microscopy, arenaviruses can be demonstrated on electron microscopy.

Clinical/Laboratory Parameters

- Infection by this arenavirus (RNA virus) causes multisystem disease, with fever, exudative pharyngitis, gastrointestinal and renal disturbances, and DIC.
- The infection is usually subclinical, and is transferred by contact with rodent excrement.
- Hepatomegaly and right upper quadrant pain and tenderness are common.
- Serum transaminases are elevated, but bilirubin is usually normal.
- Intravenous ribavirin may be effective when administered in high doses.

TABLE 3-130

Leishmaniasis (Kala Azar; *Leishmania donovani*) [564-568]

Histology

- Hepatomegaly is present and may be massive (weight up to 4 kg).
  1. In the *acute* form:
     - Hypertrophic and hyperplastic Kupffer cells and portal macrophages containing parasites (2–3 μm in diameter, ovoid with basophilic nucleus, rarely paranuclear rod-shaped kinetoplast) are present, but the parasites are rarely seen in liver cells.
     - Epithelioid granulomas as well as small clusters of macrophages containing a scanty number of parasites are seen, these granulomas sometimes exhibiting central necrosis.
     - Granulomas containing a central clear space with a fibrin ring are described.
     - Macrovesicular fatty change is common.
     - Portal and sinusoidal lymphocytic and plasma cell infiltration is present.
  2. In the *chronic* form:
     - Panacinar sinusoidal collagen deposition may be present.

Clinical/Laboratory Parameters

- Infection of humans occurs by the injection of the promastigote form of this parasite by the sandfly.
- The parasite is then taken up by the reticuloendothelial cells, where it divides by binary fission, leading to destruction of these cells.
- Organs with high concentration of reticuloendothelial cells (liver, spleen) are affected, leading to massive hepatosplenomegaly and anemia.
- Mucosal bleeding, and rarely ascites and immune dysfunction, lead to susceptibility to infections, cachexia, and in severe untreated disease, death.
- Pancytopenia, and elevations in serum alkaline phosphatase activity and transaminases are common; hyperbilirubinemia is rare.
- Diagnosis is made by detection of leishmanial forms in the bone marrow, splenic aspirate, or liver biopsy (less sensitive).
- Serologic tests using immunofluorescent antibody and enzyme immunoassays are helpful.

TABLE 3-131

Leprosy (Hansen's Disease; *Mycobacterium leprae*) [176,569-574]

Histology

- Portal and lobular granulomas are present and are of three types:
  - *Tuberculoid* (epithelioid) type: Numerous lymphocytes, histiocytes, often multinucleated giant cells, but few to no acid-fast bacillus (AFB) organisms.
  - *Lepromatous* (inflammatory) type: Foamy vacuolated macrophages, scanty lymphocytes, no multinucleated giant cells, but abundant AFB organisms within macrophages, Kupffer cells, endothelial cells, and occasionally hepatocytes.
  - *Intermediate* type: Epithelioid granulomas with few lymphocytes and no multinucleated giant cells.

Clinical/Laboratory Parameters

- Unlike tuberculosis, the liver abnormalities in leprosy are minor, although hepatic granulomas are common.
- Leprosy has two major distinct forms: the *tuberculoid* type with intense cell-mediated immunity and localized disease, and the *lepromatous* type, with little cell-mediated immunity and diffuse disease.
- Diagnosis of the different types depends on the clinical presentation, skin smear findings, and localized versus generalized nerve involvement.
- The presence of hepatic granulomas does not affect the course of disease or therapy.

TABLE 3-132

Leptospirosis (Weil's Disease; *Leptospira icterohaemorrhagica*) [143,575-577]

Histology

- Cholestasis with variable chronic inflammatory infiltration is seen within the lobules, associated with scattered acidophil body formation.
- Kupffer cell hyperplasia and hypertrophy with erythrophagocytosis is seen.
- Organisms (spirochetes 10–20 μm in diameter demonstrated by the Warthin-Starry reaction) are seen within Kupffer cells and endothelium.

Clinical/Laboratory Parameters

- These gram-negative spirochetal bacteria are shed in the urine of rodents and infrequently in pigs, dogs, and cattle and are acquired by humans when swimming in contaminated water or after exposure to animal excreta.
- After an incubation period of 7 to 10 days, a biphasic illness develops with fever, photophobia, headache, myalgia, sweating, prostration, epistaxis, and lymphadenopathy.
- Delirium, hemolysis, renal failure, anemia, thrombocytopenia, myocarditis, pericarditis, and hepatitis may follow.
- Splenomegaly is noted frequently.
- Leukocytosis, hyperbilirubinemia (partly caused by hemolysis), and moderate increases in serum transaminases and alkaline phosphatase activity are observed.
- Blood cultures are positive if obtained within the first 7 to 10 days; the organism may be identified in alkaline urine by darkfield microscopy.
- Mortality approaches 40% in severe cases, but death is not due to liver failure.

TABLE 3-133

Leukemia[61,578-582]

Histology

- The following are common features of the different types of leukemia:
  - *Acute lymphocytic:* Leukemic infiltrates are usually within the portal tracts.
  - *Acute myelogenous:* The infiltrates are usually within both the portal tracts and sinusoids.
  - *Chronic lymphocytic:* The infiltrates are usually within portal tracts, although sinusoids may also be affected.
  - *Chronic myelogenous:* Sinusoidal infiltrates are usually seen in acute blastic crises.
  - *Hairy cell leukemia:* The infiltrates are loosely cohesive mononuclear cells with moderate cytoplasm, present within portal tracts and sinusoids, and may be diffuse or focal; the cells adhere to endothelium, sometimes infiltrating into the space of Disse; peliosis may occur, and granulomas have been described.
- Some degree of sinusoidal dilatation may be seen in any type that has sinusoidal infiltrates.
- Extramedullary hematopoiesis is present when myelofibrosis of the bone marrow occurs.
- Hemosiderin is often seen within hyperplastic Kupffer cells, portal macrophages, and periportal hepatocytes secondary to hemolysis, transfusions, and/or chronic anemia.

Clinical/Laboratory Parameters

- The liver derangements seen in leukemia are related predominantly to the leukemic infiltrates in the hepatic sinusoids, regardless of the type.
- Patients present with right upper quadrant discomfort and hepatomegaly.
- In chronic leukemias, hepatosplenomegaly may be noted.
- Peripheral blood and bone marrow demonstrate the characteristic morphologic abnormalities of the leukemia.
- Serum transaminases, alkaline phosphatase activity, and bilirubin levels may be elevated to varying degrees depending on the extent of hepatic involvement.
- Serum bilirubin and alkaline phosphatase activity may also be elevated due to sepsis, which commonly occurs in these conditions.
- Hyperuricemia, an increase in lactate dehydrogenase, and hypoalbuminemia may be present.
- Hepatic abnormalities related to the chemotherapeutic agents (e.g., inducing veno-occlusive disease) or other treatments (e.g., hyperalimentation) may complicate the picture.
- Amelioration of the hepatic changes, prognosis, and outcome depend on the response of the leukemia to treatment.

TABLE 3-134
Light Chain Disease[583-588]

Histology

- Acellular eosinophilic deposits (confirmed on immunoperoxidase stains as light chains) are seen within the space of Disse and portal tracts; these deposits are strongly diPAS-positive.
- Sinusoidal dilatation and peliosis have been described.
- These deposits resemble but are *not* amyloid (negative on Congo red staining).
- The deposits have been reported to also contain heavy chains.

Clinical/Laboratory Parameters

- This plasma cell dyscrasia primarily involves the kidneys; however, the lungs, liver, and vasculature may also be involved.
- Hepatic involvement is uncommon; hepatomegaly may be present with mildly abnormal serum transaminases, good hepatic function, and rarely hyperbilirubinemia.
- Renal failure may occur.

TABLE 3-135
Listeriosis *(Listeria monocytogenes)* [143,589-592]

Histology

- Microabscess formation may be seen within the lobules.
- Granulomatous-type necrosis may be present.
- Organisms (bacilli) are often present and abundant within the abscesses.

Clinical/Laboratory Parameters

- This infection is caused by *Listeria monocytogenes* and is acquired from contaminated food or drink, particularly from cold storage of uncooked foods such as milk, milk products, and soft cheeses.
- Bacteremia accounts for fever, headache, chills, and myalgia.
- Meningitis, endocarditis, pericarditis, skin rash, peritonitis, osteomyelitis, and liver involvement are seen in severe cases.
- Hepatosplenomegaly and moderate elevation in transaminases and alkaline phosphatase activity may occur.
- Jaundice is rare except in severe infections.
- Positive blood cultures obtained early in the course of the infection confirm the diagnosis.

TABLE 3-136
Long- and Medium-Chain Acyl-CoA Dehydrogenase Deficiency[593-595]

Histology

- Severe macrovesicular fatty change is present; microvesicular fat may also be seen.
- Portal fibrosis may be seen and leads to cirrhosis in long-chain disease, but fibrosis is *not* present in medium-chain disease.

Clinical/Laboratory Parameters

- These enzymes are involved in the beta-oxidation of fatty acids; the deficiency is of autosomal recessive inheritance.
  1. In *medium-chain* deficiency:
     - Low carnitine levels are found in the plasma, skeletal muscle, and liver.
     - Recurrent hypoglycemic attacks are brought on by fasting.
     - Hepatomegaly, abnormal liver tests, and hyperammonemia are present.
  2. In *long-chain* deficiency:
     - Patients may present with a Reye's-like illness.
     - Muscle wasting and hypertrophic obstructive cardiomyopathy are common.

TABLE 3-137

Lyme Disease *(Borrelia burgdorferi)* [143,596-600]

Histology

- Microvesicular fatty change is present.
- Increased numbers of lymphocytes and neutrophils are seen within the sinusoids.
- Organisms (spirochetes 10–20 μm in diameter demonstrated by the Warthin-Starry reaction) are seen within the sinusoids and hepatocytes.

Clinical/Laboratory Parameters

- This tickborne spirochetal infection is caused by gram-negative *Borrelia burgdorferi;* the patient presents with a brief, acute illness with skin rash, arthritis, and cardiac and central nervous system symptoms.
- The initial skin lesion (erythema migrans) at the site of the tick bite develops within 8 to 9 days; late-phase illness lasts weeks to months, with musculo-skeletal and cardiac symptoms.
- Liver involvement is minor, with hepatomegaly and only mild derangement of liver tests.

TABLE 3-138

Lymphangioma[601-604]

Histology

- These tumors are solitary or multiple, and are composed of numerous dilated lymphatic channels containing proteinaceous fluid or blood.
- Typical cavernous hemangiomas may also be seen within the same liver.

Clinical/Laboratory Parameters

- This uncommon tumor may also involve other structures such as the kidneys, soft tissues, retroperitoneum, spleen, and lymph nodes.
- The ultrasonographic features and CT scan appearance may be similar to cavernous hemangiomas.
- The systemic variety usually seen in children manifests with hepatomegaly and skeletal involvement and has a poor prognosis.
- The solitary hepatic lesion has a benign course.

TABLE 3-139

Lymphoma, Hodgkin's[61,605-610]

Histology

- The liver may show diffuse microscopic involvement or exhibit variable-sized but usually small, distinct, gray mass lesions.
- The portal tracts exhibit a mixed infiltrate, depending on the subclassification of Hodgkin's disease; for instance, in the *mixed cellularity* type, lymphocytes, neutrophils, eosinophils, plasma cells, and macrophages are prominent, with Reed-Sternberg cells and atypical mononuclear cells present.
- These inflammatory cells may surround and even infiltrate into bile duct epithelium, with duct destruction and in some cases duct depletion.
- Intralobular cholestasis sometimes with mild mononuclear infiltrates may be seen; lobular infiltrates of atypical cells are also present in approximately 10% of cases.
- Variable macrovesicular fatty change may be present.
- Noncaseating epithelioid granulomas are seen predominantly within portal tracts but also within the lobules in 8 to 12% of cases.
- Peliosis and sinusoidal dilatation in the perivenular zone and midzone may be present.
- Variable portal fibrosis can occur without progression to cirrhosis.
- Hemosiderin in hyperplastic Kupffer cells, portal macrophages, and periportal hepatocytes may be seen secondary to hemolysis, transfusions, and/or chronic anemia.

Clinical/Laboratory Parameters

- Hepatic involvement in Hodgkin's disease occurs in about 5% of cases at the time of diagnosis, 30% during the course of the disease, and greater than 50% at the time of autopsy.
- The more common variants that involve the liver are nodular sclerosis and mixed cellularity types.
- In addition to clinical features of lymphadenopathy, hepatosplenomegaly, fever (Pel-Ebstein type) and pruritus, patients may have pancytopenia due to marrow involvement.
- Patients clinically present with hepatomegaly and fever; jaundice is present in approximately 14% of patients.
- The commonest hepatic abnormality is elevation in serum alkaline phosphatase activity, the frequency directly related to the severity of the disease (seen in 14% of patients with stage I and II disease, 65% with stage III, and 85% with stage IV disease).
- No cases of primary or isolated involvement of the liver have been reported.
- Elevations of lactate dehydrogenase are due to lymphoma rather than hepatic involvement.
- Although uncommon, jaundice may be due to (1) widespread involvement; (2) involvement of hilar bile ducts, mimicking bile duct obstruction; (3) severe hemolysis with bilirubin overload; and (4) perivenular cholestasis without bile duct obstruction.
- Acute liver failure has been reported, with encephalopathy and renal failure.

TABLE 3–140

Lymphoma, Non-Hodgkin's[61,581,582,609,611–617]

Histology

- This type of lymphoma may be present diffusely or as distinct mass lesions.
- The following are common features of different types of non-Hodgkin's lymphoma:
  1. *B-cell type, low grade:*
     - Small nodular deposits are seen predominantly within portal tracts, with variable spillover of these cells into the adjacent periportal regions.
     - Sinusoidal involvement by infiltrating cells may be present but is not striking.
  2. *B-cell type, high grade:*
     - Portal tracts and lobules are involved, with prominent spillover of these cells into the adjacent periportal regions; however, in some cases, sinusoidal involvement may be most obvious.
     - Portal and sinusoidal fibrosis without progression to cirrhosis can be seen but is uncommon.
     - Peliosis has been described.
  3. *T-cell type:*
     - Portal and lobular infiltrates are seen, with greater tendency for sinusoidal involvement in a chain-like fashion.
- Epithelioid granulomas have been described, and are sometimes prominent.
- Cholestasis may be seen in severe cases.
- When the infiltrate is prominent, cells may hug up against vascular endothelium, sometimes infiltrating beneath the endothelial lining, resembling endothelialitis.
- Hemosiderin deposition is often present in hyperplastic Kupffer cells, portal macrophages, and periportal hepatocytes secondary to hemolysis, transfusions, and/or chronic anemia.

Clinical/Laboratory Parameters

- Non-Hodgkin's lymphoma constitutes approximately 5.6% of all hepatic malignancies, excluding primary hepatic neoplasms.
- The spleen and abdominal lymph nodes are almost always affected when the liver is involved; however, rare cases of primary hepatic lymphomas can occur without systemic lymphoma.
- Extrahepatic bile duct obstruction may occur due to compression by enlarged hilar lymph nodes.
- An increased frequency of chronic hepatitis C has been reported to occur in this disease, but the causal relationship is not clear.
- Generally, hepatic involvement is associated with advanced disease, with the prognosis guarded.
- In the rare case of primary hepatic involvement, promising results can occur in some patients with hepatic resection and chemotherapy.

TABLE 3-141

Malaria (Plasmodium falciparum)[143,618-626]

Histology

- The liver is enlarged and dark brown.
- Abundant deposition of malaria pigment, *hemozoin* (an iron porphyrin complex, secondary to breakdown of hemoglobin, that is birefringent on polarized light and negative on iron stain), is present. The pigment is dark brown and granular and is seen in hypertrophic and hyperplastic Kupffer cells, parasitized red blood cells, and portal macrophages.
- Sinusoidal congestion may be marked, with associated circulating parasitized red blood cells hugging the sinusoidal border.
- The parasites themselves are faint clear rings with a hematoxylin-staining dot (nucleus), and are often obscured by pigment.
- When parasitemia resolves, the pigment shifts to portal macrophages and eventually is cleared.
- Portal tracts exhibit lymphocytic and plasma cell infiltrates.
- Mild macrovesicular fatty change is present.
- Stellate portal fibrosis may be seen in long-standing cases, without progression to cirrhosis.
- Variable hemosiderin deposition is seen in Kupffer cells (secondary to hemolysis) and liver cells (secondary to increased iron absorption as a result of chronic anemia).
- Prominent portal lymphocytic infiltration and sinusoidal lymphocytosis associated with Kupffer cell hyperplasia without pigment (hyperimmune reaction, *tropical splenomegaly syndrome*) may also be seen.

Clinical/Laboratory Parameters

- Infection by *Plasmodium* species is common worldwide, and is seen predominantly in tropical and subtropical regions.
- The infection is caused by four species: *P. vivax, P. ovale, P. malariae,* and *P. falciparum,* the last causing the most severe disease.
- Infection is spread by the *Anopheles* mosquita via:
  1. Inoculation of the sporozoite into the blood.
  2. Invasion into the hepatocytes (exoerythrocytic stage).
  3. Asexual development, releasing merozoites into the blood with invasion of red blood cells.
  4. Erythrocyte rupture (febrile stage), with release of the merozoites followed by invasion of other red blood cells (completed cycle, 48 to 72 hours).
- Except for *P. falciparum,* no significant liver disease is seen with the other species, although hepatosplenomegaly may be present, and mild hemolytic anemia associated with fever in endemic areas provides clues to the infection.
- In *P. falciparum* infection, modest increases in serum bilirubin (2.5 mg/dl, predominantly indirect) and mild transaminase elevations may be seen, with moderate elevations noted in about 5% of cases; the clinical course can be severe, with marked hemolysis, renal failure, coma (blackwater fever), and associated high mortality.

TABLE 3-142

Mannosidosis (Acidic Alpha-Mannosidase A and B Deficiency)[627-629]

Histology

- Liver cells contain cytoplasmic vacuoles that are PAS-negative
- Variable degrees of fatty change may be present.
- Sinusoidal collagen deposition may be seen.

Clinical/Laboratory Parameters

- In this rare autosomal recessive disorder, mannose-rich oligosaccharides accumulate in various tissues.
- Two types are recognized: *type I* occurs in the infant, with death a few years later; *type II,* with less severe disease, has onset in the late teens.
- Mental retardation, lenticular and corneal abnormalities, hearing loss, and hepatosplenomegaly are present.

TABLE 3–143

Marasmus[630]

Histology

- Fatty change is present but is mild and focal.
- The fatty change is macrovesicular, without a zonal distribution pattern.
- Peliosis has also been described.

Clinical/Laboratory Parameters

- The distinct syndrome in children, related to kwashiorkor (refer to Table 3–127), is primarily due to protein-calorie malnutrition.
- There is marked cachexia with loss of muscle mass, lethargy, a distended abdomen from an enlarged liver, and increase in susceptibility to infection.
- Liver tests are normal or mildly deranged; hypoalbuminemia is striking.
- Refeeding and restitution of protein and calories in the diet is carried out slowly to prevent diarrhea and electrolyte abnormalities.

TABLE 3–144

Marburg Virus Infection[275,283,284,631]

Histology

- Coagulative-type necrosis without inflammation is present scattered within the lobules.
- Acidophil bodies are commonly seen.
- Confluent liver cell necrosis may be present, but patchy involvement may also be present.

Clinical/Laboratory Parameters

- This severe viral hemorrhagic febrile disorder manifests with the sudden onset of fever, malaise, headache and myalgia, with shock and DIC.
- Mortality is high, with the liver a major target.

TABLE 3–145

Melioidosis *(Pseudomonas pseudomallei)*[143,632,633]

Histology

- Variable-sized abscesses are present in acute infection.
- Necrotizing granulomas may be seen within the lobules in chronic infection.

Clinical/Laboratory Parameters

- Caused by *Pseudomonas pseudomallei*, a gram-negative unencapsulated nonsporulating organism, the infection is endemic to Southeast Asia, tropical Australia, and other tropical countries.
- Most infections are subclinical.
- In patients with chronic infection, 80% have concurrent diseases such as diabetes mellitus, malnutrition, obesity, chronic renal failure, and connective tissue disease.
- The course of infection in these patients is characterized by recurring suppuration, mimicking tuberculosis or fungal infection.
- The most serious disseminated disease involves lungs, liver and spleen, with high grade fever, headache, myalgia, diarrhea, hepatosplenomegaly, and shock.
- Cultures of blood, urine, sputum, and pus are diagnostic.
- In chronic infections, serology (IgG immunofluorescent antibody titer of $\geq 1:10$) has a sensitivity of 90%.

TABLE 3-146
Mesenchymal Hamartoma[41,130,634-638]

Histology

- Solid white and firm lesions as well as multiple cystic spaces are present, the latter containing a serous or gelatinous exudate.
- Haphazard arrangement of loose edematous connective tissue is seen, admixed with dilated lymphatics and vessels.
- Numerous tortuous bile ducts and cytologically benign liver cell nodules are randomly scattered within the tumor.
- Extramedullary hematopoiesis is common.

Clinical/Laboratory Parameters

- The lesion almost always occurs in childhood between 1 and 2 years of age and manifests with progressive increase in abdominal girth.
- A mass in the liver may be palpated.
- Congestive cardiac failure has been reported due to arteriovenous shunts within the mass.
- Liver tests are not helpful, although the alkaline phosphatase activity may be elevated if the lesion is in the vicinity of the major hepatic ducts.
- Ultrasound and CT scan demonstrate the cystic nature of the lesion.

TABLE 3-147
Metachromatic Leukodystrophy (Sulfatide Lipidosis)[639-641]

Histology

- Large, foamy portal macrophages contain metachromatic granules; these granules are also seen in bile duct epithelium and less commonly in Kupffer cells and hepatocytes.

Clinical/Laboratory Parameters

- This autosomal recessive disease is caused by a deficiency of arylsulfatase A, which leads to the accumulation of galactosyl sulfate (cerebroside sulfate) in the white matter, peripheral nerves, kidneys, and gallbladder.
- There are three types: infantile, juvenile, and adult forms.
- In *multiple sulfatase deficiency*, which occurs in the infant, coarse facial features, deafness, ichthyosis, skeletal abnormalities, and hepatosplenomegaly are present.

TABLE 3-148
Microsporidiosis (*Enterocytozoon* and *Encephalitozoon* species)[143,642-645]

Histology

- Small, oval intracellular refractile spores in the cytoplasm of duct epithelium are present and are best seen on toluidine blue stain.
- In AIDS patients, duct sclerosis and eventual depletion may occur (refer to Table 3-110, Human Immunodeficiency Virus–associated Cholangiopathy).

Clinical/Laboratory Parameters

- This obligate, intracellular gram-negative protozoan parasite is recognized as a cause of opportunistic infection in patients with AIDs and organ transplants.
- Spores ingested from contaminated food and drink reach the small intestine and are internalized by macrophages after phagocytosis, allowing schizogony to occur by binary fission.
- Patients present with diarrhea, weight loss, anemia, and involvement of the biliary tract.
- Parasites can be detected in the stool or on biopsy.
- Serologic tests are not reliable.

TABLE 3-149

Mucolipidoses:[646-648] Type I, Sialidosis; Type II, I-cell Disease

Histology

- There is marked enlargement of portal macrophages and Kupffer cells, both of which have foamy cytoplasm (types I and II).
- Granulomas composed of vacuolated epithelioid cells are also seen in portal tracts (type II).

Clinical/Laboratory Parameters

- The mucolipidoses are phenotypically similar to the mucopolysaccharidoses; the patients present with mental retardation, hepatosplenomegaly, and skeletal abnormalities.
- The defect is due to a deficiency of oligosaccharide neuraminidase (sialidase), which leads to the accumulation of sialyl oligosaccharides in the tissues.

TABLE 3-150

Mucopolysaccharidoses:[649-654] Type I, Hurler's Syndrome; Type II, Hunter's Syndrome: Type III, Sanfilippo Syndrome; Type IV, Morquio Syndrome; Type VI, Maroteaux-Lamy Syndrome; Type VII, Sly Syndrome

Histology

- All classifications exhibit large, firm yellow livers.
- Hepatocytes, Kupffer cells, and rarely bile duct epithelium are swollen; the cytoplasm is faintly vacuolated and contains stored acid mucopolysaccharides within lysosomes.
- Extensive sinusoidal collagen may be seen.
- Cirrhosis has been reported.

Clinical/Laboratory Parameters

- The mucopolysaccharidoses are a group of lysosomal enzyme deficiencies; these enzymes are normally needed for stepwise degradation of glycosaminoglycans; accumulations of mucopolysaccharides in various tissues cause the manifestations of the disease types.
- There are six different phenotypic entities: types I through IV, VI and VII.
- The predominant abnormalities include coarse features, skeletal abnormalities leading to short stature, mental retardation, developmental delay, corneal opacities, and hepatosplenomegaly.
- Minor abnormalities in liver tests are noted.

TABLE 3-151

Multiple Myeloma[655-657]

Histology

- Portal tracts and sinusoids are infiltrated by numerous plasma cells and plasma cell precursors.
- The deposits may be large and focal.
- Sinusoidal amyloid may be seen in 3 to 8% of cases.

Clinical/Laboratory Parameters

- Hepatic involvement is characterized by hepatomegaly, mild increase in serum transaminases and alkaline phosphatase activity, and good hepatic synthetic function.
- Lytic bone lesions and hyperglobulinemia with identification of monoclonal proteins in serum and urine are characteristic.
- The extent of plasma cell infiltrates in the liver has little prognostic significance.

TABLE 3-152
Mycobacterium avium-intracellulare Infection[174,658-663]

Histology

- Epithelioid granulomas composed of lymphocytes, histiocytes, neutrophils, and occasional multinucleated giant cells are present within the portal tracts and lobules in the immunocompetent patient.
- In immunocompromised patients, striking well-circumscribed foamy histiocytes without multinucleated giant cells are seen within portal tracts and lobules; these cells contain abundant organisms (demonstrable on PAS and AFB stains).

Clinical/Laboratory Parameters

- *Mycobacterium avium-intracellulare* (MAI) infection is usually seen in immunocompromised patients, especially those with AIDS, but rarely may be present in immunocompetent individuals.
- Modest elevations in serum alkaline phosphatase activity may be noted, with little or no change in serum transaminases or serum bilirubin.
- In these patients, other opportunistic infections may be present, with the liver test abnormalities due to these infections rather than MAI infection.
- This organism can be cultured from blood and stool in infected patients; liver biopsy is rarely needed to confirm the diagnosis.

TABLE 3-153
Myeloproliferative Disorders[61,181,664,665]

Histology

- Sinusoidal dilatation is present, associated with variable degrees of intrasinusoidal collagen deposition.
- Portal vein thrombosis may occur.
- When hepatic vein thrombosis is present, sinusoidal acute hemorrhage may also be seen, in some instances associated with ischemic necrosis of perivenular hepatocytes, and secondary extravasation of red blood cells into the hepatic cords.
- Variable degrees of portal fibrosis may occur, but cirrhosis does not develop.
- Hemosiderin deposition is seen within Kupffer cells, portal macrophages, and periportal hepatocytes.
- Extramedullary hematopoiesis may be seen.

Clinical/Laboratory Parameters

- In these disorders, ranging from polycythemia rubra vera, myelofibrosis, and agnogenic myeloid metaplasia to essential thrombocythemia, a hypercoagulable state occurs, with propensity to hepatic and portal vein thrombosis.
- The clinical and laboratory features depend on the type of hematologic abnormality and the extent of vascular thrombosis, which may manifest itself as abdominal pain, hepatosplenomegaly, and/or ascites.
- Portal hypertension may be noted, but bleeding from esophageal varices is not frequent.

TABLE 3-154
Myoclonus Epilepsy (Lafora's Disease)[367,666-670]

Histology

- Round to oval, discrete, eosinophilic, PAS-positive cytoplasmic inclusions (Lafora bodies), occasionally surrounded by a clear halo, are seen in periportal hepatocytes, and stain positively with methenamine silver and colloidal iron stains.
- The inclusions have a "ground-glass" appearance on H&E stain.
- Portal and periportal fibrosis may occur without progression to cirrhosis.

Clinical/Laboratory Parameters

- In this rare autosomal recessive disorder, patients present predominantly with progressive neurologic symptoms of intractable myoclonus, leading to death from aspiration and pulmonary complications.
- Lafora bodies (intraneuronal inclusions) are identified in the brain and liver of these patients.
- Liver tests are normal or only mildly elevated.

TABLE 3-155
Neonatal Hepatitis[314,671-675]

Histology

- Giant cell transformation of perivenular liver cells is characteristic, the cells containing anywhere from 4 to more than 50 nuclei.
- These giant cell changes may involve all three zones, but may be accentuated in the perivenular zone.
- Neutrophils are occasionally present surrounding the giant cells.
- Cholestasis with variable lobular mononuclear inflammation is seen.
- Variable sinusoidal collagen deposition is often present.
- Portal tracts exhibit variable lymphocytic infiltration.
- Extramedullary hematopoiesis may occur.
- Hemosiderin in liver cell cytoplasm may be seen.
- Depending on the etiology (e.g., alpha$_1$-antitrypsin deficiency), fibrosis and biliary cirrhosis may occur.

Clinical/Laboratory Parameters

- Jaundice in the neonatal period (1 week – 2 months) is characteristic, and hepatosplenomegaly is usually present.
- Hyperbilirubinemia and moderate elevation of serum transaminases are common.
- Decrease in serum albumin and prolongation of the prothrombin time is usually mild to moderate.
- Positive antibodies to *t*oxoplasma, *o*ther infections, *r*ubella, *c*ytomegalovirus, and *h*erpesvirus (TORCH) as well as serologic testing for the hepatotropic viruses (types A, B, C) may provide an etiology.
- Alpha$_1$-antitrypsin deficiency, various metabolic disorders, and biliary tract diseases, particularly extrahepatic biliary atresia, need exclusion.

TABLE 3-156
Niemann-Pick Disease, Types B and C (Sphingomyelin-Cholesterol Lipidosis)[676-682]

Histology

- Large, vacuolated to foamy, hypertrophic, PAS-negative Kupffer cells and portal macrophages are present, which are oil red O–positive for fat on frozen section.
- Kupffer cells may also exhibit lipochrome pigment.
- In the neonate, changes of neonatal hepatitis (refer to Table 3–155) may be present.
- Intrasinusoidal collagen deposition may be seen, with liver cell atrophy.
- Cirrhosis has been reported (type B disease).
- Paucity of ducts may be seen (type C disease).

Clinical/Laboratory Parameters

- A deficiency of sphingomyelinase, a lysosomal enzyme that hydrolyses sphingomyelin, leads to the accumulation of sphingomyelin and nonesterifed cholesterol in the brain, liver, and other organs.
- Five types have been reported with varying degrees of severity.
- The predominant presentation is failure to thrive, mental retardation, and hepatosplenomegaly.
- Death usually occurs within 5 years.

TABLE 3-157
Nocardiosis (*Nocardia asteroides* and *N. brasiliensis*)[143,683-686]

Histology

- Microabscesses are present and may coalesce.
- A surrounding fibrinoid granulomatous reaction may be seen at the periphery of the abscesses.
- Organisms may be seen within neutrophils and appear as gram-positive beaded bacilli that are weakly AFB-positive and best seen by Grocott silver stain.

Clinical/Laboratory Parameters

- The skin and subcutaneous tissues are involved primarily by the formation of abscesses and draining sinuses.
- Involvement of the lungs with cavitary lesions resembles tuberculosis.
- In immunocompromised patients (usually with *N. asteroides*) other organs such as the liver, spleen, kidneys, and brain may be involved.

TABLE 3–158

Nodular Regenerative Hyperplasia[41,48,343,446,687–690]

Histology

- The liver contains numerous small, firm, and diffusely scattered white nodules ranging from 0.1 to 1.0 cm in diameter (rarely larger nodules have been described).
- Histologically the nodules are composed of cytologically benign hydropic hepatocytes bulging and expanding into the parenchyma.
- Obliterative vascular changes may be seen secondary to thrombosis and recanalization of terminal hepatic and portal veins.
- Extramedullary hematopoiesis and bile plugs have been reported, but are uncommon.

Clinical/Laboratory Parameters

- This disorder usually occurs in the adult population, and presents with features of portal hypertension (ascites, esophageal variceal hemorrhage).
- Associated disorders include myeloproliferative disease, leukemia and lymphoma, congestive heart failure, subacute bacterial endocarditis, and various autoimmune diseases (e.g., Felty's syndrome, rheumatoid arthritis).
- Physical examination may demonstrate splenomegaly.
- Liver tests are only mildly abnormal and not helpful.
- Although complications of portal hypertension require therapy, the major therapeutic approach is the treatment of the underlying disease.

TABLE 3–159

Nonalcoholic Steatohepatitis[691–699]

Histology

- Predominantly a macrovesicular fatty change is present, usually involving over 75% of hepatocytes, with no zonal distribution pattern.
- Microvesicular fat may also be seen.
- Mallory bodies are sometimes present, either in the perivenular zone or randomly distributed within the lobules, and may be surrounded by neutrophils (satellitosis).
- Both a neutrophilic and lymphocytic infiltrate is seen within the lobules, associated with mild necroinflammatory changes.
- Sinusoidal collagen deposition is usually seen, and often accentuated in the perivenular zone, sometimes associated with inflammation of the terminal hepatic venular endothelium.
- Glycogenated nuclei of hepatocytes are often present, predominantly in periportal liver cells.
- Rarely megamitochondria of hepatocytes may be present.
- Portal tracts show variable lymphocytic infiltration; although occasional neutrophils may be seen, they are uncommon.
- Variable degrees of portal fibrosis are present, with eventual progression to a micronodular cirrhosis in a minority of cases.
- Patients with diabetes mellitus may have well or poorly formed regenerative nodules in the cirrhotic stage, while patients status post jejunoileal bypass surgery usually have sharply demarcated nodules in end-stage disease.
- Noncaseating granulomas may be seen in the lobules in up to 7% of cases status post jejunoileal bypass surgery.

Clinical/Laboratory Parameters

- Although considered a disease with female preponderance, recent studies suggest that men are also affected.
- Patients may be asymptomatic, or they may complain of right upper quadrant discomfort.
- Obesity may be seen, although the disease may also develop in patients of normal weight.
- Hepatomegaly is common.
- Hyperlipidemia, diabetes mellitus (sometimes insulin-resistant), and mild iron overload may be present.
- Liver test abnormalities include mild to moderate increases in serum transaminases, with ALT almost always higher than AST (unless cirrhosis is present).
- There is normal hepatic synthetic function, usually with normal alkaline phosphatase activity and serum bilirubin (although hyperbilirubinemia may be seen in advanced disease).
- Therapy is related to the underlying condition.
- Ursodeoxycholic acid may improve liver tests, although fibrosis on biopsy remains unchanged.
- Although the course of the disease is often benign, nonetheless up to 40% of patients may develop progression of the fibrosis, with cirrhosis occurring in from 10% to 15% of patients over many years.

TABLE 3–160

Nonspecific Reactive Hepatitis[61,700]

Histology

- Portal tracts exhibit variable lymphocytic infiltration not uniformly involving all portal tracts, without piecemeal necrosis.
- Plasma cells and eosinophils can occasionally be seen within the portal structures but are not common.
- The parenchyma shows generally mild focal necrosis and hepatocytolysis; the inflammatory cells are chiefly lymphocytes, with macrophages in areas of necrosis (positive on diPAS stain).
- At times the lymphocytes may have a back-to-back arrangement within the sinusoids.
- Small microgranulomas not exhibiting multinucleated giant cells may occasionally be seen.
- Variable macrovesicular fatty change is usually present.

Clinical/Laboratory Parameters

- This entity is a secondary response of the liver to numerous extrahepatic and often systemic disorders.
- There are no distinct clinical symptoms related to the associated disorder.
- Although serum transaminases may be mildly elevated, other liver tests are normal.

TABLE 3–161

Paracoccidioidomycosis (South American Blastomycosis; *Paracoccidioides brasiliensis*)[143,704]

Histology

- Epitheliod granulomas are seen predominantly within portal tracts.
- Budding yeast forms 5 to 60 μm in diameter can be seen within the granulomas.
- Portal fibrosis may be seen without progression to cirrhosis.

Clinical/Laboratory Parameters

- Infection is recognized in rural areas of Mexico and South America.
- Humans are infected by inhalation of conidia, which are present with the soil.
- Two patterns of involvement may occur: reticuloendothelial, with hepatosplenomegaly (juvenile form), and respiratory (adult form).
- Disseminated disease involves the skin, lymph nodes, oropharynx, liver, spleen, and adrenal glands.

TABLE 3–162

Partial Nodular Transformation[48,705–708]

Histology

- Firm white nodules ranging from 3 to 40 mm in diameter are present at the hilum of the liver.
- The nodules are entirely composed of cytologically benign hydropic liver cells exhibiting prominent bulging (regeneration).

Clinical/Laboratory Parameters

- This uncommon lesion is seen in adulthood, and presents with features of portal hypertension (ascites, esophageal variceal hemorrhage).
- Serum aminotransferases may be normal, although there may be a slight rise in the alkaline phosphatase activity.
- Treatment of the portal hypertension forms the mainstay of management.

TABLE 3–163

Paucity of Intrahepatic Ducts (Intrahepatic Biliary Atresia)[709–717]: Syndromatic (Alagille's) and Nonsyndromatic

Histology

Both Syndromatic and Nonsyndromatic

- Interlobular bile ducts are absent.
- Giant cell transformation of hepatocytes is seen in the early stages.
- An increase in copper and copper-binding protein is present in periportal hepatocytes.
- Extramedullary hematopoiesis may be present.
- Portal lymphocytic infiltration is present but mild.

Syndromatic

- Destruction of interlobular ducts by lymphocytes can be see in the first 3 to 6 months.
- Cholestasis in zone 3 with mononuclear inflammatory infiltrates is present and is most prominent by 1 year.
- Portal fibrosis may occur with time, but does *not* progress to cirrhosis.

Nonsyndromatic

- Cholestasis in zone 3 with mild mononuclear inflammatory infiltrate is present within the first 90 days.
- Diffuse interstitial fibrosis may occur.
- Portal fibrosis progressing to biliary cirrhosis may occur.

Clinical/Laboratory Parameters

- Also termed *arteriohepatic dysplasia,* paucity of duct syndrome presents during the first few months of life with jaundice and pruritus, the latter often intense.
- Hepatomegaly is common.
- Hyperbilirubinemia, with slight elevation of the serum transaminases, and hypercholesterolemia are present.
- In the *syndromatic* form, extrahepatic manifestations are distinctive, with broad forehead, hypertelorism, vertebral arch defects, peripheral pulmonic stenosis, short stature, and renal abnormalities.
- The *nonsyndromatic* form does not have the described clinical features; in some cases, there may be rapid progression to cirrhosis.

TABLE 3–164

Peliosis Hepatis[154,156,630,689,718–722]

Histology

- Lysis of reticulin fibers occurs randomly within the lobules, with predominantly microcyst formation. The cysts are filled with red blood cells and communicate with adjacent dilated sinusoids containing variable atrophic liver cells.
- Fibrin may initially be present along the cyst walls, which are partially devoid of endothelial cells; new vessel formation within the fibrin stroma may be seen.
- In patients with AIDS, bacillary angiomatosis (refer to Table 3–35) can occur; in these patients, the cysts may become larger (up to 2 cm in diameter) and are detectable on imaging.
- In rare instances, microcalcifications may be seen.
- Peliotic cysts may be seen in various neoplasms (e.g., liver cell adenoma, fibrolamellar hepatocellular carcinoma).

Clinical/Laboratory Parameters

- Peliosis hepatis is a relatively benign condition seen in association with the use of androgenic and anabolic steroids, with chronic debilitating diseases such as tuberculosis and AIDS, and in patients after renal transplantation.
- Splenic cysts may also be present.
- Liver tests are normal except when associated with steroid therapy, in which hyperbilirubinemia, mild transaminase elevations, and hypoalbuminemia have been observed.
- Most patients are asymptomatic, with hepatomegaly sometimes seen.
- In rare instances death may occur due to rupture and secondary intra-abdominal hemorrhage.

TABLE 3-165
Penicilliosis *(Penicillium marneffei)*[143,723-725]

Histology

- Epithelioid granulomas may be present within the parenchyma.
- A diffuse form may also be seen, with nonbudding organisms 5 × 2 μm in diameter within hypertrophic Kupffer cells and histiocytes.

Clinical/Laboratory Parameters

- This infection, caused by molds (hyalohyphomycosis), is prevalent in Southeast Asia and is increasingly seen in patients with AIDS and those receiving cancer chemotherapy.
- The majority (75%) of patients develop a variety of skin lesions ranging from umbilicated papules mistaken for molluscum contagiosum, ecthymiform lesions, folliculitis, subcutaneous nodules, and morbilliform eruptions.
- The liver and spleen are involved in disseminated disease.

TABLE 3-166
Pentastomiasis *(Armillifer [Porocephalus] armillatus)*[143,726-728]

Histology

- Fibrotic calcified and rarely cystic nodules 5 to 10 mm in diameter enclosing dead parasites are seen.

Clinical/Laboratory Parameters

- This larva, referred to as tongue worm, is present in rodents and herbivorous animals that ingest *Armillifer* eggs, with the deposition of larvae in the animal's muscles and other organs.
- Humans are infected by drinking water contaminated by these eggs, or by consuming raw tissues of herbivorous hosts.
- Encysted larvae are found in the mesentery, lung, liver, and peritoneal cavity.

TABLE 3-167
Perivenular Fibrosis, Alcoholic Etiology[21,31,32,36,729]

Histology

- Sinusoidal collagen deposition within the perivenular region is seen to various degrees in all forms of alcoholic liver disease.
- A thin rim of collagen involving at least two thirds of the terminal hepatic venules, with variable intimal fibrosis, is present; occasionally endothelial inflammation of the venules is seen.
- Variable periportal sinusoidal collagen deposition is also seen.
- Macrovesicular fatty change is usually present.

Clinical/Laboratory Parameters

- Patients with alcoholic perivenular fibrosis have a greater propensity to develop ascites since there is a physiologic hepatic venous outflow block.
- Physical examination may demonstrate stigmata of chronic liver disease, with hepatomegaly and infrequently splenomegaly.
- Serum transaminases are usually mildly elevated with the AST greater than the ALT, but both usually below 100 IU/L.
- In active alcoholic patients, decompensation may be manifested by elevated serum bilirubin, hypoalbuminemia, and prolongation of the prothrombin time.

TABLE 3-168

Pneumocystis carinii Infection[143,730–735]

Histology

- In AIDS patients, focally widened sinusoids with patchy liver cell necrosis but little inflammation are present.
- Focal areas of frothy eosinophilic material containing small, pale cysts with a few basophilic dots are seen on hematoxylin-eosin stain; the organisms are best demonstrated as oval or cup-shaped folded cysts 4 to 6 μm in diameter on methenamine silver stain.

Clinical/Laboratory Parameters

- *Pneumocystis* is a eukaryotic microbe with morphologic features similar to fungi, but it is neither a true fungus nor a protozoan.
- The ubiquitous organism is acquired by the airborne route.
- Fever, nonproductive cough, and shortness of breath are characteristic.
- Slight increase in serum aminotransferases may be present with liver involvement.
- Lymph nodes, heart, pancreas, liver, spleen, brain, thyroid, and kidneys may be involved in disseminated disease (usually in patients with low CD4 counts) with multiorgan failure and death often occurring.

TABLE 3-169

Polyarteritis Nodosa[690,736–739]

Histology

- Segmental and destructive fibrinoid necrosis of small and medium-sized hepatic arteries is present.
- A mixed acute and chronic inflammatory infiltrate including eosinophils is present within portal tracts, primarily involving the vascular wall and lumen of the medium-sized arteries, often with vascular thrombosis.
- Granulomatous vasculitis with giant cells may be present.
- Cholestasis, secondary involvement of portal vein branches, and lobular ischemic necrosis may also be seen in severe cases.
- Fibrointimal fibrosis with eventual scarring occurs in advanced end-stage lesions.
- The small arterioles within the portal tracts are usually spared.

Clinical/Laboratory Parameters

- Polyarteritis nodosa is an inflammatory, necrotizing process seen in a variety of rheumatologic and autoimmune diseases.
- An association with chronic hepatitis B infection has been reported that appears to be of low frequency.
- Manifestations of the disease include skin rash, arthritis or arthralgia, and fatique.
- Renal involvement is characterized by proteinuria and an active urinary sediment.
- Mild increases in serum transaminases and modest increases in alkaline phosphatase activity are noted.
- Serum bilirubin is not usually elevated unless the underlying disease process is active.
- Autoimmune markers (antinuclear antibody, rheumatoid factor, anti-DNA) may be variably positive.
- Arteriography of the hepatic vasculature may demonstrate pseudoaneurysms.

TABLE 3-170

Polymyalgia Rheumatica[740–744]

Histology

- Portal lymphocytic infiltration is present and may be prominent, with mild focal necrosis and predominantly macrovesicular fatty change within the lobules.
- Granulomas have been reported.

Clinical/Laboratory Parameters

- This vasculitic disorder is seen in the elderly population, who develop pain and stiffness of the proximal upper limbs and shoulders.
- A minority of patients may have increased alkaline phosphatase activity.
- Temporal arteritis and central retinal venous occlusion are associated.

TABLE 3-171

Porphyria Cutanea Tarda[304,745-750]

Histology

- Needle-shaped birefringent cytoplasmic inclusions (uroporphyrin) are seen in hepatocytes on hematoxylin-eosin stain, best identified under polarized light using unstained paraffin sections.
- Intense red autofluorescence of uroporphyrin on frozen sections is present.
- There are variable degrees of macrovesicular fatty change
- Hemosiderin in periportal hepatocytes is often seen.
- Portal tracts may exhibit prominent lymphocytic infiltration surrounding but not infiltrating ducts.
- Focal lobular necrosis and mononuclear inflammation is common but usually mild.
- Fibrosis progressing to micronodular cirrhosis can be seen, in some instances secondary to chronic alcoholism or chronic HCV infection.

Clinical/Laboratory Parameters

- An inherited or acquired defect of uroporphyrinogen decarboxylase, the disease manifests with photosensitivity and uroprophyrinuria.
- The skin is fragile, with vesiculations, hypo- and hyperpigmentation, sclerodermatous change, and facial hypertrichosis.
- Excessive iron accumulation in the liver, use of certain drugs such as estrogen or chloroquine, chronic alcoholism, or chronic hepatitis type C may exacerbate the uroporphyrinuria and clinical manifestations.
- Phlebotomy ameliorates the photosensitivity and correlates with decline in uroporphyrin levels.

TABLE 3-172

Primary Biliary Cirrhosis[151,152,506,751-757]

Histology

- Nonsuppurative, destructive interlobular duct lesions are present, primarily involving ducts 40 to 80 μm in diameter, with lymphocytes surrounding and invading ducts showing cytoplasmic vacuolization, nuclear pyknosis, and occasional epithelial hyperplasia.
- Neutrophils, plasma cells, and occasional eosinophils can also be seen within portal tracts; in rare instances, neutrophils may invade duct epithelium, resembling acute cholangitis.
- Although portal inflammatory cells often spill over into the adjacent periportal zones, in approximately 15% of cases true piecemeal necrosis can be seen.
- Epithelioid granulomas are seen in 25% of cases, more frequently in the early stage; the granulomas are often adjacent to or surrounding injured ducts.
- Lobules with variable lymphocytic infiltration and focal necrosis are present, the inflammation more common in the periportal zones.
- At the fibrotic stage, interlobular ducts disappear, associated with prominent atypical cholangiolar proliferation characterized by scanty to absent lumen, epithelial flattening, nuclear hyperchromasia, and serpentine growth pattern.
- Bridging fibrosis eventually occurs, leading to cirrhosis (biliary type with jigsaw growth pattern of the regenerative nodules) associated with severe ductopenia.
- Cholestasis is unusual until later stages of the disease, where bile plugs often appear in the periportal zone and within dilated cholangioles.
- Mallory bodies may be present in periportal hepatocytes, especially in the later stage of the disease.
- Prominent amounts of copper and copper-binding protein are present in periportal and periseptal hepatocytes in late-stage disease.

Clinical/Laboratory Parameters

- A chronic cholestatic disease of uncertain etiology, this disease primarily affects middle-aged women who frequently are asymptomatic, but may initially present with pruritus and fatigue.
- Bone pain with osteopenia, symptoms related to associated CREST (calcinosis, Raynaud's phenomenon, esophageal dysmotility, sclerodactyly, telangiectasias) and sicca syndromes, and steatorrhea may be present.
- Hepatosplenomegaly and xanthelasmas may be present on physical examination; with advancing disease, portal hypertension, ascites, bleeding esophageal varices, and encephalopathy develop.
- Jaundice is noted in advanced disease with increasing levels indicative of poor prognosis.
- Isolated moderate to marked elevation of alkaline phosphatase activity with or without mild increase in serum transaminases provides clues to the diagnosis, which is confirmed by positive antimitochondrial antibody (AMA), normal bile ducts on endoscopic retrograde cholangiopancreatography, and elevated serum cholesterol, fasting bile acid, and IgM levels.
- Since AMA has been shown to be positive in other liver diseases (e.g., autoimmune hepatitis, primary sclerosing cholangitis), depending on the mode of testing, its further characterization into the M2 fraction shows this to be most specific for primary biliary cirrhosis in some, but not all, series.
- Although there are cases of patients with primary biliary cirrhosis with normal or near-normal alkaline phosphatase activity, this feature is not common.
- Management includes various drugs such as ursodeoxycholic acid; liver transplantation is the definitive treatment in advanced disease.

TABLE 3-173

Primary Sclerosing Cholangitis[151,212,506,755,758-766]

Histology

- Fibro-obliterative "onion skin" periductal fibrosis is seen primarily involving large to medium-sized ducts, with degeneration and atrophy of duct epithelium, and eventual replacement of ducts by fibrous tissue.
- Smaller ducts may also be involved, either in conjunction with larger ducts or alone (small duct lesions), with cytologic atypia of duct epithelium.
- Portal tracts exhibit lymphocytic infiltration with occasional plasma cells and eosinophils; these inflammatory cells are often oriented around ducts.
- Piecemeal necrosis may be seen in a minority of patients.
- Segmental involvement of ducts may be present, and responsible for some ducts exhibiting changes characteristic of obstruction, with acute cholangitis and cholangiolitis; in addition, only one main hepatic duct may be involved, resulting in focal hepatic involvement (hemicirrhosis).
- Lobules may exhibit mononuclear inflammatory changes, which when present are usually periportal.
- Variable degrees of macrovesicular fatty change may be present.
- Cholestasis is present, at first perivenular, then periseptal in later stages of disease.
- As the disease progresses, portal fibrosis occurs with loss of interlobular ducts associated with variable cholangiolar proliferation.
- Eventually bridging fibrosis occurs with biliary cirrhosis and severe ductopenia.
- Mallory bodies, copper, and copper-binding protein are present in periportal and periseptal hepatocytes as the disease progresses.
- In the extraheaptic bile ducts and large intrahepatic ducts at the hilum, variable duct damage occurs, with fibrosis, saccular dilatation, ulceration, xanthomatous proliferation, and bile impregnation.
- Acquired variants are seen with AIDS (CMV infection), status post rupture of hydatid cysts, and certain drugs (e.g., fluorodeoxyuridine).
- Cholangiocarcinoma is a known complication.

Clinical/Laboratory Parameters

- This chronic cholestatic disorder affects predominantly young to middle-aged men, associated in 50 to 75% of cases with chronic ulcerative colitis.
- The clinical course is punctuated by recurrent episodes of jaundice, fever, abdominal pain, and pruritus.
- The diagnosis is confirmed by the characteristic segmental obliteration (beading) of the intra- and extrahepatic bile ducts on endoscopic retrograde cholangiopancreatography.
- During episodes of cholangitis, increases in serum bilirubin and alkaline phosphatase activity are common.
- Hepatic synthetic function is well preserved unless the disease is advanced.
- Hepatosplenomegaly is a frequent finding.
- Other associated diseases include pancreatitis, rheumatoid arthritis, Sjögren's syndrome, systemic lupus erythematosus, and bronchiectasis.
- The development of portal hypertension, ascites, and bleeding esophageal varices indicates advanced disease.
- Management includes operative or endoscopic stenting of biliary tract strictures.
- The risk of cholangiocarcinoma is increased, and occurs in up to 15% of patients, especially in those with coexisting chronic ulcerative colitis.
- Liver transplantation is the definitive therapy in advanced or clinically intractable disease.

TABLE 3–174

Progressive Familial Intrahepatic Cholestasis (Byler's Syndrome)[712,767–772]

Histology

- Cholestasis in the perivenular zone is present in the early stage, with rosette formation and syncytial giant cell transformation of hepatocytes.
- Bile duct proliferation is seen in the early stages, with eventual progression to duct loss. Ducts that are present may exhibit epithelial damage without accompanying inflammation.
- Biliary fibrosis eventually occurs with progression to secondary biliary cirrhosis.
- An increase in copper and copper-binding protein is seen in periportal and periseptal hepatocytes.

Clinical/Laboratory Parameters

- First described in Amish kindred (Byler) and of unknown etiology, this disorder is characterized by pruritus, jaundice, hepatosplenomegaly, and steatorrhea occurring between 1 and 10 months of age.
- Growth retardation and mental retardation have been reported.
- Rickets can be present in undiagnosed cases but xanthomas do not occur.
- Laboratory tests confirm elevated serum bilirubin and alkaline phosphatase activity, but the serum cholesterol is not increased.
- Prolongation of prothrombin time also occurs that is not corrected by vitamin K in advanced disease.
- Most patients die between 2 and 15 years of age; hepatocellular carcinoma has been reported.
- Liver transplantation is the definitive therapy.

TABLE 3–175

Progressive Perivenular Alcoholic Fibrosis[21,37,773]

Histology

- Sinusoidal fibrosis in zone 3 is dense, with virtual obliteration of the vascular lumen of the terminal hepatic venules; the adjacent hepatocytes are arranged in straight cords, without regenerative activity.
- Occasionally endothelial inflammation of the venules is seen.
- Variable degrees of periportal intrasinusoidal collagen deposition are seen.
- Macrovesicular fatty change is usually present.

Clinical/Laboratory Parameters

- Also termed *chronic sclerosing hyaline necrosis* in the older literature, this chronic alcoholic liver disease may follow acute attacks, but more often is indolent.
- Patients present with manifestations of chronic liver disease, including ascites that usually is not responsive to diuretic therapy, esophageal varices, muscle wasting, and eventual hepatic and renal failure *(hepatorenal syndrome)*.

TABLE 3–176

Pylephlebitis[774–777]

Histology

- The portal veins are surrounded and infiltrated by neutrophils, often with portal vein thrombosis.
- Endothelial swelling and sloughing of affected portal veins may also be seen.
- Microabscess formation involving portal tracts and lobules may be present in severe or untreated cases.

Clinical/Laboratory Parameters

- Pylephlebitis is a thrombophlebitis of the portal vein and its intrahepatic branches, and occurs as a consequence of intra-abdominal sepsis, intrahepatic infections and abscesses, or infection involving the umbilical veins, which extend into the left portal vein and its radicles.
- Patients are febrile and jaundiced and may develop septic shock.
- Hyperbilirubinemia is common and may be marked.
- Modest increases in serum transaminases, hypoalbuminemia, and prolongation of the prothrombin time are observed.
- Elevation in alkaline phosphatase activity is usually moderate but may be marked (up to 1000 IU/L).

TABLE 3–177

Pyogenic Abscesses[116,117,778–782]

Histology

- In severe cases of bacterial sepsis (refer to Table 3–36), microabscesses may be present initially within the portal tracts; however, eventual involvement of the lobules in untreated cases may occur with confluent lobular necrosis and enlarged pyogenic abscess formation.
- Portal tracts adjacent to the abscesses may often show acute cholangitis.
- Organisms in some cases may be demonstrable in the abscess on Gram stain.

Clinical/Laboratory Parameters

- Patients may present with jaundice, elevations of serum alkaline phosphatase activity, and mild increases in transaminases.
- Hypoalbuminemia, anemia, and leukocytosis are frequent.
- The severity of hyperbilirubinemia is greater than seen with amebic abscess formation.
- The lesion is easily demonstrable on imaging.

TABLE 3–178

Q Fever *(Coxiella burnetii)*[174,783–788]

Histology

- Granulomas are present in both portal tracts and lobules, and are composed of lymphocytes, histiocytes, and occasional eosinophils and neutrophils. Epithelioid cells and multinucleated giant cells can occasionally be seen but are not common.
- Typically the "doughnut" lesion *(ring granuloma)* is present and consists of a granuloma with a central fat vacuole or clear space surrounded by a fibrin ring (phosphotungstic acid–hematoxylin [PTAH]-positive).
- Granulomas are often present without central fat vacuoles.
- Coalescence of granulomas may occur.
- Moderate portal lymphocytic and plasma cell infiltration is present; mild lobular necrosis and lymphocytic infiltration in addition to granuloma formation may also be seen.
- Resolution of granulomas may lead to fibrous scarring.
- A moderate degree of macrovesicular fatty change is present.
- Note that ring granulomas, although characteristic of Q fever, may also be seen in Epstein-Barr virus and cytomegalovirus infections, leishmaniasis, staphylococcal bacteremia, certain types of lymphoma, and allopurinol hepatotoxicity.

Clinical/Laboratory Parameters

- This worldwide infection is caused by *Coxiella burnetii,* a pleomorphic intracellular rickettsial organism.
- The organisms are transferred by a tick vector, but infection is most often acquired by inhalation and less commonly by ingestion of infected food products derived from livestock (cattle, goats, sheep) and birds.
- The majority of infections are symptomatic and self-limited; fever, hepatitis, and pneumonitis may be present to variable degrees.
- In significant infections, high-grade fever, endocarditis, hepatosplenomegaly, moderate increases in serum transaminases and alkaline phosphatase activity, and mild increase in serum bilirubin values are seen.
- Diagnosis is confirmed by serologic studies (antibody titers to phase 1 and 2 antigens).

TABLE 3–179

Recurrent Cholestasis with Lymphedema (Norwegian Cholestasis)[789,790]

Histology

- Cholestasis in the perivenular zone is present in the early stage, associated with rosette formation and syncytial giant cell transformation of hepatocytes.
- Although bile duct proliferation is seen in the early stages, eventual progression to ductopenia occurs; the remaining ducts may show epithelial damage without accompanying inflammation.
- Biliary fibrosis eventually occurs with progression to secondary biliary cirrhosis.
- An increase in copper and copper-binding protein is seen in periportal and periseptal hepatocytes.

Clinical/Laboratory Parameters

- This disorder of unknown mechanism was first described in Norwegian infants born to consanguineous parents.
- Patients present with jaundice, failure to thrive, rickets, anemia, bleeding tendencies, and lymphedema involving the lower extremities.
- Cholestasis fluctuates after the first 6 years of life.
- Serum bilirubin and alkaline phosphatase activity are elevated with decrease in prothrombin time.
- Serum cholesterol and triglycerides are also elevated.
- Lymphangiography demonstrates an absence of deep lymphatics.

TABLE 3–180

Recurrent Intrahepatic Cholestasis of Pregnancy[22,26,29,791–794]

Histology

- Cholestasis is seen in the perivenular zone, in some instances accompanied by a mild mononuclear inflammatory infiltrate.
- Syncytial giant cell transformation of hepatocytes may be seen, which is more prominent in the perivenular zone.
- Portal tracts exhibit a mild lymphocytic infiltration.

Clinical/Laboratory Parameters

- This disorder is characterized by the development of pruritus during pregnancy, usually during the third trimester.
- The pruritus spontaneously resolves following delivery.
- These patients develop similar symptoms on oral contraceptives.
- Mild elevations of serum transaminases and alkaline phosphatase activity may be seen but hepatic synthetic function is normal.

TABLE 3–181

Recurrent Pyogenic Cholangiohepatitis[795–799]

Histology

- Dilated intra- and extrahepatic bile ducts are present and often prominent.
- These duct changes may be diffuse or focal (segmental).
- Parasitic infestation of large ducts (most notably *Ascaris* and *Clonorchis*) may also be present, with secondary sclerosing cholangitis and segmental narrowing of the common bile duct.
- Pylephlebitis of the portal vein may occur, rarely associated with lobular infarction.
- Calculi are common, associated with secondary changes of large duct obstruction, including duct proliferation and ectasia, acute cholangitis, periductal fibrosis, cholestasis, and abscess formation.

Clinical/Laboratory Parameters

- This disease is common in Asia and associated frequently with the liver fluke *Clonorchis sinensis* (refer to Table 3–55); the clinical course is characterized by repeated episodes of jaundice, fever, and abdominal pain due to acute cholangitis.
- The disease is also seen in other geographic areas not endemic for *Clonorchis;* ascariasis has also been implicated.
- During episodes, leukocytosis, hyperbilirubinemia, elevated alkaline phosphatase activity, and mild increases in serum transaminases are noted.
- Cholangiography demonstrates strictures of the intrahepatic bile ducts.
- Liver abscesses occur frequently, and atrophy of the liver lobes, usually the left, has been reported.

TABLE 3–182

Reye's Syndrome[800–806]

Histology

- The liver is grossly yellow, with panacinar micro-vesicular fatty change involving virtually all hepato-cytes.
- The liver cells may microscopically appear swollen and vacuolated, whereby the fat may not be appreciated on H&E stain, especially during the first 24 hours; these cells, however, are strongly positive for lipid on the oil red O and Sudan black B stains (performed on frozen sections of fresh or formalin-fixed tissue).
- The fat droplets may be smaller in zone 3.
- The liver cell nuclei are centrally located due to diffuse fat within the cytoplasm.
- Liver cell necrosis and portal inflammation are minimal to absent.
- Irregular cytoplasmic inclusions may be present, representing distorted mitochondria.

Clinical/Laboratory Parameters

- Reye's syndrome is seen in association with viral influenza epidemics and is perhaps potentiated by aspirin use.
- This disorder usually affects children but does not exclude young adults.
- The syndrome develops after a prodromal viral-type illness followed by vomiting and alteration of sensorium, and may progress rapidly to coma, seizures, and death.
- Elevation of serum transaminases (AST, ALT), prolongation of prothrombin time, hypoglycemia, and hyperammonemia are typical laboratory findings.
- The cerebrospinal fluid is usually normal.
- Mortality is about 40%; liver transplantation is life-saving in patients with liver failure.

TABLE 3–183

Rheumatoid Arthritis[807–811]

Histology

- Portal lymphocytic infiltration is seen, with associated mild lobular mononuclear inflammatory infiltration; in Felty's syndrome, prominent sinusoidal lymphocytosis may also be seen.
- Variable, predominantly macrovescular fatty change is present.
- Sinusoidal dilatation may also be seen.
- Lipogranulomas have been described in association with gold therapy (pigmented gold particles in granuloma).
- Arteritis may be seen, with secondary infarction and hemorrhage within the lobules.
- Nodular regenerative hyperplasia (refer to Table 3–158) has been reported but is uncommon.

Clinical/Laboratory Parameters

- Most patients with rheumatoid arthritis do not have hepatic manifestations, although approximately 10% of patients may have enlarged livers with abnormal alkaline phosphatase activity (biliary origin).
- The serum transaminases are almost always normal; however, when elevated, the cause relates to drugs used in therapy of rheumatoid arthritis rather than the arthritis itself.
- In Felty's syndrome, hepatomegaly is common, and patients may have some evidence of portal hypertension (ascites, esophageal varices).

TABLE 3–184

Rubella Virus Infection[143,812–815]

Histology

- Features of neonatal hepatitis (refer to Table 3–155) may be present.
- In mild cases, nonspecific focal necrosis, cholestasis, and lymphocytic infiltration may be seen.
- Massive hepatic necrosis may occur but is uncommon.
- Ductopenia has been described but is infrequent.

Clinical/Laboratory Parameters

- This RNA virus causes a benign, self-limited infection in humans that is manifested by mild fever, suboccipital lymphadenopathy, and skin rash.
- Congenital rubella syndrome from intrauterine infection causes growth and mental retardation, deafness, congenital heart disease, corneal opacities, cataracts, retinopathy, and meningoencephalitis; late manifestations include immunodeficiency.
- Hepatic manifestations include hepatosplenomegaly and modest increase in serum transaminases with normal or mild increase in serum bilirubin.
- Serologic diagnosis is made by the presence of acute and convalescent hemagglutination inhibition antibodies.

TABLE 3–185

Rubeola Virus Infection[816,817]

Histology

- Variable degrees of portal lymphocytic infiltration are seen.
- Lobular mononuclear inflammation and focal necrosis are present but are generally mild.
- Fatty change may be present.
- Syncytial giant cells and viral inclusions are rare but have been reported; however, inclusions are not typically seen in patients with AIDS.

Clinical/Laboratory Parameters

- This highly contagious RNA virus causes an exanthematous infection with fever, cough, coryza, and conjunctivitis developing after an incubation period of 8 to 12 days.
- In severe hemorrhagic measles, seizures, mucosal bleeding, and DIC can occur.
- Transient anicteric hepatitis characterized by mild to moderate increases in serum transaminases may develop, with rare hyperbilirubinemia.
- Serologic tests by complement fixation, hemagglutination inhibition, and enzyme immunoassays confirm the diagnosis.

TABLE 3–186

Salmonellosis (Typhoid Fever; *Salmonella typhi*)[818–823]

Histology

- Portal lymphocytic infiltration is present and may be prominent.
- Bile ducts may rarely show acute cholangitis.
- Clusters of well to poorly formed granulomas consisting of histiocytes and Kupffer cells are seen within the lobule *(typhoid nodule)*; sometimes larger granulomas undergo central necrosis.
- The granulomas are randomly distributed within the lobule, but may have a slight periportal accentuation.
- Sinusoidal lymphocytosis is seen.
- Focal necrosis is present within the lobule, but is generally mild.
- Prominent hypertrophic and hyperplastic Kupffer cells are present, sometimes exhibiting erythrophagocytosis.
- Microvesicular fatty change may be seen.
- Endothelialitis of portal, terminal hepatic, or sublobular veins may be present.

Clinical/Laboratory Parameters

- The infection caused by the gram-negative aerobic organism *Salmonella typhi* is acquired by ingesting food and water contaminated by this organism.
- The incubation period is 14 days; the infection can last 2 to 3 weeks and is characterized by fever, headache, malaise, prostration, diarrhea (in the first week), and delirium or rarely coma.
- An evanescent skin rash (rose spots) may develop in the second week.
- Intestinal hemorrhage and perforation in the 2nd to 3rd weeks and encephalopathy are associated with a poor prognosis.
- Rarely, pneumonia, meningitis, myocarditis, and osteomyelitis (in patients with sickle cell disease) may be seen.
- Splenomegaly is seen in 60 to 75% of cases; hepatomegaly is mild and liver tests are modestly abnormal.
- The diagnosis is confirmed by blood culture in the first week and positive serologic tests (Widal reaction) with high titers of antibodies against somatic O antigen.

TABLE 3–187
Sarcoidosis[174,176,464,512,824–828]

Histology

- Epithelioid granulomas are present, composed of transformed activated macrophages, occasional multinucleated giant cells, and scattered lymphocytes.
- The granulomas may be seen diffusely throughout the lobules, but are usually more prominent within portal tracts and periportal regions.
- The granulomas may contain Schaumann bodies (concentric basophilic laminations) and asteroid bodies (spindly radiating star-like structures within epithelioid cells).
- Central fibrinoid necrosis may be seen but is not common.
- The granulomas may coalesce, forming small mass lesions that can be visualized on imaging.
- Fibrous bands can surround and infiltrate into the granulomas, forming septate divisions, a feature characteristic of sarcoidosis but unusual in other causes of granulomas.
- Eventually resolution of granuloma with scar tissue can occur.
- The portal tracts exhibit variable degrees of lymphocytic infiltration.
- The lobules may exhibit mild focal necrosis and lymphocytic infiltration.
- Endothelial damage of outflow vessels may be seen but is uncommon.
- Cholestasis may be present but is uncommon; however, nonsuppurative lesions resembling those seen in primary biliary cirrhosis (refer to Table 3–172) can occur, with eventual biliary cirrhosis and ductopenia; note that these patients are negative for antimitochondrial antibody.
- Portal fibrosis (21% of cases) and cirrhosis (6% of cases) may occur.

Clinical/Laboratory Parameters

- A systemic inflammatory disease of uncertain etiology, sarcoidosis is characterized by epithelioid granulomas in many organs, chiefly the lung and liver, with a predilection for this disease among African American women.
- The clinical presentation is variable, ranging from the asymptomatic patient with elevated alkaline phosphatase activity to the febrile patient with hepatomegaly, hypercalcemia, hilar lymphadenopathy, interstitial lung disease, and rarely jaundice and features of portal hypertension.
- The commonest liver test abnormality is the elevation of serum alkaline phosphatase (approximately six times normal), with mild elevation in transaminases.
- Serum bilirubin is normal or mildly elevated except in a small subset of patients in whom marked hyperbilirubinemia has been observed.
- Hepatic synthetic function is usually well preserved.
- The presence of uveal findings on slit lamp examination and positive angiotensin-converting enzyme may be helpful in the diagnosis in some patients.

TABLE 3–188

Schistosomiasis (Schistosoma mansoni, S. japonicum, and S. mekongi) [143,174,464,829–836]

Histology

- The liver is firm with a thickened outer capsule; "clay-pipestem" fibrosis is characterized by thickened white stellate tracts involving the larger portal structures.
- *S. mansoni* is 60 × 140 μm in diameter with a lateral spine, while *S. japonicum* and *S. mekongi* are smaller with a lateral knob. These features are often seen on routine H & E sections.
- Rarely an adult worm may be demonstrated in the portal vein.
- In the early lesion, live eggs in portal venous radicles are surrounded by eosinophils forming an abscess (which may demonstrate Charcot-Leyden crystals); eventually these are replaced by an epithelioid granuloma with eosinophils at the periphery.
- Gray-black pigment (resembling hemozoin) is seen within the eggs but also within the macrophages of the granuloma, portal macrophages, and Kupffer cells.
- After a few weeks the eggs die, degenerate, and become empty shells that may calcify without inflammation.
- Portal fibrosis eventually occurs, with prominent perigranulomatous lamellar-type fibrosis ("pipestem" lesion); the granulomas eventually disappear and are replaced by fibrous scar.
- Ova and granuloma may occur within portal veins (endophlebitis), with thrombosis, fibrous obliteration, and decrease in portal venous radicals.
- As the ova disappear, the collagen in the portal tracts becomes dense, with variable periportal sinusoidal collagen deposition, without development of cirrhosis.

Clinical/Laboratory Parameters

- Humans are the definitive hosts for these helminths, which reside in the intestinal tributaries of the portal venous system.
- Eggs are laid and shed either through the urinary bladder (*S. japonicum*) or stool (*S. mansoni*).
- Larvae hatched from eggs in the water (rivers and streams contaminated by effluents) enter snails (intermediate host) and form sporocysts from which cercariae develop and eventually break out of the snail into the water.
- The cercariae eventually penetrate the skin of humans (who swim or bathe in these waters) and travel the lymphatics to the lungs and the liver, where they enter the portal venous system and eventually end in the tributaries by retrograde migration.
- Eggs in the tissues provoke a host immune response with granuloma formation and fibrosis.
- Patients with acute infection (Katayama disease) present with fever, chills, hepatomegaly, lymphadenopathy, and eosinophilia.
- A small percentage of these patients may go on to develop chronic liver disease, with melena, esophageal varices, ascites, and hepatosplenomegaly.
- Minor elevations in serum transaminases and alkaline phoshatase activity may be seen.
- The diagnosis is confirmed by recognition of the eggs in stool or biopsy specimens and by serologic tests.

TABLE 3–189

Sickle Cell Anemia [837–842]

Histology

- Aggregates of clumped, crescent-shaped, red blood cells admixed with fibrin thrombi are present within the sinusoids, this feature most prominent in the perivenular zone. In severe cases, coagulative necrosis of perivenular hepatocytes may occur.
- Perivenular sinusoidal congestion and dilatation are present; this feature may at times, however, be diffuse.
- Variable sinusoidal collagen deposition may be seen with time in the perivenular zone secondary to numerous episodes of hepatic venous outflow obstruction from sludged red blood cells within terminal hepatic venules.
- Hepatic vein thrombosis may also occur.
- Hemosiderin is seen in hyperplastic Kupffer cells, portal macrophages, and periportal hepatocytes.
- Macrovesicular fatty change is occasionally seen.
- Extramedullary hematopoiesis may be present secondary to chronic hemolysis.

Clinical/Laboratory Parameters

- Sickle cell anemia (homozygous HbSS) is a severe, genetically inherited hemolytic disorder that usually first manifests in childhood.
- Patients may develop hepatic crises related to sickling of the red blood cells within the hepatic sinusoids, characterized by right upper quadrant abdominal pain, fever, hyperbilirubinemia (may be marked with indirect predominance), and moderate to marked increases in the serum transaminases (due to ischemia).
- Hepatic synthetic function is mildly abnormal, but in severe cases progression to liver failure has been reported.
- Other associated disorders include cholecystitis and choledocholithiasis (usually due to pigmented stones), jaundice (due to sepsis), and hemosiderosis.
- Rarely hepatic vein thrombosis has been reported.

TABLE 3-190

Solitary Nonparasitic Cyst[65,843-847]

Histology

- The cysts are usually unilocular (95% cases), round to oval, well-encapsulated, rarely pedunculated, and contain considerable (up to 17 L reported) fluid (serous, mucoid, bile-stained, and purulent [secondary to superinfection]).
- The right lobe is involved twice as often as the left lobe.
- The cysts are lined by a single layer of cuboidal to flattened duct epithelium with adjacent well-demarcated fibrous bands.
- The cyst wall may contain macrophages, hemosiderin, cholesterol crystals, and foreign body giant cells.
- Cysts may collapse, the smaller resembling corpora atretica of the ovary.
- Von Meyenberg complexes may be present adjacent to the cyst.
- Multilocular cysts occur in 5% of cases.
- Microcalcifications may occur.

Clinical/Laboratory Parameters

- The lesions are discovered incidentally by scanning modalities or when hepatomegaly is detected on abdominal examination.
- Patients are usually asymptomatic except when the cyst is extremely large, when bleeding into the cyst develops, or when spontaneous rupture occurs.
- Management is conservative.

TABLE 3-191

Spontaneous Rupture in Pregnancy[848-850]

Histology

- Focal but predominantly subcapsular acute hemorrhage occurs with rupture.
- Secondary ischemic coagulative necrosis of hepatocytes in hemorrhagic regions are often present.

Clinical/Laboratory Parameters

- This rare but potentially fatal condition is seen in pregnancy-induced hypertension, may be associated with the HELLP syndrome, or may be idiopathic.
- Patients usually in the third trimester of pregnancy present with an acute onset of severe right upper quadrant or epigastric abdominal pain; anemia followed by hypotension, shock, and death will occur without treatment.
- Abdominal tenderness, guarding, and distention related to blood in the peritoneal cavity may be present.
- Ultrasound and CT scans of the abdomen confirm the presence of a large subcapsular hematoma of the liver with free blood in the peritoneal cavity.
- Emergent cesarean section if presentation occurs prior to delivery, and efforts to stem bleeding from the liver (including hepatic lobectomy), may be necessary.
- Recovery occurs if rupture is managed expediently, with no apparent risk of recurrence in subsequent pregnancies.

TABLE 3–192

Strongyloidiasis *(Strongyloides stercoralis)* [143,851,852]

Histology

- Larvae (600 × 16 μm in diameter) are present in small portal veins and sinusoids, with or without an inflammatory reaction.
- When inflammation is present, a granulomatous response with multinucleated giant cells and eosinophils is seen.

Clinical/Laboratory Parameters

- This female nematode, called threadworm, is endemic worldwide.
- The adult parasite hatches eggs in the small intestinal mucosa from which rhabditiform larvae hatch.
- These then pass into the feces, where they mature to filariform larvae, which have the propensity to penetrate skin and infect barefoot humans.
- These larvae migrate to the lungs from the peripheral circulation, penetrate the alveoli, and escape into the tracheobronchial tree where they migrate cephalad and eventually enter the small intestine after being swallowed.
- The skin (site of entry), pulmonary (migration), and gastrointestinal tracts are the main targets of infection.
- In disseminated disease, seen in immunosuppressed individuals, pneumonitis, septicemia, ulcerative enteritis and colitis, meningitis, peritonitis, and hepatic involvement can be seen, referred to as hyperinfection syndrome, with mortality exceeding 50%.

TABLE 3–193

Surgical Hepatitis[853,854]

Histology

- Clusters of neutrophils are centered in the perivenular zone with involvement of the terminal hepatic venules, and histologically mimic microabscesses.
- Neutrophils are also seen involving Glisson's capsule.
- In severe cases, neutrophils may be seen scattered throughout all zones.
- This feature is usually focal, and does not involve all lobules equally.
- The adjacent hepatocytes are normal; however, in prolonged surgery, the hepatocytes adjacent to the neutrophils may exhibit ischemia without liver cell dropout.

Clinical/Laboratory Parameters

- In prolonged surgical procedures involving manipulation of the liver, an inflammatory component may be seen in liver tissue which is artifactually induced and *not* related to a primary liver disease.

TABLE 3-194

Syphilis *(Treponema pallidum)*[855–862]

Histology

- Three different subtypes may be seen:
  1. *Congenital*
     - Neonatal hepatitis with giant cells occur, with large areas of focal necrosis associated with numerous spirochetes (demonstrable on Warthin-Starry reaction).
     - Small granulomas may be seen.
     - As the disease progresses, portal fibrosis and diffuse interstitial fibrosis may be seen.
  2. *Secondary*
     - Epithelioid granulomas, acute cholangitis, and vasculitis involving small arterioles and venules are present, these vessels often undergoing obliterative changes.
     - Organisms may be seen but are not common.
  3. *Tertiary*
     - Gumma formation occurs, demonstrated as single or multiple tuberculoid-type granulomas with central necrosis resembling caseation, with plasma cell infiltration.
     - Eventual dense scarring of these granulomas may develop, forming broad bands and "potato-like" nodules *(hepar lobatum)* with microcalcifications rarely present.
     - Endarteritis with obliteration of the vascular lumen may be seen.

Clinical/Laboratory Parameters

- Syphilis is a highly infectious venereal disorder caused by the obligate anaerobe spirochete *Treponema pallidum*.
- The organisms can be identified by darkfield microscopy of smears from the primary chancre sore.
- Women acquiring infection during the third trimester of pregnancy may transmit the virus in utero, leading to *congenital* syphilis characterized by hyperbilirubinemia, mild increases in serum transaminases and alkaline phosphatase activity, hepatosplenomegaly, skin rash, anemia, and central nervous system abnormalities.
- In the *secondary* stage (which develops approximately 4 to 6 weeks after the primary infection), hepatosplenomegaly occurs in a minority of patients, with generalized lymphadenopathy and anemia; hyperbilirubinemia may also occur, with modest elevations in aminotransferases and alkaline phosphatase activity.
- In *tertiary* syphilis, hepatic gummas develop, with the irregularities of the liver surface grossly suggesting cirrhosis; however, there is no distinct nodularity and no evidence of portal hypertension.

TABLE 3-195

Systemic Carnitine Deficiency[863–866]

Histology

- Fatty change is present and is often diffuse; the fat is predominantly macrovesicular but it can also be microvesicular in the presence of acute illness.
- The fat within the hepatocytes may disappear when patients develop a steady state, the fat then appearing only in sinusoidal lining cells.
- Portal fibrosis may occur, but cirrhosis does not develop.

Clinical/Laboratory Parameters

- L-Carnitine is involved in the transport of long-chain fatty acid acyl coenzyme A important for the oxidation of fats; it is not clear if this condition is caused by excessive renal loss of L-carnitine.
- Deficiency of L-carnitine leads to a syndrome that resembles Reye's syndrome; patients present with hypoglycemia (hypoketotic), lethargy, skeletal muscle weakness, and elevated serum transaminases.
- Administration of L-carnitine is the treatment of choice.

TABLE 3–196

Systemic Lupus Erythematosus[867–871]

Histology

- Mild macrovesicular fatty change is usually seen, with mild focal necrosis and lymphocytic infiltration within the lobules.
- Sinusoidal congestion and cholestasis may also be seen.
- Granulomas have been reported, sometimes exhibiting a peripheral fibrin ring.
- Arteritis has been described with secondary infarction and hemorrhage within the lobules.
- Peliosis may also be seen.

Clinical/Laboratory Parameters

- Systemic lupus erythematosus (SLE) is associated with hepatomegaly and mildly abnormal liver tests in a minority of patients, with hyperbilirubinemia uncommon.
- Although cirrhosis has in the past been described, further studies have not supported this finding, as SLE in the clinical setting may mimic autoimmune hepatitis (both disorders occurring in young women with positive antinuclear antibody), which is well known to progress to cirrhosis in untreated patients.

TABLE 3–197

Tangier's Disease (Familial High-density Lipoprotein Deficiency)[872–874]

Histology

- Kupffer cells and portal macrophages have foamy cytoplasm containing needle-shaped birefringent cholesterol crystals seen under polarized light on frozen section.
- Cirrhosis may occur.

Clinical/Laboratory Parameters

- This disease is characterized by an absence or severe deficiency of high-density lipoproteins (HDL) and leads to the accumulation of cholesteryl esters in the tonsils, spleen, and peripheral nerves.
- The defect is considered to be related to rapid catabolism of apolipoprotein A-1 (1–3% of normal) and HDL.
- Serum cholesterol is decreased but triglycerides may be normal or increased.
- Patients present with mild lymphadenopathy, mild to moderate hepatomegaly, splenomegaly, and neuropathy.

TABLE 3–198

Toxemia of Pregnancy (Eclampsia)[22,26,29,406,875–881]

Histology

- Periportal sinusoidal dilatation, congestion, and intrasinusoidal fibrin deposition are seen, associated with focal coagulative liver cell necrosis.
- Hepatic arteries and arterioles exhibit endothelial damage with fibrin deposition within the lumen.
- Fibrin thrombi may be seen within the portal veins.
- Acute hemorrhage, predominantly subcapsular, may be present; in these instances, rupture may occur.
- In severe cases, multilobular confluent necrosis, collapse, and infarction may result.

Clinical/Laboratory Parameters

- Preeclampsia is a multisystem disorder that complicates anywhere from 3 to 10% of all pregnancies, is not unique to primiparae, and is manifested by pregnancy-induced hypertension, edema, and proteinuria.
- In progressive or severe cases (eclampsia), accelerated hypertension and seizures occur and require urgent management, including early termination of pregnancy.
- Mild to moderate elevations of serum transaminases, hypoalbuminemia, hyperuricemia, and in severe cases hyperbilirubinemia and prolonged prothrombin time are seen.
- Elevations in alkaline phosphatase in the third trimester is not wholly of liver origin with contribution from the placenta.
- Rarely, severe liver injury can lead to liver failure.

TABLE 3-199
Toxic Shock Syndrome[882,883]

Histology

- Perivenular cholestasis is present, with variable lobular acute and chronic inflammatory infiltration.
- Acute cholangitis, with variable portal neutrophilic infiltration may be seen.
- Microvesicular fatty change is present.
- Pylephlebitis of portal veins, and arteritis have been described.

Clinical/Laboratory Parameters

- Toxic shock syndrome is caused by staphylococcal exotoxin and develops in women who used tampons contaminated with the toxin.
- Salient findings include hyperbilirubinemia, mild elevations of serum transaminases, mild to moderate increase in alkaline phosphatase activity, increased serum bile salt concentrations, and hypoalbuminemia.

TABLE 3-200
Toxoplasmosis *(Toxoplasma gondii)*[884-888]

Histology

- Neonatal hepatitis (refer to Table 3–155) with syncytial giant cells may occur in infection in the neonate.
- In immunocompromised patients, small inflammatory granulomas containing parasitized liver cells are present; the parasites are seen as microscopic cysts containing numerous pinpoint merozoites.
- Epithelioid granulomas have been described.

Clinical/Laboratory Parameters

- *Toxoplasma gondii* is a parasite that infects humans when cysts containing merozoites are ingested in uncooked or mostly raw meats, and less commonly by exposure to cat feces.
- Asymptomatic infection occurs in about 50% of the infected population, and increasingly this infection is seen in immunodeficient (AIDS) patients.
- In congenital infection, hepatosplenomegaly, jaundice, purpura, chorioretinitis, seizures, hydrocephalus, and intracerebral calcifications may occur.
- Hepatitis is uncommon, with only mild increases in serum bilirubin, transaminases, and alkaline phosphatase activity.

TABLE 3-201
Tuberculosis *(Mycobacterium tuberculosis)*[174,176,824,889-891]

Histology

- Portal and lobular epithelioid granulomas containing Langhans' giant cells are present.
- The granulomas are usually small and most often are negative on AFB stain; however, in active disease, central caseous necrosis may be seen, and the granulomas are often positive on AFB stain.
- Larger coalescent granulomas may become grossly visible (*tuberculoma,* which may measure several centimeters in diameter).
- Variable macrovesicular fatty change is present, and tends to be periportal in chronically ill patients.
- Portal fibrosis may occur in cases of healed granulomas, which then tend to become sclerosed, with occasional microcalcifications.
- In severe cases, a mixed lymphocytic and neutrophilic portal infiltrate with destruction of ducts and acute cholangitis may occur.
- In AIDS, the granulomas may lack epithelioid cells, and characteristically contain abundant AFB-positive organisms.

Clinical/Laboratory Parameters

- Hepatic involvement by miliary *Mycobacterium tuberculosis* infection is one of the most common causes of granulomatous hepatitis and is responsible for up to 25% of all cases in a study at the University of Southern California (USC) Liver Unit.
- Within 1 year after exposure, 3 to 5% of patients may develop clinical disease, while the majority are asymptomatic with positive skin tests.
- The biliary tract may be involved in countries (e.g., the Philippines) where the disease is endemic and may present with biliary tract obstruction or features similar to sclerosing cholangitis.
- Fever is common during active infection and is associated with weight loss, anorexia, and night sweats.
- Mild splenomegaly may be seen in about 30% of cases.
- Leukocytosis (leukemoid reaction), leukopenia, anemia, and thrombocytopenia may suggest granulomas in the bone marrow.
- The predominant abnormality in liver tests is the elevation of serum alkaline phosphatase activity, with minor increases in serum transaminases and bilirubin.

TABLE 3–202

Tyrosinemia[892–897]

Histology

- Intracanalicular cholestasis with bile plugs may be associated with pseudoacinar transformation of liver cells.
- Both large cell and small cell dysplasia of liver cells is often present.
- Extramedullary hematopoiesis may be present.
- Variable degrees of intrasinusoidal collagen deposition are seen.
- Macrovesicular fatty change is present.
- Variable hemosiderosis is often identified.
- Both macronodular and micronodular cirrhosis occurs, with large macroregenerative nodules occasionally seen.
- Hepatocellular carcinoma is a well-known complication.

Clinical/Laboratory Parameters

- An inborn metabolic defect of fumarylacetoacetase in the metabolic pathway of phenylalanine and tyrosine, this disorder leads to elevated levels of tyrosine and its metabolites.
- The disease may present either acutely or in a chronic form, with failure to thrive, vomiting, diarrhea, hepatosplenomegaly, ascites, edema, prolongation of prothrombin time, jaundice, and mental retardation.
- Renal tubular defects may also occur, with glucosuria, hyperphosphaturia, aminoaciduria, and proteinuria.
- The *acute* form presents in the neonate and leads to liver failure and death within the first 3 to 9 months.
- In the *chronic* form hepatocellular carcinoma occurs in up to 35% of patients who survive beyond the age of 2 years.
- Liver transplantation is the curative treatment of choice.

TABLE 3–203

Ulcerative Colitis[61,208,245,246,898,899]

Histology

- Macrovesicular (1+ to 2+) fatty change is present in up to 50% of cases.
- Portal lymphocytic infiltration is seen, sometimes associated with piecemeal necrosis.
- Mild focal necrosis and lymphocytic infiltration are seen within the lobules.
- Periductal fibrosis and sclerosis may occur (1–5% of cases) with associated biliary fibrosis and eventual biliary cirrhosis.
- Macronodular cirrhosis may also be seen without the above-described duct lesions.
- Cholangiocarcinoma is a known complication (0.4–1.4% of cases).

Clinical/Laboratory Parameters

- Liver dysfunction is seen in up to 10% of patients with either ulcerative colitis or Crohn's disease (refer to Table 3–59).
- Primary sclerosing cholangitis (PSC; refer to Table 3–173) can be seen in up to 5% of patients; in fact, two-thirds of patients with PSC have coexisting ulcerative colitis.
- A serious complication of patients with both PSC and ulcerative colitis is cholangiocarcinoma.
- Chronic liver disease with progression to cirrhosis may also occur but is infrequent.

TABLE 3-204

Veno-occlusive Disease[177,182,375,900-904]

Histology

Acute

- Early lesions exhibit subintimal edema, acute hemorrhage, and fibrin deposition involving small hepatic veins (<300 μm in diameter).
- Associated sinusoidal congestion and hemorrhage are present, with secondary perivenular liver cell ischemic necrosis.
- Red blood cells may be seen beneath the space of Disse and within the hepatic cords, replacing ischemic hepatocytes *(red blood cell–trabecular lesion)*.
- Cholestasis may be seen in the perivenular zone but is not common.

Chronic

- Concentric or eccentric intimal fibrosis and narrowing of terminal hepatic venules occurs, with eventual fibrous obliteration of the lumen.
- Endothelial proliferation may be seen, with recanalization of the fibrotic vascular lumen.
- Over time there is atrophy of perivenular hepatocytes with variable sinusoidal dilatation accompanied by sinusoidal fibrosis.
- Obliteration of small portal veins may also be seen.
- Eventual bridging fibrosis between terminal hepatic venules occurs, with development of a *cardiac cirrhosis* (reverse lobulation with portal tract sparing).
- In advanced cases, bridging fibrosis also occurs between terminal hepatic venules and portal tracts, leading to micronodular cirrhosis.

Clinical/Laboratory Parameters

- This nonthrombotic occlusion of small hepatic veins (<300 μm in diameter) may be produced by ingestion of pyrrolizidine alkaloids *(bush tea)*, alkylating cancer chemotherapeutic agents, bone marrow and kidney transplantation, hepatic irradiation, urethane therapy, or exposure to arsenicals and vinyl chloride monomer, and is initiated by vascular endothelial injury.
- This disorder is endemic in parts of Africa, the Middle East, and India; in Jamaica, up to 30% of patients with chronic liver disease may have chronic veno-occlusive disease.
- In the *acute* presentation patients may develop jaundice, abdominal pain, hepatomegaly, ascites or unexplained increase in weight, the occurrence of which after bone marrow transplant is diagnostic.
- Hyperbilirubinemia is usually present, associated with a modest elevation of the serum transaminases; in severe cases, thrombocytopenia may occur.
- Resolution occurs with recognition and withdrawal of the offending drug.
- In the *chronic* form, the onset is insidious, occurring months to years after exposure to the inciting agent, with ascites, esophageal varices, and hepatomegaly usually present.

TABLE 3–205

Viral Hepatitis, Acute, Classic Type (Generally Seen for All Hepatotropic Viruses)[905-910]

Histology

- Portal lymphoid infiltration and hyperplasia is usually prominent, with slight variation from one portal tract to the next; neutrophils can also be seen in portal tracts in the early stage, without orientation to ducts or vessels.
- Spillover of inflammatory cells into the adjacent periportal regions is usually seen; although piecemeal necrosis may be present, this feature is uncommon.
- Hepatocytes are swollen, with eventual dropout and replacement by macrophages and hypertrophic Kupffer cells.
- Liver cells may also shrink and become deeply eosinophilic, with pyknotic nuclei *(apoptosis, acidophil [Councilman] bodies)* and with eventual extrusion into the sinusoids with phagocytosis.
- Lobular inflammatory infiltrate is chiefly lymphocytic with occasional plasma cells; in the early stages, the inflammation and liver cell necrosis are more prominent in the perivenular zone, sometimes associated with mild perivenular collapse in more severe cases.
- Cholestasis may be seen and is usually accentuated in the perivenular zone, associated with variable bile duct proliferation.
- Pigment-laden Kupffer cells are seen in areas of focal necrosis and may contain lipochrome pigment and sometimes bile and hemosiderin, and they may stain diPAS-positive (increase in lysozomal activity).
- Kupffer cell hyperplasia and hypertrophy are present and usually prominent.
- Giant cell transformation may be present in neonates and the younger age group (refer to Table 3–155, Neonatal Hepatitis); in adults this feature is uncommon.
- With resolution, spotty clusters of pigment-laden histiocytes are present within the lobule (*tombstone* lesions, diPAS-positive) associated with mild portal lymphocytic infiltration for months after the acute episode, which slowly and completely resolves.

Clinical/Laboratory Parameters

- Patients with acute viral hepatitis typically present after the incubation period with acute onset of malaise, anorexia, vomiting, and right upper quadrant pain; less frequently they present with low-grade fever, headache, myalgia, and diarrhea.
- Jaundice is often present except in mild and asymptomatic cases.
- Physical examination is otherwise usually nondescript and unremarkable; in some patients, tenderness over a soft, enlarged liver may be noted.
- Splenomegaly can be seen in about 10% of cases.
- The peripheral white blood count may be normal with lymphocytosis.
- Serum transaminase elevations vary from moderate to marked, ranging usually from 500 to 5000 IU/L, ALT usually higher than AST.
- Alkaline phosphatase activity may be mildly or moderately elevated.
- Hyperbilirubinemia is usually present.
- Lactate dehydrogenase activity may rarely be elevated.
- Serum albumin and prothrombin time are usually normal or minimally abnormal except in severe cases.
- Diagnosis of acute viral hepatitis is confirmed by serologic tests (refer to the following tables for the different hepatotropic viruses).
- Recovery is the rule; however, in approximately 1% of cases, fulminant hepatitis may develop with an overall poor prognosis (refer to Table 3–213, Viral Hepatitis, Acute, with Bridging Necrosis; Table 3–215, Viral Hepatitis, Acute, with Panacinar Necrosis), and may necessitate liver transplantation.
- Chronic hepatitis may occur, depending on the virus involved and the age of the patient (refer to the following tables for chronic viral hepatitis).

TABLE 3–206
Viral Hepatitis, Acute, Type A[911–916,1016]

Histology

- Acute viral hepatitis type A shows the basic histo-pathology seen in the classic form (refer to Table 3–205, Viral Hepatitis, Acute, Classic Type), with the following features:
  - Periportal inflammation and necrosis may occasionally be more prominent than in the perivenular zone.
  - Portal plasma cell infiltration may be prominent.
  - Perivenular cholestasis may be striking, and often is associated with only a mild degree of lobular inflammation and necrosis.

Clinical/Laboratory Parameters

- Acute viral hepatitis type A is caused by the RNA hepatitis A virus (HAV), which is a Picornavirus and is transmitted by the fecal-oral route.
- The incubation period ranges from 15 to 45 days.
- The hepatitis may be asymptomatic (frequently in children) or symptomatic.
- Acute type A viral hepatitis may be transmitted among intravenous addicts from HAV-contaminated heroin.
- Patients are not infectious at the time symptoms appear.
- The diagnosis is confirmed serologically by positive anti-HAV IgM.
- *Passive* immunization should be offered to family members and sexual partners.
- This infection can also be prevented by *active* immunization using two doses of recombinant vaccine administered intramuscularly 6 months apart.

TABLE 3–207
Viral Hepatitis, Acute, Type B[906–908,917–919,1017]

Histology

- Acute viral hepatitis type B shows the basic histo-pathology seen in the classic form (refer to Table 3–205, Viral Hepatitis, Acute, Classic Type), with the following features:
  - Lymphocytes within the lobules may be in close contact with damaged liver cells, and sometimes may be seen within liver cell cytoplasm *(emperi-polesis)*.

Clinical/Laboratory Parameters

- Acute viral hepatitis type B is caused by the DNA hepatitis B virus (HBV) transmitted sexually or parenterally, with an incubation period ranging from 3 to 6 months.
- The diagnosis of acute infection is confirmed by positive HBsAg and anti-HBc IgM.
- Acute reactivation of chronic hepatitis B should be excluded in the differential diagnosis by determining the hepatitis B virus DNA (HBV-DNA) level, which is usually low or nonmeasurable in acute type B viral hepatitis.
- In symptomatic adult patients, recovery is common and chronic disease occurs in only 2 to 5% of patients; however, in neonates who are infected at the time of delivery from HBsAg-positive mothers, the disease is usually asymptomatic but chronicity may develop in up to 90% of cases.

TABLE 3-208

Viral Hepatitis, Acute, Type B + Delta[920-922,1018]

Histology

- Acute viral hepatitis type B + delta shows the basic histopathology seen in the classic form (refer to Table 3-205, Viral Hepatitis, Acute, Classic Type), with the following features:
  - The degree of lobular inflammation and necrosis is more prominent than with HBV infection alone, and may be associated with perivenular collapse.
  - Variable microvesicular fatty change may be present.
  - The delta antigen can be demonstrated in the majority of liver cell nuclei on immunoperoxidase stain.

Clinical/Laboratory Parameters

- The hepatitis D (delta) virus (HDV) is a putative virus that requires HBV for acute infection and replication.
- The infection occurs most frequently in intravenous drug addicts and can present either as coinfection, in which both HBV and HDV are transmitted concurrently, or as a superinfection, in which HDV infects a chronic, usually nonreplicative (hepatitis B e [HBe] antibody–positive) HBV carrier.
- In *coinfection,* severe hepatitis develops, sometimes manifesting as a biphasic illness; with recovery, both HBV and HDV are cleared but because of the severity of the disease, 20 to 50% of patients may develop fulminant hepatic failure.
- In *superinfection,* acute hepatitis develops in a chronic HBV carrier and results in chronic delta infection in 90% of cases; superinfection must be distinguished from reactivation of HBV or infection with other hepatitis viruses.
- The diagnosis of acute infection is confirmed by positive high titer of anti-delta IgM compared with low-titer anti-delta IgG, and positive HDV RNA.

TABLE 3-209

Viral Hepatitis, Acute, Type C[923-928,1015]

Histology

- Acute viral hepatitis type C shows the basic histopathology seen in the classic form (refer to Table 3-205, Viral Hepatitis, Acute, Classic Type), with the following features:
  - Hepatocytes may show less cytologic damage than with HBV infection.
  - Occasionally sinusoidal lymphocytosis is present.
  - Bile ducts may be surrounded and infiltrated by lymphocytes, with variable but only mild cytologic atypia.
  - Portal lymphocytic infiltration may be quite prominent, sometimes demonstrating lymphoid follicles with germinal centers (worry about progression to chronicity in these cases).

Clinical/Laboratory Parameters

- Hepatitis C virus (HCV) is an RNA virus related to the flaviviruses and pestiviruses and is transmitted primarily by parenteral and rarely by sexual routes.
- The incubation period ranges from 15 to 150 days.
- Acute viral hepatitis type C is usually mild and patients are frequently asymptomatic.
- Fulminant hepatic failure is very rare.
- Serum transaminases are usually modestly elevated and hyperbilirubinemia is uncommon.
- Diagnosis of acute hepatitis is confirmed with positive hepatitis C virus RNA by nested polymerase chain reaction (qualitative), since hepatitis C virus antibody may arise late during the course of the acute infection.
- There are 6 recognized genotypes (1 through 6) and over 80 subtypes; genotype 1 is the commonest type worldwide (40–80% of all cases) and is responsible for over 70% of cases in the United States.
- Chronicity develops in from 60 to 80% of cases.

TABLE 3–210

Viral Hepatitis, Acute, Type E[909,929–933,1019]

Histology

- Acute viral hepatitis type E shows the basic histopathology seen in the classic form (refer to Table 3–205, Viral Hepatitis, Acute, Classic Type), with the following features:
  - Periportal cholangiolar proliferation, ectasia, neutrophilic infiltration, and bile plug formation are present.
  - Acinar-type lobular changes of liver cells are seen, these acini often containing bile.

Clinical/Laboratory Parameters

- Hepatitis E virus (HEV) is an RNA virus of the Calcivirus family, transmitted by fecal-oral spread, endemic in developing countries, and indistinguishable clinically from other types of acute hepatitis.
- The clinical course is different in pregnant women, in whom mortality approaches 25% during the acute infection.
- Hyperbilirubinemia with elevations in alkaline phosphatase and pruritus suggest biliary tract obstruction in the differential diagnosis.
- The diagnosis is considered in travelers from nonendemic countries to developing countries and can be confirmed by positive anti-HEV IgM and/or IgG, and presence of HEV RNA.
- There is no known treatment, and chronic liver disease does not occur.

TABLE 3–211

Viral Hepatitis, Acute, Type G[934–938,1020]

Histology

- Acute viral hepatitis type G shows the basic histopathology seen in the classic form (refer to Table 3–205, Viral Hepatitis, Acute, Classic Type), with the following features:
  - Portal and lobular inflammatory changes are quite mild, especially when compared with the other hepatotropic viruses.
- Note that it is important to rule out coinfection with one of the other hepatotropic viruses when portal and lobular activity is prominent.

Clinical/Laboratory Parameters

- Hepatitis G virus (HGV) is an RNA virus of the Flaviviridae family with 25% homology with hepatitis C virus.
- It is transmitted parenterally and is commonly found in blood donors.
- Hepatitis G virus infection occurs frequently in patients with chronic hepatitis C, especially genotype 3a.
- A mild nonspecific hepatitis has been described for HGV infection with no risk of progression to chronic liver disease.
- Diagnosis can be made by positive HGV RNA.
- This viral infection has little clinical significance; in fact, there is no convincing evidence that HGV is a primary hepatotropic virus.

TABLE 3–212

Viral Hepatitis, Acute, Type Non A-G[936,939–942]

Histology

- Acute viral hepatitis type non A-G shows the basic histopathology seen in the classic form (refer to Table 3–205, Viral Hepatitis, Acute, Classic Type), with the following features:
  - Giant cell transformation of liver cells may be seen, which is sometimes prominent, and associated with paramyxovirus-like inclusions seen by electron microscopy.

Clinical/Laboratory Parameters

- Hepatitis not due to the known hepatitis viruses, drugs or toxins, and in which other liver diseases such as autoimmune hepatitis and Wilson's disease can be ruled out, are designated hepatitis non A-G by a process of exclusion.
- It is not known if infection is due to a single or multiple viruses, although paramyxoviruses have been implicated as a possible cause of the liver injury.
- A few cases of severe hepatitis requiring liver transplantation have been reported; however, it is not clear if this viral infection should be considered as the etiology of the liver disease in these patients.

TABLE 3-213

Viral Hepatitis, Acute, with Bridging Necrosis (Submassive Hepatic Necrosis)[943-948]

Histology	Clinical/Laboratory Parameters
■ Perivenular confluent liver cell dropout and collapse is seen with merging (bridging) into periportal zones associated with cholestasis in viable lobules. ■ Variable lymphocytic infiltration is seen within the lobules and is associated with prominent Kupffer cell hyperplasia and hypertrophy. ■ Portal tracts show moderate lymphocytic infiltration and hyperplasia. ■ In areas of portal to perivenular bridging necrosis, cholangiolar proliferation and ectasia is present and often striking, with neutrophilic exudation often seen *(acute cholangiolitis)*.	■ These patients have more severe disease than typical acute viral hepatitis, with development of liver failure after 12 weeks from onset of symptoms. ■ The clinical presentation is characterized by the development of hypoalbuminemia, prolongation of the prothrombin time, hyperbilirubinemia, and the development of ascites, encephalopathy, and/or renal failure. ■ Portal hypertension can develop acutely and is the explanation for ascites formation. ■ Serum transaminases decrease as the disease progresses and are not correlated with improvement. ■ Recovery occurs in about 50% of patients, with liver transplantation offered for patients who progress.

TABLE 3-214

Viral Hepatitis, Acute, with Impaired Regeneration[943,949,950]

Histology	Clinical/Laboratory Parameters
■ Prominent collapse in the perivenular zone is seen with adjacent viable liver cells forming distinct straight cords *without* regenerative activity. ■ Variable focal necrosis and lymphocytic infiltration are seen in the lobules. ■ Cholestasis is present and most prominent in the later stage of the disease. ■ Prominent cholangiolar proliferation and ectasia are seen associated with bile plugs and adjacent neutrophils. ■ Portal lymphocytic infiltration is present to a moderate degree.	■ Older patients who develop acute viral hepatitis have a delayed recovery with persistent hyperbilirubinemia and pruritus. ■ Alkaline phosphatase may be mildly to moderately elevated. ■ Serum transaminases initially are moderately elevated but return to normal; however, the bilirubin remains elevated or continues to rise, and is associated with prolonged prothrombin time in the more severe cases. ■ The clinical course is usually prolonged, with resolution after 6 to 12 months. ■ Although there is no evidence that the disease may progress to chronicity, continued deterioration with hepatic failure signals a poor outcome.

TABLE 3-215

Viral Hepatitis, Acute, with Panacinar Necrosis (Massive Hepatic Necrosis)[946-948]

Histology	Clinical/Laboratory Parameters
■ Liver cell necrosis, dropout, and collapse are present diffusely involving all hepatocytes in all zones, associated with prominent Kupffer cell hyperplasia, hypertrophy, and lobular lymphocytic infiltration. ■ Portal tracts show moderate lymphocytic infiltration and hyperplasia. ■ Periportal cholangiolar proliferation (transformed hepatocytes), ectasia, and neutrophilic infiltration with bile plugs may be striking the longer the time period from the initial onset.	■ These patients are considered to have fulminant hepatic failure with symptoms of liver failure developing within 8 weeks of the initial onset. ■ Patients rapidly develop encephalopathy, marked prolongation of prothrombin time, ascites, and functional renal failure *(hepatorenal syndrome)* in the context of acute viral hepatitis. ■ Sepsis, bleeding from gastric erosions, hypoglycemia, hypovolemia, DIC, and adult respiratory distress syndrome are recognized complications. ■ Liver transplantation is the treatment of choice and is life-saving; however, this may not be possible if patients rapidly develop cerebral edema and herniate.

TABLE 3-216

Viral Hepatitis, Chronic, Classic Type
(Generally Seen for Types B, B + Delta, C, Non A-G)[74,149,906–908,910,951]

Histology

- With time, variable degrees of portal and lobular fibrosis occur, with bridging fibrosis and eventual fibrous bands with regenerative nodule formation *(cirrhosis)*.
- The cirrhosis is generally macronodular (the nodules >3 mm in diameter) in the early stages, but with advanced disease both macro- and micronodules are usually seen.
- The portal tracts exhibit variable lymphocytic infiltration.
- Piecemeal necrosis, defined as spillover of inflammatory cells from the portal tracts into the adjacent periportal regions, surrounding individual and small groups of hepatocytes *(trapped hepatocytes)*, is present, and often varies from one portal tract to the next.
- Mononuclear lobular inflammation with acidophil body formation is present, but it varies from one lobule to the next.
- Dysplastic changes of liver cell nuclei may be seen, predominantly in the periportal or periseptal zones.
- Occasional periportal or periseptal hepatocytes may have a uniformly intensely eosinophilic cytoplasm resembling inclusions *(oncocytic change)*.
- When the degree of lobular activity is minimal, the hepatocytes may appear hydropic and have a "cobblestoning" type appearance due to regeneration.
- *Reactivation* (associated with active viral replication) is manifested by diffuse necroinflammatory changes within the lobules, sometimes associated with focal lobular collapse (seen more frequently in chronic HBV infection than HCV infection; it is not certain if it occurs with non A-G infection).
- Cholastasis may be present but is generally uncommon except in reactivation or advanced disease with hepatic failure.
- In intravenous drug users, expanded portal tracts containing particulate polarizable material used in injection are sometimes seen and are located free or within portal macrophages; this material may also be visualized less commonly within Kupffer cells.

Clinical/Laboratory Parameters

- Chronic viral hepatitis is loosely defined as persistently abnormal liver tests or clinical confirmation of liver disease for at least 6 months after acute onset of the infection.
- Patients regardless of the etiology present with chronic elevation of serum transaminases, which range from 50 to 500 IU/L and often fluctuate, with little correlation between the height of the transaminases and symptoms or severity of the liver disease.
- On physical examination, stigmata of chronic liver disease such as spider angiomas and palmar erythema may be noted; as the disease progresses, ascites and esophageal varices may also occur.
- Serum albumin and bilirubin are usually normal except in the more severe or advanced cases, or when reactivation occurs.
- Mild prolongation of the prothrombin time is observed.
- In more advanced cases, thrombocytopenia and leukopenia suggest the development of hypersplenism.
- The natural history and modes of therapy relate to the specific virus involved.

TABLE 3–217

Viral Hepatitis, Chronic, Type B[367,436,437,906–908,952–956,1017]

Histology

- Chronic viral hepatitis type B shows the basic histopathology seen in the classic form (refer to Table 3–216, Viral Hepatitis, Chronic, Classic Type), with the following features:
  - "Ground-glass" cells (positive on orcein stain and immunoperoxidase stain for HBsAg) are seen scattered within the lobules in from 50 to 75% of cases.
  - Immunoperoxidase stains for HBcAg may be positive in liver cell nuclei and occasionally within the cytoplasm.
  - Plasma cell infiltration within portal tracts and fibrous bands may be prominent.
  - There is a high incidence of hepatocellular carcinoma in both cirrhotic and noncirrhotic livers.
- Note that the degree of expression of nuclear HBcAg and membranous HBsAg vary directly with the degree of active viral replication.

Clinical/Laboratory Parameters

- Chronic hepatitis B develops in from 2 to 5% of adult patients following acute hepatitis B, but in up to 90% of neonates who are infected at time of delivery from HBsAg-positive mothers.
- The course fluctuates with periods of replication and nonreplicative phases of the virus.
- The replicative state is identified by positive HBe antigen and high concentrations of hepatitis B virus DNA (HBV DNA), whereas the nonreplicative state is associated with positive HBe antibody and low or absent levels of HBV DNA.
- The progression is characterized by a decrease in serum albumin, prolongation of the prothrombin time, leukopenia, and thrombocytopenia.
- Progression to cirrhosis occurs, although the time frame varies considerably depending on reactivation (exacerbation of the disease) and response to therapy.
- The risk of developing hepatocellular carcinoma is approximately 50 to 200 times greater in HBsAg-positive versus HBsAg-negative patients.
- The mode of therapy includes alpha-interferon, in which positive predictors include high pretreatment ALT levels, low HBV DNA levels, adult-acquired disease, and active necroinflammatory changes on biopsy.
- Alpha-interferon therapy allows conversion from the replicative to nonreplicative state in 40% of cases.
- Although lamivudine also inhibits viral replication, relapses with discontinuation are common and thus its role in long-term therapy is not clear.

TABLE 3–218

Viral Hepatitis, Chronic, Type B + Delta[920,921,957–959,1018]

Histology

- Chronic viral hepatitis type B + delta shows the basic histopathology seen in the classic form (refer to Table 3–216, Viral Hepatitis, Chronic, Classic Type), with the following features:
  - The degree of piecemeal necrosis and lobular activity is greater than with HBV infection alone.
  - Occasional microvesicular fat may be present.
  - The delta antigen is often demonstrated within liver cell nuclei on immunoperoxidase stain.
  - Progression to cirrhosis in some cases may be rapid.
  - As opposed to chronic HBV infection alone, the incidence of hepatocellular carcinoma is low.

Clinical/Laboratory Parameters

- A more severe course of chronic hepatitis B develops after superinfection with the delta virus (HDV).
- Hepatitis B virus is usually in the nonreplicative state (positive anti-HBe, low titer or negative HBV DNA) with chronic HDV infection; this may be an explanation for the low recurrence of HBV after liver transplantation in patients with HBV and HDV cirrhosis.
- The diagnosis of chronic HDV infection is confirmed by high-titer anti-HDV IgG and positive HDV RNA.
- In approximately 80% of cases, chronic HDV infection progresses to cirrhosis in 5 to 10 years.
- There is a significant decline of HDV infection in the Western world.
- Since HBV is usually nonreplicative in chronic B and delta infection, interferon therapy is generally not effective.

TABLE 3–219

Viral Hepatitis, Chronic, Type C[150,923–928,960–962,1015]

Histology

- Chronic viral hepatitis type C shows the basic histopathology seen in the classic form (refer to Table 3–216, Viral Hepatitis, Chronic, Classic Type), with the following features:
  - Portal lymphoid aggregates are present and often prominent, with or without germinal centers.
  - Plasma cells within the portal tracts may occasionally be seen.
  - Bile ducts are often surrounded and partially infiltrated by lymphocytes, with little cytologic atypia of duct epithelium.
  - Ductopenia may be seen involving some portal tracts, although this feature is uncommon.
  - Sinusoidal lymphocytic infiltration is frequent.
  - Variable degrees of macrovesicular fatty change (1–2+) are seen in over 75% of cases.
  - Glycogenated nuclei of liver cells located in the periportal zone may be present.
  - Variable degrees of sinusoidal collagen deposition are seen, with no distinct zonal distribution.
  - An increase in hemosiderin may be seen in periportal hepatocytes.
  - The incidence of hepatocellular carcinoma is high, and occurs almost exclusively in the cirrhotic liver.

Clinical/Laboratory Parameters

- Chronic HCV infection is the most common cause of chronic hepatitis in the United States and the leading cause for liver transplantation.
- Approximately 70 to 80% of patients with acute hepatitis C develop chronic hepatitis.
- Patients with genotype 1 are more likely to develop severe chronic hepatitis and seem less responsive to therapy.
- Patients are generally asymptomatic, with only 6% having symptoms of chronic liver disease.
- The serum ALT values are only mildly elevated, although there is a wide variability and fluctuation over time.
- A decline in serum albumin levels, prolongation of the prothrombin time, and thrombocytopenia confirm progression to more advanced disease.
- The rate of progression to cirrhosis is dependent in part on the rate of disease activity: less than 10% progress within 10 years when activity is mild on initial biopsy, but 44 to 100% progress when the activity is moderate to severe; other cofactors, such as alcohol intake and infection at an older age, also play a role in disease progression.
- Diagnosis is confirmed by positive anti-HCV antibody and HCV RNA.
- Treatment with interferon and ribavirin has resulted in sustained viral remission in 45% of patients.
- The incidence of hepatocellular carcinoma (HCC) in the cirrhotic stage is quite high, where in Europe and Japan as many as 50 to 75% of patients with HCC have detectable anti-HCV.

TABLE 3–220

Viral Hepatitis, Chronic, Type G[934,935,937,938,963,1020]

Histology

- Chronic viral hepatitis type G shows minimal portal and lobular inflammatory changes.
- Fibrosis or cirrhosis is *not* seen in chronic HGV infection alone.

Clinical/Laboratory Parameters

- Chronic hepatitis G (HGV) is frequently seen in association with chronic hepatitis C, although coinfection does not adversely influence the course of chronic hepatitis C or affect response of HCV to therapy.
- There is no convincing evidence that chronic HGV alone is a primary hepatotropic virus and causes liver disease.

TABLE 3–221

Viral Hepatitis, Chronic, Type Non A-G[940,941]

Histology

- Chronic viral hepatitis type non A-G shows the basic histopathology seen in the classic form (refer to Table 3–216, Viral Hepatitis, Chronic, Classic Type), with the following features:
  - Giant cell transformation of hepatocytes similar to those seen in the acute phase has been described.

Clinical/Laboratory Parameters

- Approximately 15 to 20% of chronic hepatitis has no known cause.
- The possibility of a not yet identified hepatotropic virus (or viruses) must be considered.
- The clinical course and outcome cannot properly be assessed at this time.

TABLE 3–222

Visceral Larva Migrans (Toxocariasis; *Toxocara canis*)[143,964–969]

Histology

- A granulomatous reaction is seen throughout the lobules, with central fibrinous necrosis, infiltration by eosinophils, and giant cell reaction.
- The granulomas may become large, with multiple mass lesions seen on imaging.

Clinical/Laboratory Parameters

- *Toxocara canis,* an intestinal parasite (roundworm) of dogs, has a life cycle similar to ascariasis (refer to Table 3–31) with extraintestinal migratory phases; however, the changes are more florid, with formation of eosinophilic abscesses and later granulomas.
- Other involved organs include the heart, lymphatic system, central nervous system, and the eye.
- The migratory episodes may present with fever, urticarial rash, wheezing, and rhinorrhea.
- Children tend to have more severe disease with failure to thrive, weight loss, and hepatomegaly.
- Leukocytosis and eosinophilia may be marked, serum transaminases are mildly elevated, and bilirubin is normal or only mildly increased.
- Serologic tests, using the larval antigen and enzyme immunoassays, are positive in over 85% of infected patients.

TABLE 3–223

Waldenström's Macroglobulinemia[689,970–972]

Histology

- Portal tracts and sinusoids are infiltrated by numerous plasma cells and plasma cell precursors.
- Sinusoidal amyloid may also be seen; however, eosinophilic nonamyloid deposits (light chains) within the space of Disse have also been reported.
- Peliosis hepatis and nodular regenerative hyperplasia have been reported.

Clinical/Laboratory Parameters

- This plasma cell dyscrasia characteristically produces high concentrations of IgM monoclonal antibodies, and in many ways is similar to multiple myeloma (refer to Table 3–151) and non-Hodgkin's lymphoma (refer to Table 3–140).

TABLE 3–224

Weber-Christian Disease[973–975]

Histology

- Macrovesicular fatty change is present and may be prominent, sometimes associated with a lymphocytic and neutrophilic infiltration within the lobules.
- Mallory body formation may also be present.

Clinical/Laboratory Parameters

- This uncommon disorder is characterized by the presence of numerous subcutaneous nodules with associated inflammation (*panniculitis*).
- Hepatomegaly may be striking.

TABLE 3–225

Whipple's Disease[976–980]

Histology

- Foamy macrophages that are diPAS-positive are often seen within portal tracts and hypertrophic Kupffer cells.
- Epithelioid granulomas have also been described.

Clinical/Laboratory Parameters

- This uncommon bacterial infection (Whipple's bacilli) of the small intestine is associated with marked infiltration of the intestinal mucosa by foamy macrophages.
- The liver is usually involved, with good hepatic function.

TABLE 3–226

Wilson's Disease (Hepatolenticular Degeneration)[981–991]

Histology

- In the early stages this disorder may present with histologic features similar to those seen in acute viral hepatitis (refer to Table 3–205, Viral Hepatitis, Acute, Classic Type).
- Variable portal inflammation is present, chiefly lymphocytes with occasional plasma cells, often with piecemeal necrosis.
- Focal necrosis and hepatocytolysis are present to variable degrees; when the disease is more active, syncytial giant cells may be seen.
- Fulminant hepatitis with bridging (submassive) hepatic necrosis and extensive lobular collapse may also occur.
- Variable degrees of macrovesicular and occasionally microvesicular fatty change are present with no zonal distribution.
- Glycogenated nuclei of hepatocytes are seen in the periportal zones.
- Lipochrome pigment is often increased in periportal liver cells; these granules are large, clumped, and often vacuolated.
- Liver cell dysplasia may also be present.
- Kupffer cells may be hypertrophied, often containing hemosiderin (secondary to hemolysis) or small amounts of copper (secondary to hepatocytolysis).
- Mallory bodies are sometimes seen in periportal liver cells, especially in more advanced disease.
- An increase in copper (rubeanic acid stain) and copper-binding protein (orcein stain) is present in periportal liver cells but also can be seen diffusely throughout the lobules; this pigment is more common in earlier-stage disease and irregularly distributed within cirrhotic nodules.
- Eventually progression to macronodular or micronodular cirrhosis with sinusoidal collagen deposition occurs.

Clinical/Laboratory Parameters

- An autosomal recessive disorder with a disease incidence of 1:30,000 and gene frequency of 1:200, the disease is due to a mutation on the long arm of chromosome 13.
- Progressive accumulation of copper in liver, brain, cornea, and kidneys accounts for the manifestations of the disease.
- There is a slight male predominance, with initial manifestations of liver disease between 3 and 33 years of age.
- Patients may present either with chronic hepatitis with elevated serum transaminases, bilirubin, and globulin, or with established cirrhosis, portal hypertension, bleeding varices, and liver failure.
- Psychiatric and/or neuromotor abnormalities (disturbances in gait, speech) are the first presenting signs in approximately 45% of cases.
- Rarely, fulminant liver failure may be the initial presentation, with marked jaundice, hemolytic anemia, renal failure, hypouricemia, encephalopathy, and progression to death unless liver transplantation is performed.
- Diagnosis is confirmed if decreased serum ceruloplasmin is associated with increased urinary copper and the presence of Kayser-Fleischer rings on slit lamp examination of the cornea.
- D-Penicillamine, trientine chelation, and zinc therapy for maintenance may result in improvement.

TABLE 3-227
Wolman's Disease[992-996]

Histology

- Enlarged hypertrophic foamy diPAS-positive Kupffer cells and portal macrophages contain birefringent crystals on frozen section, with positive oil red O staining for neutral fat.
- Liver cells exhibit both macrovesicular and often microvesicular fatty change.
- Sinusoidal collagen deposition and portal fibrosis may occur.
- Cirrhosis has been described but is rare.

Clinical/Laboratory Parameters

- An isolated deficiency of acid hydrolase activity, this disorder resembles cholesterol ester storage disease (refer to Table 3-52), but is more severe, with accumulation of cholesterol esters and triglycerides in the liver, spleen, lymph nodes, and adrenal glands.
- Patients usually die within the first year, and symptoms develop within the first 2 weeks of life, with vomiting, diarrhea, failure to thrive, hepatosplenomegaly, and lymphadenopathy.
- Anemia, peripheral blood lymphocytes with intracytoplasmic and intranuclear vacuolization, and hyperbilirubinemia are seen.
- Calcification of the adrenal glands is frequently seen on imaging of the abdomen.

TABLE 3-228
Yellow Fever[275,284,997-999]

Histology

- Confluent midzonal coagulative-type necrosis with numerous acidophil bodies but mild lobular inflammation is present.
- Rarely the liver cells demonstrate intranuclear eosinophilic inclusions *(Torres bodies)*.
- Liver cells may exhibit syncytial multinucleated giant cell formation.
- Portal lymphocytic infiltration and hyperplasia are present but not striking.
- Mild microvesicular fatty change may be present.

Clinical/Laboratory Parameters

- This systemic viral infection develops after an incubation period of 3 to 6 days, and clinically ranges from mild infection to a fulminant course.
- Fever, headache, myalgia, nausea, and vomiting are followed by a toxic phase often with bradycardia, jaundice, hematemesis, hemorrhagic manifestations, renal failure, and sometimes coma leading to death in about 20% of cases.
- Leukopenia, hyperbilirubinemia, moderate to marked increases in serum transaminases, prolongation of the prothrombin time, and elevated blood urea nitrogen and creatinine levels are seen in severe cases.
- The diagnosis is made by positive neutralizing antibodies, hemagglutination inhibition antibody, or virus inoculations.

TABLE 3-229
Zellweger's Syndrome (Refsum's Disease)[1000-1005]

Histology

- Sinusoidal collagen deposition is present.
- Cholestasis with focal necrosis may be seen.
- Hemosiderin deposition is present, predominantly in Kupffer cells but also may be seen within hepatocytes.
- Paucity of ducts have been described.
- Micronodular cirrhosis has been reported.

Clinical/Laboratory Parameters

- The absence of functional peroxisomes is the key characteristic of this disease.
- Hepatomegaly, jaundice, hypoprothrombinemia, mental retardation, renal cysts, characteristic facies, corneal opacities, cataracts, and glaucoma are clinical features.
- Death occurs usually in infancy.

TABLE 3-230

Zygomycosis (*Mucor* species)[143,1006–1010]

Histology

- Necrotizing granulomas up to 1 cm in diameter are present, with prominent coagulative necrosis containing hyphae.

Clinical/Laboratory Parameters

- Numerous fungi including *Mucor* species contribute to this ubiquitous disease, which is seen more frequently in diabetics and patients on immunosuppressive therapy.
- Inhalation of spores infects sinuses and the lower respiratory tract.
- Infection of surgical and other wounds allows the organism to travel across tissue planes with invasion of blood vessels.
- The liver is involved in disseminated disease, with hepatic injury often secondary to vascular involvement with resultant ischemia.

CHAPTER 4

Drug-Induced and Toxic Liver Cell Injury

This chapter is organized into tables listing various drugs and toxins that may produce liver cell injury either by direct hepatotoxicity or hypersensitivity reaction.[1011-1014] The drugs and toxins are listed according to the type of liver cell injury that is manifested. It is fairly common for drugs to produce a wide variety of changes or mixed patterns. For instance, phenytoin may cause spotty necrosis with inflammation, confluent necrosis, cholestasis with inflammation, or granulomas. Each table also refers to the appropriate table in Chapter 2 that lists other liver diseases causing similar histologic features.

TABLE 4–1

Lobular Necrosis with Minimal to Absent Inflammation (refer to Table 2–17)

Perivenular (Zone 3)

Acetaminophen	Ethionamide	Propylthiouracil
Aflatoxin B1	Halogenated hydrocarbons	Pyrrolizidine alkaloids
Alpha-methyldopa	Ketoconazole	Tannic acid
Carbon tetrachloride	Metoprolol	Tetrachloroethylene
Chloroform	Mithramycin	Tricrynafen
Copper	Mushrooms	Urethane
Dimethylnitrosamine	Phalloidin	

Midzonal (Zone 2)

Beryllium	Dioxane

Periportal (Zone 1)

Allyl formate	Ferrous sulfate	Phosphorus
Endotoxin from *Proteus vulgaris*		

Perivenular or Periportal

Cocaine

Diffuse Confluent

Galactosamine	2-Nitropropane	Tetrachloroethane
Halogenated hydrocarbons	Phenelzine	Trinitrotoluene
Mushrooms		

TABLE 4–2

Lobular Necrosis with Inflammation (refer to Table 2–16)

Alpha-methyldopa	Etretinate	Nitrofurantoin	Propylthiouracil
Aspirin	Glyburide	Oxacillin	Rifampin
Benzarone	Halogenated hydrocarbons	Oxyphenisatin	Sulfadoxine
Chlorpromazine	Indomethacin	Papaverine	Sulfasalazine
Dantrolene	Isoniazid	Para-aminosalicylic acid	Sulfonamides
Dapsone	Lisinopril	Perhexiline maleate	Suloctidil
Diclofenac	Methotrexate	Phenylbutazone	Ticrynafen
Disulfiram	Naproxen	Phenytoin	Toxic oil (rapeseed)
Ethanol	Niacin	Pirprofen	

TABLE 4–3

Lobular Confluent Necrosis (refer to Table 2–18)

Allopurinol	Ethionamide	Niacin	Probenecid
Alpha-methyldopa	Halogenated hydrocarbons	Nicotinic acid	Prochlorperazine
Captopril	Hydralazine	Nitrofurantoin	Propylthiouracil
Carbamazepine	Indomethacin	Pemoline	Sulfamethoxazole
Chlordiazepoxide	Iproclozide	Phenelzine sulfate	Sulfonamides
Cimetidine	Isoniazid	Phenylbutazone	Ticrynafen
Dacarbazine	Ketoconazole	Phenytoin	Troglitazone
Erythromycin	Mithramycin	Piroxicam	Valproic acid
Ethacrynic acid	Mitomycin		

TABLE 4–4

Cholestasis with Inflammation (refer to Table 2–16)

Acetaminophen	Cimetidine	Isocarboxazid	Quinethazone
Acetohexamide	Cisplatin	Isoniazid	Ranitidine
Allopurinol	Clorazepate dipotassium	Meprobamate	Rifampin
Alpha-methyldopa	Cyclosporine	6-Mercaptopurine	Sulfasalazine
Aminoglutethimide	Dacarbazine	Naproxen	Sulfonamides
Aminosalicylic acid	Dantrolene	Nicotinic acid	Sulindac
Amitriptyline	Diazepam	Nifedipine	Tamoxifen
Amoxicillin–clavulanic acid	Diclofenac	Nitrofurantoin	Thiabendazole
Aprindine	Disopyramide phosphate	Nomifensine	Thiopental
Atenolol	Enalapril	Oxacillin	Thioridazine
Azathioprine	Erythromycin	Oxyphenisatin	Tocainide
Benoxaprofen	Ethchlorvynol	Papaverine	Tolazamide
Captopril	Ethionamide	Para-aminosalicylic acid	Tolbutamide
Carbamazepine	Fluoxymesterone	Penicillamine	Total parenteral nutrition
Carbarsone	Fluphenazine	Penicillin	Toxic oil (rapeseed)
Carbimazole	Flurazepam	Perphenazine	Tranylcypromine sulfate
Carisoprodol	Flutamide	Phenobarbital	Triazolam
Cefadroxil monohydrate	Glibenclamide	Phenylbutazone	Trifluoperazine
Cefazolin	Gold sodium thiomalate	Phenytoin	Trimethobenzamide hydrochloride
Chlorambucil	Griseofulvin	Piperazine	Trimethoprim-sulfamethoxazole
Chlordiazepoxide	Halogenated hydrocar-	Piroxicam	Tripelennamine
Chlorothiazide	bons	Pizotyline	Troleandomycin
Chlorpromazine	Haloperidol	Polythiazide	Valproic acid
Chlorpropamide	Imipramine	Prajmalium bitartrate	Verapamil
Chlortetracycline	Indomethacin	Prochlorperazine	Zimeldine
Chlorthalidone	Iodipamide meglumine	Propoxyphene	

TABLE 4–5

Cholestasis, Simple (refer to Table 2–8)

Cyclosporin A	Mestranol	Norethindrone	Piroxicam
Ethchlorvynol	Methandrostenolone	Norethynodrel	Prochlorperazine
Fluoxymesterone	Methimazole	Norgestrel	Warfarin
Gold sodium thiomalate	Methyltestosterone		

TABLE 4–6

Bile Ducts: Inflammation by Neutrophils (refer to Table 2–2)

Allopurinol	Chlorpropamide	Hydralazine
Chlorpromazine	Chlorothiazide	Sulindac

TABLE 4-7

Bile Ducts: Inflammation by Lymphocytes (refer to Table 2–3); Ductopenia (refer to Table 2–6)

Acetaminophen	Chlorpromazine	Methyltestosterone	Thiabendazole
Ajmaline (alkaloid isolated from	Cromolyn	Phenylbutazone	Tiopronin
Rauwolfia serpentina)	Diazepam	Piroxicam	Tolbutamide
Ampicillin	Haloperidol	Prochlorperazine	Toxic oil (rapeseed)
Arsenicals	Imipramine	Sulfonylurea agents	Trifluoperazine
Chlorothiazide	Methylenediamine		

TABLE 4-8

Bile Ducts: Periductal Fibrosis (refer to Table 2–5)

Flurodeoxyuridine (by endoscopic retrograde cholangiopancreatography)

TABLE 4-9

Portal Fibrosis (refer to Table 2–28)

Cirrhosis, or Portal Fibrosis with Progression to Cirrhosis on Serial Biopsies

Acetaminophen	Dantrolene	Methotrexate	Phenylbutazone
Acetohexamide	Diclofenac	Methyltestosterone	Tamoxifen
Alpha-methyldopa	Ethanol	Nitrofurantoin	Thiabendazole
Amiodarone	Ferrous fumarate	Oxyphenisatin	Total parenteral nutrition
Chlorothiazide	Isoniazid	Papaverine	Valproic acid
Chlorpromazine	Mercaptopurine	Perhexiline maleate	

Portal Fibrosis Without Progression to Cirrhosis

Arsenic	Thorotrast (thorium dioxide)	Vinyl chloride

TABLE 4-10

Fatty Change (refer to Table 2–12)

Macrovesicular

Acetaminophen	Corticosteroids	Hydrazine	Organic solvents
Alpha-methyldopa	Cyanamide	Ibuprofen	Perhexiline maleate
Amanitin	Dantrolene	Indomethacin	Phosphorus
Asparaginase	Dichloroethylene	Isoniazid	Rifampin
Azidothymidine (AZT)	Dimethylformamide	Methimazole	Sulfasalazine
Bleomycin	Ethanol	Methotrexate	Sulindac
Borates	Ethyl chloride	Methyl bromide	Tamoxifen
Cadmium	Etretinate	Methyl chloride	Tannic acid
Chromate	Floxuridine	Minocycline	Total parenteral nutrition
Cisplatin	Flurazepam	Mitomycin	Warfarin
Clometacin	Gold sodium thiomalate	Mushrooms	
Cocaine	Halogenated hydrocarbons	Nitrofurantoin	

Microvesicular

Aflatoxin	Desferrioxamine	Ketoprofen	Piroxicam
Amiodarone	Didanosine	Margosa oil	Pyrrolizidine alkaloids
Antiemetics	Dimethylformamide	Methyl salicylate	Tetracycline
Aspirin	Ethanol	Mushrooms	Tolmetin
Camphor	Ethionine	Pentenoic acid	Valproic acid
Chlortetracycline	Hypoglycin A	Phalloidin	
Cocaine	Ibuprofen	Phosphorus	

TABLE 4-11

Sinusoids: Peliotic Lesions (refer to Table 2-31)

Androgenic/anabolic steroids	Estrone sulfate	Methyltestosterone	Tamoxifen
Arsenic	Fluoxymesterone	Oxymetholone	6-Thioguanine
Azathioprine	6-Mercaptopurine	Phalloidin	Thorotrast (thorium dioxide)
Danazol	Methandrostenolone	Steroids, endogenous production	Vitamin A
Diethylstilbestrol	Methotrexate	(adrenal tumor)	

TABLE 4-12

Sinusoids: Dilatation, Congestion, and Hemorrhage (refer to Table 2-30)

Metoclopramide   Oral contraceptives

TABLE 4-13

Hepatic Venous Outflow Obstruction (Budd-Chiari Syndrome) (refer to Table 2-32 and Table 2-37); Veno-occlusive Disease (refer to Table 2-37)

Actinomycin D	Dacarbazine	6-Mercaptopurine	Thorotrast (thorium dioxide)
Adriamycin	Danazol	Mestranol	Urethane
Aflatoxin	Daunorubicin	Methyltestosterone	Valproic acid
Arsenicals	Dimethylbusulfan	Mitomycin	Vinblastine
Azathioprine	Estrogens	Norethindrone	Vincristine
Busulfan	Ethanol	Pyrrolizidine alkaloids	Vinyl chloride
Carmustine	Ethinyl estradiol	Tamoxifen	Vitamin A
Cysteamine	5-Fluoro-2'-deoxyuridine	6-Thioguanine	
Cytosine arabinoside			

TABLE 4-14

Vasculitis (refer to Table 2-36)

Allopurinol	Chlorpropamide	Phenytoin	Sulfonamides
Chlorothiazide	Penicillin	Phenylbutazone	

TABLE 4-15

Granulomas (refer to Table 2-13)

Allopurinol	Dimethicone	Oxacillin	Ranitidine
Alpha-methyldopa	Disopyramide	Oxyphenbutazone	Silica
Aspirin	Feprazone	Oxyphenisatin	Succinylsulfathiazole
Bacille Calmette-Guérin therapy or vaccination	Glibenclamide	Papaverine	Sulfadiazine
Barium	Gold sodium thiomalate	Penicillin	Sulfadimethoxine
Beryllium	Green-lipped mussel (Seatone)	Phenazone	Sulfadoxine-pyrimethamine
Carbamazepine	Halogenated hydrocarbons	Phenprocoumon	Sulfanilamide
Carbutamide	Hydralazine	Phenylbutazone	Sulfasalazine
Cephalexin	Isoniazid	Phenytoin	Sulfathiazole
Chlorpromazine	Mestranol	Polyvinyl pyrrolidone	Sulfonamides
Chlorpropamide	Metolazone	Prajmalium	Sulfonylurea agents
Copper	Mineral oil	Procainamide	Thorotrast (thorium dioxide)
Dapsone	Nitrofurantoin	Procarbazine	Tocainide
Diazepam	Norethindrone	Pronestyl	Tolbutamide
Diltiazem	Norethynodrel	Quinidine	Trichlormethiazide
	Norgestrel	Quinine	Trimethoprim-sulfamethoxazole

TABLE 4–16

Neoplasms (refer to Tables 2–20 and 2–21)

Benign

Liver Cell Adenoma

Anabolic steroids	Oral contraceptives	Toxic oil (rapeseed)

Focal Nodular Hyperplasia

Estrogens

Nodular Regenerative Hyperplasia

Anabolic steroids	Corticosteroids	Oral contraceptives	Toxic oil (rapeseed)
Copper	Ethanol	Thorotrast (thorium dioxide)	Vinyl chloride

Malignant

Hepatocellular Carcinoma

Aflatoxin	Arsenic	Methotrexate	Thorotrast (thorium dioxide)
Anabolic steroids	Ethanol	Oral contraceptives	Vinyl chloride

Angiosarcoma

Anabolic steroids	Copper	Oral contraceptives	Thorotrast (thorium dioxide)
Arsenic	Diethylstilbestrol	Phenelzine	Vinyl chloride

Cholangiocarcinoma

Alpha-methldopa	Isoniazid	Oral contraceptives	Thorotrast (thorium dioxide)
Anabolic steroids			

TABLE 4–17

Inclusions: Hepatocytes (refer to Table 2–14)

Cytoplasmic

Procainamide

Nuclear

Lead

"Ground Glass"–like Hepatocytes

Chlorpromazine	Cyanamide	Phenytoin	Phenobarbital

TABLE 4–18

Inclusions: Kupffer Cells and Portal Macrophages (refer to Table 2–15)

Polyvinyl pyrrolidone	Silicone rubber (damaged cardiac prosthetic valves)	Talc, particulate material	Thorotrast (thorium dioxide)

TABLE 4–19

Pigments (refer to Table 2–22)

Lipochrome

Aminopyrine	Chlordecone (Kepone)	Phenacetin	Phenothiazines
Cascara sagrada	Chlorpromazine		

Hemosiderin

Cimetidine	Ethanol	Iron, oral and parenteral

Radiopaque

Thorotrast (thorium dioxide)

TABLE 4–20

Mallory Bodies (refer to Table 2–19)

Amiodarone	Estrogens	Methotrexate	Tamoxifen
Collidine	Ethanol	Nicardipine	Tetracycline
4,4,4-Diethylaminoethoxyhexestrol	Glucocorticoids	Nifedipine	Valproic acid
Diethylstilbestrol	Griseofulvin	Perhexiline maleate	Vitamin A
Diltiazem			

CHAPTER 5

References

1. Ludwig J, Batts KP. Practical Liver Biopsy Interpretation: Diagnostic Algorithms. 2nd ed. ASCP Press: Chicago, 1998.
2. Snover DC. Biopsy Diagnosis of Liver Diseases. Williams & Wilkins: Baltimore, 1992.
3. Scheuer PJ, Lefkowitz JH. Liver Biopsy Interpretation. WB Saunders: London, 1994.
4. MacSween RNM, Anthony PP, Scheuer PJ, et al. Pathology of the Liver. 3rd ed. Churchill Livingston: Edinburgh, 1994.
5. Klatskin G, Conn HO. Histopathology of the Liver. Oxford University Press: New York, 1993.
6. Wight DGD. Atlas of Liver Pathology. Kluwer Academic Publications: Boston, 1993.
7. Patrick RS, McGee J O'D. Biopsy Pathology of the Liver. 2nd ed. Chapman and Hall: London, 1988.
8. Schiff ER, Sorrell MF, Maddrey WC. Schiff's Diseases of the Liver. 8th ed. Lippincott-Raven: Philadelphia, 1999.
9. Ruebner BH, Montgomery CK, French SW. Diagnostic Pathology of the Liver and Biliary Tract. 2nd ed. Hemisphere Publications: New York, 1991.
10. Phillips MJ, Poucell S, Patterson J, et al. The Liver. An Atlas and Text of Ultrastructural Pathology. Raven Press: New York, 1987.
11. Peters RL, Craig JR. Liver Pathology. Churchill Livingstone: New York, 1986.
12. Craig JR, Peters RL, Edmondson HA. Tumors of the liver and intrahepatic bile ducts. AFIP fascicle 26, 2nd series. Armed Forces Institute of Pathology: Washington, DC, 1988.
13. Partin JS, Partin JC, Schubert WK, et al. Liver ultrastructure in abetalipoproteinemia: Evolution of micronodular cirrhosis. Gastroenterology 1974;67:107–118.
14. Avigan MI, Ishak KG, Gregg RE, et al. Morphologic features of the liver in abetalipoproteinemia. Hepatology 1984;4:1223–1226.
15. Kane JP, Havel RJ. Disorders of the biogenesis and secretion of lipoproteins containing the β-apolipoproteins. In Scriver CR, Beaudet AL, Sly WS, et al, eds. The Metabolic Basis of Inherited Disease. 6th ed. McGraw-Hill: New York, 1989, pp 1139–1164.
16. Putman HC, Dockerty MB, Waugh JM. Abdominal actinomyces: An analysis of 122 cases. Surgery 1993;28:781–790.
17. Kazmi KA, Rab SM. Primary hepatic actinomycosis: A diagnostic problem. Am J Trop Med Hyg 1989;40:310–311.
18. Meade RH. Primary hepatic actinomycosis. Gastroenterology 1980;78:355–359.
19. Randall B. Sudden death and hepatic fatty metamorphosis. JAMA 1980;243:1723–1725.
20. Randall B. Fatty liver and sudden death: A review. Hum Pathol 1980;11:147–153.
21. Edmondson HA. Alcoholic liver disease. In Peters RL, Craig JR, eds. Liver Pathology. Churchill Livingstone: New York, 1986, pp 255–283.
22. Knox TA, Olans LB. Liver disease in pregnancy. N Engl J Med 1996;335:569–576.
23. Pockros PJ, Peters RL, Reynolds TB. Idiopathic fatty liver of pregnancy: Findings in ten cases. Medicine 1984;63:1–11.
24. Rolfes DB, Ishak KG. Acute fatty liver of pregnancy: A clinicopathologic study of 35 cases. Hepatology 1985;5:1149–1158.
25. Kaplan MM. Acute fatty liver of pregnancy. N Engl J Med 1985;313:367–370.
26. Rolfes DB, Ishak KG. Liver disease in pregnancy. Histopathology 1986;10:555–570.
27. Batey RG. Acute fatty liver of pregnancy: Is it genetically predetermined? Am J Gastroenterol 1996;91:2262–2264.
28. Usta IM, Sibai BM. Acute fatty liver of pregnancy. J Med Liban 1995;43:186–193.
29. Riely CA. Hepatic disease in pregnancy. Am J Med 1994;96 (1A):18S–22S.
30. Reyes H, Sandoval L, Wainstein A, et al. Acute fatty liver of pregnancy: A clinical study of 12 episodes in 11 patients. Gut 1994;35:101–106.
31. MacSween RNM, Burt AD. Histologic spectrum of alcoholic liver disease. Semin Liv Dis 1986;6:221–232.
32. French SW, Nash J, Shitabata P, et al. Pathology of alcoholic liver disease. Semin Liv Dis 1993;13:154–169.
33. Edmondson HA, Peters RL, Reynolds TB, et al. Sclerosing hyaline necrosis of the liver in the chronic alcoholic. Ann Intern Med 1963;59:646–673.
34. Maddrey WC. Alcoholic hepatitis: Clinicopathologic features and therapy. Semin Liv Dis 1988;8:91–102.
35. Pares A, Caballeria J, Bruguera M, et al. Histologic course of alcoholic hepatitis: Influence of abstinence, sex, and extent of hepatic damage. J Hepatol 1986;2:33–42.
36. Okanoue T, Burbige EJ, French SW. The role of the Ito cell in perivenular and intralobular fibrosis in alcoholic hepatitis. Arch Pathol Lab Med 1982;107:459–463.
37. Edmondson HA. Pathology of alcoholism. Am J Clin Pathol 1980;74:725–742.
38. Sorensen TIA, Orholm M, Bentsen KD, et al. Prospective evaluation of alcohol abuse and alcoholic liver injury in men as predictors of development of cirrhosis. Lancet 1984;2:241–244.
39. Allaire GS, Rabin L, Ishak KG, et al. Bile duct adenoma: A study of 152 cases. Am J Surg Pathol 1988;12:708–715.
40. Govindarajan S, Peters RL. The bile duct adenoma: A lesion distinct from Meyenburg complex. Arch Pathol Lab Med 1984; 108:922–924.
41. Anthony PP. Tumours and tumour-like lesions of the liver and biliary tract. In MacSween RNM, Anthony PP, Scheuer PJ, et al, eds. Pathology of the Liver. 3rd ed. Churchill Livingstone: Edinburgh, 1994, pp 635–711.
42. Bhathal PS, Hughes NR, Goodman ZD. The so-called bile duct adenoma is a peribiliary gland hamartoma. Am J Surg Pathol 1996;20:858–864.
43. Edmondson HA, Henderson B, Benton B. Liver-cell adenomas associated with use of oral contraceptives. N Engl J Med 1976; 294:470–472.
44. Kerlin P, Davis GL, McGill DB, et al. Hepatic adenoma and focal nodular hyperplasia: Clinical, pathologic, and radiologic features. Gastroenterology 1983;84:994–1002.
45. Poe R, Snover DC. Adenomas in glycogen storage disease type 1: Two cases with unusual histologic features. Am J Surg Pathol 1988;12:477–483.
46. Korula J, Yellin A, Kanel G, et al. Hepatocellular carcinoma coexisting with hepatic adenoma: Incidental discovery after long-term oral contraceptive use. West J Med 1991;155:416–418.
47. Foster JH, Berman MM. The benign lesions: Adenoma and focal nodular hyperplasia. Major Probl Clin Surg 1977;22:138–178.
48. Petrovic LM. Benign hepatocellular tumors and tumor-like lesions. In Ferrell LD, ed. Diagnostic Problems in Liver Pathology. Hanley & Belfus: Philadelphia, 1994, pp 119–139.
49. DeCarlis L, Pirotta V, Rondinara GF, et al. Hepatic adenoma and focal nodular hyperplasia: Diagnosis and criteria for treatment. Liver Transpl Surg 1997;3:160–165.
50. Cherqui D, Rahmouni A, Charlotte F, et al. Management of focal nodular hyperplasia and hepatocellular adenoma in young women: A series of 41 patients with clinical, radiological, and pathological correlations. Hepatology 1995;22:1674–1681.
51. Labrune P, Trioche P, Duvaltier I, et al. Hepatocellular adenomas in glycogen storage disease type I and III: A series of 43 patients and review of the literature. J Pediatr Gastroenterol Nutr 1997;24:276–279.
52. Bianchi L. Glycogen storage disease I and hepatocellular tumors. Eur J Pediatr 1993;152 (Suppl 1):S63–S70.
53. Furuya K, Nakamura M, Yamamoto Y, et al. Macroregenerative nodule of the liver. A clinicopathologic study of 345 autopsy cases of chronic liver disease. Cancer 1988;61:99–105.
54. Nakanuma Y, Terada T, Ueda K, et al. Adenomatous hyperplasia of the liver as a precancerous lesion. Liver 1993;13:1–9.
55. Ferrell L. Hepatocellular nodules in the cirrhotic liver: Diagnostic features and proposed nomenclature. In Ferrell LD, ed. Diagnostic Problems in Liver Pathology. Hanley & Belfus: Philadelphia, 1994, pp 105–117.
56. Varki NM, Bhuta S, Drake T, et al. Adenovirus hepatitis in two successive liver transplants in a child. Arch Pathol Lab Med 1990;114:106–109.
57. Carmichael GP, Zahradnik JM, Moyer GH, et al. Adenovirus hepatitis in an immunosuppressed adult patient. Am J Clin Pathol 1979;71:352–355.

58. Krilov LR, Rubin LG, Frogel M, et al. Disseminated adenovirus infection with hepatic necrosis in patients with human immunodeficiency virus infection and other immunodeficiency states. Rev Infect Dis 1990;12:303–307.

59. Saad RS, Demetris AJ, Lee RG, et al. Adenovirus hepatitis in the adult allograft liver. Transplantation 1997;64:1483–1485.

60. Gerber MA, Thung SN, Bodenheimer HC, et al. Characteristic histologic triad in liver adjacent to metastatic neoplasm. Liver 1986;6:85–88.

61. MacSween RNM, Burt AD. Liver pathology associated with diseases of other organs. *In* MacSween RNM, Anthony PP, Scheuer PJ, et al, eds. Pathology of the Liver. 3rd ed. Churchill Livingstone: Edinburgh, 1994, pp 713–764.

62. Melnick PJ. Polycystic liver. Arch Pathol 1955;59:162–172.

63. Kwok MK, Lewin KJ. Massive hepatomegaly in adult polycystic liver disease. Am J Surg Pathol 1988;12:321–324.

64. Ramos A, Torres VE, Holley KE, et al. The liver in autosomal dominant polycystic kidney disease. Arch Pathol Lab Med 1990;114:180–184.

65. Keda T, Nakanuma Y, Terada T. Cystic dilatation of peribiliary glands in livers with adult polycystic disease and livers with solitary nonparasitic cysts: An autopsy study. Hepatology 1992;16:334–340.

66. Lieber CS, Schmid R. Stimulation of hepatic fatty acid synthesis by ethanol. Am J Clin Nutr 1961;9:436–438.

67. Hall P de la M. Alcoholic liver disease. *In* MacSween RNM, Anthony PP, Scheuer PJ, et al, eds. Pathology of the Liver. 3rd ed. Churchill Livingstone: Edinburgh, 1994, pp 317–348.

68. Lieber CS, Jones DP, DeCarli LM. Effects of prolonged ethanol intake: Production of fatty liver despite adequate diets. J Clin Invest 1965;44:1009–1021.

69. Lieber CS, DeCarli LM. Hepatotoxicity of ethanol. J Hepatol 1991;12:394–401.

70. Lieber CS. Biochemical and molecular basis of alcohol-induced injury to liver and other tissues. N Engl J Med 1988;319:1639–1650.

71. Uchida T, Kao H, Quispe-Sjogren M, et al. Alcoholic foamy degeneration—a pattern of acute alcoholic injury of the liver. Gastroenterology 1983;84:683–692.

72. Montull S, Pares A, Bruguera M, et al. Alcoholic foamy degeneration in Spain: Prevalence and clinico-pathological features. Liver 1989;9:79–85.

73. Koyama K, Kanayama M, Uchida T, et al. Serial liver biopsies of two patients with alcoholic foamy degeneration. Jpn J Hepatol 1984;25:657–665.

74. Wada K, Kondo F, Kondo Y. Large regenerative nodules and dysplastic nodules in cirrhotic livers: A histopathologic study. Hepatology 1988;6:1684–1688.

75. Anthony PP, Ishak KG, Nayak NC, et al. The morphology of cirrhosis. J Clin Pathol 1978;31:395–414.

76. Lee FI. Cirrhosis and hepatoma in alcoholics. Gut 1966;7:77–85.

77. Gluud C, Henrickson JH, Nielsen G. Prognostic indicators in alcoholic cirrhotic men. Hepatology 1988;8:222–227.

78. Hart J, Lewin KJ. Liver allograft pathology. *In* Ferrell LD, ed. Diagnostic Problems in Liver Pathology. Hanley & Belfus: Philadelphia, 1994, pp 207–250.

79. Ludwig J. Histopathology of the liver following transplantation. *In* Maddrey WC, Sorrell MF, eds. Transplantation of the Liver. Appleton & Lange: Norwalk, CT, 1995, pp 267–295.

80. Demetris AJ, Batts KP, Dhillon AP, et al. Banff schema for grading liver allograft rejection: An international consensus document. Hepatology 1997;25:658–663.

81. International Working Party: Terminology for hepatic allograft rejection. Hepatology 1995;22:648–654.

82. Demetris AJ, Seaberg EC, Batts KP, et al. Reliability and predictive value of the National Institute of Diabetes and Digestive and Kidney Diseases Liver Transplantation Database nomenclature and grading system for cellular rejection of liver allografts. Hepatology 1995;21:408–416.

83. Rizkalla KS, Asfar SK, McLean CA, et al. Key features distinguishing post-transplantation lymphoproliferative disorders and acute liver rejection. Mod Pathol 1997;10:708–715.

84. Demetris AJ. Immune cholangitis: Liver allograft rejection and graft-versus-host disease. Mayo Clin Proc 1998;73:367–379.

85. Wiesner RH, Demetris AJ, Belle SH, et al. Acute hepatic allo-

86. Datta Gupta S, Hudson M, Burroughs AK, et al. Grading of cellular rejection after orthotopic liver transplantation. Hepatology 1995;21:46–57.

87. Demetris AJ, Qian SG, Sun H, et al. Liver allograft rejection: An overview of morphologic findings. Am J Surg Pathol 1990; 14 (Suppl 1):49–63.

88. McVicar JP, Kowdley KV, Bacchi CE, et al. The natural history of untreated focal allograft rejection in liver transplant recipients. Liver Transpl Surg 1996;2:154–160.

89. Deschenes M, Belle SH, Krom RA, et al. Early allograft dysfunction after liver transplantation: A definition and predictors of outcome. National Institute of Diabetes and Digestive and Kidney Diseases Liver Transplantation Database. Transplantation 1998;66:302–310.

90. Van Hoek B, Wiesner RH, Krom RAF, et al. Severe ductopenic rejection following liver transplantation: Incidence, time of onset, risk factors, treatment, and outcome. Semin Liver Dis 1992;12:41–50.

91. Demetris AJ, Seaberg EC, Batts KP, et al. Chronic liver allograft rejection: A National Institute of Diabetes and Digestive and Kidney Diseases interinstitutional study analyzing the reliability of current criteria and proposal of an expanded definition. National Institute of Diabetes and Digestive and Kidney Disease Liver Transplantation Database. Am J Surg Pathol 1998;22:28–39.

92. Rubin R, Munoz SJ. Clinicopathologic features of late hepatic dysfunction in orthotopic liver transplants. Hum Pathol 1993; 24:643–651.

93. Davies SE, Portmann BC, O'Grady JG, et al. Hepatic histological findings after transplantation for chronic hepatitis B virus infection, including a unique pattern of fibrosing cholestatic hepatitis. Hepatology 1991;13:150–157.

94. Harrison RF, Davies MH, Goldin RD, et al. Recurrent hepatitis B in liver allografts: A distinctive form of rapidly developing cirrhosis. Histopathology 1993;23:21–28.

95. Goldstein NS, Hart J, Lewin KJ. Diffuse hepatocyte ballooning in liver biopsies from orthotopic transplant patients. Histopathology 1991;18:331–338.

96. Ng IOL, Burroughs AK, Rolles K, et al. Hepatocellular ballooning after liver transplantation: A light and electronmicroscopic study with clinicopathological correlation. Histopathology 1991;18:323–330.

97. Ludwig J, Batts KP, MacCarty RL. Ischemic cholangitis in hepatic allografts. Mayo Clin Proc 1992;67:519–526.

98. Randhawa PS, Jaffe R, Demetris AJ, et al. Expression of Epstein-Barr virus-encoded small RNA (by the EBER-1 gene) in liver specimens from transplant recipients with post-transplantation lymphoproliferative disease. N Engl J Med 1992;327: 1710–1714.

99. Nalesnik MA. Posttransplantation lymphoproliferative disorders (PTLD): Current perspectives. Semin Thorac Cardiovasc Surg 1996;8:139–148.

100. Manez R, Breinig MC, Linden P, et al. Posttransplant lymphoproliferative disease in primary Epstein-Barr virus infection after liver transplantation: The role of cytomegalovirus disease. J Infect Dis 1997;176:1462–1467.

101. Egawa H, Inomata Y, Uemoto S, et al. Lymphoproliferative disorders in patients undergoing living-related liver transplantation. Transplant Proc 1998;30:136–137.

102. Liu G, Butany J, Wanless IR, et al. The vascular pathology of human allografts. Hum Pathol 1993;24:182–188.

103. Huttenlocher PR, Solitaire GB, Adams G. Infantile diffuse cerebral degeneration with hepatic cirrhosis. Arch Neurol 1975;33: 186–192.

104. Harding BN, Egger J, Portmann B, et al. Progressive neuronal degeneration of childhood with liver disease. Brain 1986;109: 181–206.

105. Narkewicz MR, Sokol RJ, Beckwith B, et al. Liver involvement in Alpers' disease. J Pediatr 1991;119:260–267.

106. Eriksson S, Lindmark B, Lilja H. Familial alpha$_1$-antichymotrypsin deficiency. Acta Med Scand 1986;220:447–453.

107. Lindmark B, Millward-Sadler H, Callea F, et al. Hepatocyte inclusions of α_1-antichymotrypsin in a patient with partial defi-

ciency of α_1-antichymotrypsin and chronic liver disease. Histopathology 1990;16:211–225.

108. Morse JO. Alpha$_1$-antitrypsin deficiency. N Engl J Med 1978; 299:1099–1105.

109. Bradfield JW, Blenkinsopp WK. Alpha$_1$-antitrypsin globules in the liver and PiM phenotype. J Clin Pathol 1977;30:579–584.

110. Talbot IC, Mowat AP. Liver disease in infancy: Histological features and relationship to α_1-antitrypsin phenotype. J Clin Pathol 1975;28:559–563.

111. Malone M, Mieli-Vergani G, Mowat AP, et al. The fetal liver in PiZZ α_1-antitrypsin deficiency: A report of five cases. Pediatr Pathol 1989;9:923–931.

112. Rubel LR, Ishak KG, Benjamin SB, et al. α_1-Antitrypsin deficiency and hepatocellular carcinoma: Association with cirrhosis, copper storage and Mallory bodies. Arch Pathol Lab Med 1982;106:678–681.

113. Psacharopoulos HT, Mowat AP, Cook PJL, et al. Outcome of liver disease associated with α_1-antitrypsin deficiency (PiZ). Arch Dis Child 1983;58:882–887.

114. Perlmutter DH. Liver disease associated with alpha$_1$-antitrypsin deficiency. Prog Liver Dis 1993;11:139–165.

115. Knight R. Hepatic amebiasis. Semin Liv Dis 1984;4:277–292.

116. Reynolds TB. Liver abscess. In Kaplowitz N, ed. Liver and Biliary Diseases. 2nd ed. Williams & Wilkins: Baltimore, 1996, pp 463–468.

117. Barnes PF, De Cock KM, Reynolds TB, et al. A comparison of amebic and pyogenic abscess of the liver. Medicine 1987;66: 472–483.

118. Brandt H, Perez Tamayo R. Pathology of human amebiasis. Hum Pathol 1970;1:351–385.

119. Sharma MP, Dasarathy S, Verma N, et al. Prognostic markers in amebic abscess: A prospective study. Am J Gastroenterol 1996;91:2584–2588.

120. Ralls PW, Coletti PM, Quinn MF, et al. Sonographic findings in hepatic amebic abscess. Radiology 1982;145:123–126.

121. Levine RA. Amyloid disease of the liver: Correlation of clinical, functional and morphologic features in forty-seven patients. Am J Med 1962;33:349–357.

122. Kyle RA, Bayrd ED. Amyloidosis: Review of 236 cases. Medicine (Baltimore) 1975;54:271–299.

123. Chopra S, Rubinow A, Koff RS, et al. Hepatic amyloidosis: A histopathologic analysis of primary (AL) and secondary (AA) forms. Am J Pathol 1984;115:186–193.

124. Kanel GC, Uchida T, Peters RL. Globular hepatic amyloid—an unusual morphologic presentation. Hepatology 1981;1:647–652.

125. Glenner GG. Amyloid deposits and amyloidosis: The β-fibrilloses. N Engl J Med 1980;302:1283–1292, 1333–1343.

126. Rubinow A, Koff RS, Cohen AS. Severe intrahepatic cholestasis in primary amyloidosis. Am J Med 1978;64:937–946.

127. Looi L-M, Sumithran E. Morphologic differences in the pattern of liver infiltration between systemic AL and AA amyloidosis. Hum Pathol 1988;19:732–735.

128. Gertz MA, Kyle RA. Hepatic amyloidosis: Clinical appraisal in 77 patients. Hepatology 1997;25:118–121.

129. Gertz MA, Kyle RA. Hepatic amyloidosis: The natural history in 80 patients. Am J Med 1988;85:73–80.

130. Craig JR. Mesenchymal tumors of the liver: Diagnostic problems for the surgical pathologist. In Ferrell LD, ed. Diagnostic Problems in Liver Pathology. Hanley & Belfus: Philadelphia, 1994, pp 141–160.

131. Goodman ZD, Ishak KG. Angiomyolipomas of the liver. Am J Surg Pathol 1984;4:745–750.

132. Nonomura A, Mizukami Y, Kadoya M. Angiomyolipoma of the liver: A collective review. J Gastroenterol 1994;29:95–105.

133. Hoffman AL, Emre S, Verham RP, et al. Hepatic angiomyolipoma: Two case reports of caudate-based lesions and review of the literature. Liver Transpl Surg 1997;3:46–53.

134. Messiaen T, Lefebvre C, Van Beers B, et al. Hepatic angiomyo(myelo)lipoma: Difficulties in radiological diagnosis and interest of fine needle aspiration biopsy. Liver 1996;16:338–341.

135. Kanel GC, Korula J, Liew CT, et al. Atypical diffuse angiosarcoma of the liver. West J Med 1987;146:482–485.

136. Locker GY, Doroshow JH, Zwelling LA, et al. The clinical features of hepatic angiosarcoma: A report of four cases and a review of the English literature. Medicine 1979;58:48–64.

137. Popper H, Thomas LB, Telles NC, et al. Development of hepatic angiosarcoma in man induced by vinyl chloride, Thorotrast, and arsenic: Comparison with cases of unknown etiology. Am J Pathol 1978;92:349–376.

138. Saleh HA, Tao LC. Hepatic angiosarcoma: Aspiration biopsy cytology and immunocytochemical contributions. Diagn Cytopathol 1998;18:208–211.

139. Khuroo M, Zargar SA, Mahajan R. Hepatobiliary and pancreatic ascariasis in India. Lancet 1990;1:1503–1506.

140. Gayotto LCDC, Muszkat RML, Souza IV. Hepatobiliary alterations in massive biliary ascariasis: Histopathological aspects of an autopsy case. Rev Inst Med Trop São Paulo 1990;32:91–95.

141. Khuroo MS, Zargar SA. Biliary ascariasis: A common cause of biliary and pancreatic disease in an endemic area. Gastroenterology 1985;88:418–423.

142. Walsh TJ, Hamilton SR: Disseminated aspergillosis complicating hepatic failure. Arch Intern Med 1983;143:1189–1191.

143. Lucas SB. Other viral and infectious diseases and HIV-related liver diseases. In MacSween RNM, Anthony PP, Scheuer PJ, et al, eds. Pathology of the Liver. 3rd ed. Churchill Livingstone: Edinburgh, 1994, pp 269–315.

144. Manns M. Autoantibodies in liver disease—updated. J Hepatol 1989;9:272–280.

145. Heathcote EJ. Autoimmune cholangitis. Clin Liver Dis 1998;2: 303–312.

146. McFarlane IG. Autoimmunity and hepatotropic viruses. Semin Liv Dis 1991;11:223–233.

147. Johnson PJ, McFarlane IG, Eddleston ALWF. The natural course and heterogeneity of autoimmune-type chronic active hepatitis. Semin Liver Dis 1991;11:187–196.

148. Poulsen H, Christoffersen P. Abnormal bile duct epithelium in chronic aggressive hepatitis and cirrhosis: A review of morphology and clinical, biochemical, and immunologic features. Hum Pathol 1972;3:217–225.

149. Bianchi L, Gudat F. Chronic hepatitis. In MacSween RNM, Anthony PP, Scheuer PJ, et al, eds. Pathology of the Liver. 3rd ed. Churchill Livingstone: Edinburgh, 1994, pp 349–395.

150. Bach N, Thung SN, Schaffner F. The histological features of chronic hepatitis C and autoimmune chronic hepatitis: A comparative analysis. Hepatology 1992;15:572–577.

151. Czaja AJ. Frequency and nature of the variant syndromes of autoimmune liver disease. Hepatology 1998;28:360–365.

152. Chazouilleres O, Wendum D, Serfaty L, et al. Primary biliary cirrhosis—autoimmune hepatitis overlap syndrome: Clinical features and response to therapy. Hepatology 1998;28:296–301.

153. Entrican JH, Williams H, Cook IA, et al. Babesiosis in man: Report of a case from Scotland with observations on the infecting strain. J Infect 1979;1:227–234.

154. Slater LN, Welch DF, Min KW. *Rochalimaea henselae* causes bacillary angiomatosis and peliosis hepatis. Arch Intern Med 1992;152:602–606.

155. Steeper TA, Rosenstein H, Weiser J, et al. Bacillary epithelioid angiomatosis involving the liver, spleen, and skin in an AIDS patient with concurrent Kaposi's sarcoma. Am J Clin Pathol 1992;97:713–718.

156. Perkocha LA, Geaghan SM, Yen TSB, et al. Clinical and pathological features of bacillary peliosis hepatis in association with human immunodeficiency virus infection. N Engl J Med 1990; 323:1581–1586.

157. Carcana JA, Montes M, Camara DS, et al. Functional and histopathological changes in the liver during sepsis. Surg Gynecol Obstet 1982;154:653–656.

158. Barnes PF, Arevalo C, Chan LS, et al. A prospective evaluation of bacteremic patients with chronic liver disease. Hepatology 1988;8:1099–1103.

159. Schmid M, Heft ML, Gattiker R, et al. Benign postoperative intrahepatic cholestasis. N Engl J Med 1965;272:545–550.

160. Collins JD, Bassendine MF, Ferner R, et al. Incidence and prognostic importance of jaundice after cardiopulmonary bypass surgery. Lancet 1983;2:1119–1129.

161. Hayes PC, Bouchier IAD. Postoperative jaundice. Baillieres Clin Gastroenterol 1989;3:485–505.

162. Marcellin P, Erlinger S. Benign recurrent cholestasis. Gastroenterol Clin Biol 1985;9:679–684.

163. Brenard R, Geubel AP, Benhamou J-P. Benign recurrent intrahepatic cholestasis: A report of 26 cases. J Clin Gastroenterol 1989;11:546–551.

164. Biempica L, Gutstein S, Arias IM. Morphological and biochemical studies of benign recurrent cholestasis. Gastroenterology 1967;52:521–535.

165. Chung EB. Multiple bile-duct hamartomas. Cancer 1970;25:287–296.

166. Judge DM, Samuel I, Perine PL, et al. Louse-borne relapsing fever in man. Arch Pathol Lab Med 1974;97:136–140.

167. Guardia J, Martinez-Vazquez JM, Moragas A. The liver in boutonneuse fever. Gut 1974;15:549–551.

168. Walker DH, Staiti A, Mansueto G, et al. Frequent occurrence of hepatic lesions in boutonneuse fever. Acta Trop 1986;43:175–181.

169. Cascio A, Dones P, Romano A, et al. Clinical and laboratory findings of boutonneuse fever in Sicilian children. Eur J Pediatr 1998;157:482–486.

170. Williams RK, Crossley K. Acute and chronic hepatic involvement of brucellosis. Gastroenterology 1982;83:455–458.

171. Cervantes F, Bruguera M, Carbonell, J et al. Liver disease in brucellosis: A clinical and pathological study of 40 cases. Postgrad Med 1982;58:346–350.

172. Spink WW, Hoffbauer FW, Walker EE, et al. Histopathology of the liver in human brucellosis. J Lab Clin Med 1949;34:40–58.

173. Bruguera M, Cervantes F. Hepatic granulomas in brucellosis. Ann Intern Med 1980;92:571–572.

174. Kanel GC, Reynolds TB. Hepatic granulomas. *In* Kaplowitz N, ed. Liver and Biliary Diseases. 2nd ed. Williams & Wilkins: Baltimore, 1996, pp 455–462.

175. Vallejo JG, Stevens AM, Dutton RV, et al. Hepatosplenic abscesses due to *Brucella melitensis:* Report of a case involving a child and review of the literature. Clin Infect Dis 1996;22:485–489.

176. Sabharwal BD, Malhotra N, Garg R, et al. Granulomatous hepatitis: A retrospective study. Indian J Pathol Microbiol 1995;38:413–416.

177. Simpson IW. Budd-Chiari syndrome and veno-occlusive disease. *In* Peters RL, Craig JR, eds. Liver Pathology. Churchill Livingstone: New York, 1986, pp 299–314.

178. Rector WG, Xu Y, Goldstein L, et al. Membranous obstruction of the inferior vena cava in the United States. Medicine 1985;64:134–143.

179. Tavill AS, Wood EJ, Kreel L, et al. The Budd-Chiari syndrome: Correlation between hepatic scintigraphy and the clinical, radiological, and pathological findings in nineteen cases of hepatic venous outflow obstruction. Gastroenterology 1975;68:509–518.

180. Tanaka M, Wanless IR. Pathology of the liver in Budd-Chiari syndrome: Portal vein thrombosis and the histogenesis of veno-centric cirrhosis, veno-portal cirrhosis, and large regenerative nodules. Hepatology 1998;27:488–496.

181. Usui T, Kitano K, Midorikawa T, et al. Budd-Chiari syndrome caused by hepatic vein thrombosis in a patient with myeloproliferative disorder. Intern Med 1996;35:871–875.

182. Liew CT. A comparative histopathological study of hepatic venous outflow obstruction in veno-occlusive disease and Budd-Chiari's syndrome. Chang Keng I Hsueh 1990;13:167–181.

183. Simson IW. The causes and consequences of chronic hepatic venous outflow obstruction. S Afr Med J 1987;72:11–14.

184. Mitchell MC, Boitnott JK, Kaufman S, et al. Budd-Chiari syndrome: Etiology, diagnosis and management. Medicine 1982;61:199–218.

185. Klein AS, Sitzmann JV, Coleman J, et al. Current management of the Budd-Chiari syndrome. Ann Surg 1990;212:144–149.

186. Johnson TL, Barnett JL, Appelman HD, et al. Candida hepatitis: Histopathologic diagnosis. Am J Surg Pathol 1988;12:716–720.

187. Haron E, Feld R, Tuffnell P, et al. Hepatic candidiasis: An increasing problem in immunocompromised patients. Am J Med 1987;83:17–26.

188. Lewis JH, Patel HR, Zimmerman HJ. The spectrum of hepatic candidiasis. Hepatology 1982;1:479–487.

189. Bondestam S, Jansson S, Kivisaari L, et al. Liver and spleen candidiasis: Imaging and verification by fine-needle aspiration biopsy. BMJ 1981;282:1514–1515.

190. Attah EB, Nagarajan S, Obineche EN, et al. Hepatic capillariasis. Am J Clin Pathol 1983;79:127–130.

191. Choe G, Lee HS, Seo JK, et al. Hepatic capillariasis: First case report in the Republic of Korea. Am J Trop Med Hyg 1993;48:610–625.

192. Caroli J. Diseases of the intrahepatic biliary tree. Clin Gastroenterol 1973;2:147–161.

193. Marchal GJ, Desmet VJ, Proesmans WC, et al. Caroli's disease: High-frequency US and pathologic findings. Radiology 1986;158:507–511.

194. Phinney PR, Austin GE, Kadell BM. Cholangiocarcinoma arising in Caroli's disease. Arch Pathol Lab Med 1981;105:194–197.

195. Taylor AC, Palmer KR. Caroli's disease. Eur J Gastroenterol Hepatol 1998;10:105–108.

196. Barros JL, Polo JR, Sanabia J, et al. Congenital cystic dilatation of the intrahepatic bile ducts (Caroli's disease): Report of a case and review of the literature. Surgery 1979;85:589–592.

197. Rizkallah MF, Meyer L, Ayoub EM. Hepatic and splenic abscesses in cat-scratch disease. Pediatr Infect Dis J 1988;7:191–195.

198. Delbeke D, Sandler MP, Shaff MI, et al. Cat-scratch disease: Report of a case with liver lesions and no lymphadenopathy. J Nucl Med 1988;29:1454–1456.

199. Lamps LW, Gray GF, Scott MA. The histologic spectrum of hepatic cat scratch disease. A series of six cases with confirmed Bartonella henselae infection. Am J Surg Pathol 1996;20:1253–1259.

200. Dandman BC, Albanese BA, Kacica MA, et al. Cat scratch disease in two children presenting with fever of unknown origin: Imaging features and association with a new causative agent, *Rochalimaea henselae.* Pediatrics 1995;95:767–771.

201. Schwartz SI, Husser WC. Cavernous hemangioma of the liver. A single institution report of 16 resections. Ann Surg 1987;205:456–465.

202. Hobbs KEF. Hepatic haemangiomas. World J Surg 1990;14:468–471.

203. Gandolfi L, Leo P, Solmi L, et al. Natural history of hepatic haemangiomas: Clinical and ultrasound study. Gut 1991;32:677–680.

204. Yamashita Y, Ogata I, Urata J, et al. Cavernous hemangioma of the liver. Pathologic correlation with dynamic CT findings. Radiology 1997;203:121–125.

205. Iyer CP, Stanley P, Mahour GH. Hepatic hemangiomas in infants and children: A review of 30 cases. Am Surg 1996;62:356–360.

206. Alpert LI, Zak FG, Werthamer S, et al. Cholangiocarcinoma: A clinicopathologic study of five cases with ultrastructural observations. Hum Pathol 1974;5:709–728.

207. Klatskin G. Adenocarcinoma of the hepatic duct at its bifurcation within the porta hepatis: An unusual tumor with distinctive clinical and pathological features. Am J Med 1965;38:241–256.

208. Rosen CB, Nagorney DM. Cholangiocarcinoma complicating primary sclerosing cholangitis. Semin Liv Dis 1991;11:26–30.

209. Wee A, Ludwig J, Coffey RJ, et al. Hepatobiliary carcinoma associated with primary sclerosing cholangitis and chronic ulcerative colitis. Hum Pathol 1985;16:719–726.

210. Nakajima T, Kondo Y, Miyazaki M, et al. A histopathologic study of 102 cases of intrahepatic cholangiocarcinoma. Hum Pathol 1988;19:1228–1234.

211. Kaczynski J, Hansson G. Wallerstedt S. Incidence, etiologic aspects and clinicopathologic features in intrahepatic cholangiocellular carcinoma—a study of 51 cases from a low-endemicity area. Acta Oncol 1998;37:77–83.

212. Bergquist A, Glaumann H, Persson B, et al. Risk factors and clinical presentation of hepatobiliary carcinoma in patients with primary sclerosing cholangitis: A case-control study. Hepatology 1998;27:311–316.

213. Sinawat P, Hemsrichart V. A histopathologic study of 61 cases of peripheral intrahepatic cholangiocarcinoma. J Med Assoc Thai 1991;74:448–453.

214. Alonso-Lej F, Rever WB, Pessagno DJ. Congenital choledochal

cyst, with a report of two, and an analysis of 94 cases. Surg Gynecol Obstet 1959;108:1–30.

215. Ando H, Ito T, Sugito T. Histological study of the choledochal cyst wall. Jap J Gastroenterol 1987;84:1797–1801.

216. Fieber SS, Nance FC. Choledochal cyst and neoplasm: A comprehensive review of 106 cases and presentation of two original cases. Am Surg 1997;63:982–987.

217. Schiff L, Schubert WK, McAdams AJ, et al. Hepatic cholesterol ester storage disease: A familial disorder. Am J Med 1968;44: 538–546.

218. DiBisceglie AM, Ishak KG, Rabin L, et al. Cholesterol ester storage disease: Hepatopathology and effect of therapy with lovastatin. Hepatology 1990;11:764–772.

219. Beauder AL, Ferry GD, Nichols BL, et al. Cholesterol ester storage disease: Clinical, biochemical and pathological studies. J Pediatr 1997;90:910–914.

220. Tylki-Szymanska A, Rujner J, Lugowska A, et al. Clinical, biochemical and histological analysis of seven patients with cholesterol ester storage disease. Acta Paediatr Jpn 1997;39:643–646.

221. Bridges RA, Berendes H, Good RA. A fatal granulomatous disease of childhood. Am J Dis Child 1959;97:387–408.

222. Nakhleh RE, Glock M, Snover DC. Hepatic pathology of chronic granulomatous disease of childhood. Arch Pathol Lab Med 1992;116:71–75.

223. Tauber AI, Borregaard N, Simons, et al. Chronic granulomatous disease. Medicine (Baltimore) 1983;62:286–309.

224. White JR, Martin LD. Hepatic failure in an infant with chronic granulomatous disease. J Clin Gastroenterol, 1998;26:89–91.

225. Terada T, Nakamura Y, Kono N, et al. Ciliated hepatic foregut cyst: A mucus histological, immunohistochemical, and ultrastructural study in three cases in comparison with normal bronchi and intrahepatic bile ducts. Am J Surg Pathol 1990;14: 356–363.

226. Wheeler DA, Edmondson HA. Ciliated hepatic foregut cyst. Am J. Surg Pathol 1984;8:467–470.

227. Sun T. Pathology and immunology of *Clonorchis sinensis* infection of the liver. Ann Clin Lab Sci 1984;14:208–215.

228. Hou PC. The pathology of *Clonorchis sinensis* infestation of the liver. J Pathol 1955;70:53–64.

229. Ho JK, Lau WY, Liu K, et al. Liver infested with *Clonorchis sinensis* in orthotopic liver transplantation: A case report. Transplant Proc 1994;26:2269–2271.

230. Liu LX, Harinasuta KT. Liver and intestinal flukes. Gastroenterol Clin North Am 1996;25:627–636.

231. Bronnimann DA, Adam RD, Galgiani JN, et al. Coccidioidomycosis in the acquired immunodeficiency syndrome. Ann Intern Med 1987;106:372–379.

232. Ampel NM, Ryan KJ, Carry PJ, et al. Fungemia due to *Coccidioides immitis:* An analysis of 16 episodes in 15 patients and a review of the literature. Medicine (Baltimore) 1986;65:312–321.

233. Dodd LG, Nelson SD. Disseminated coccidioidomycosis detected by percutaneous liver biopsy in a liver transplant recipient. Am J Clin Pathol 1990;93:141–144.

234. Sommerschild HC, Langmark F, Maurseth K. Congenital hepatic fibrosis: Report of two new cases and review of the literature. Surgery 1973;73:53–58.

235. Kerr DNS, Harrison CV, Sherlock S, et al. Congenital hepatic fibrosis. Q J Med 1960;30:91–117.

236. De Vos BF, Cuvelier C. Congenital hepatic fibrosis. J Hepatol 1988;6:222–228.

237. McCarthy LJ, Baggenstoss AH, Logan GB. Congenital hepatic fibrosis. Gastroenterology 1966;49:27–36.

238. Nathan M, Batsakis JG. Congenital hepatic fibrosis. Surg Gynecol Obstet 1969;128:1033–1041.

239. Summerfield JA, Nagafuchi Y, Sherlock S, et al. Hepatobiliary fibropolycystic disease: A clinical and histological review of 51 patients. J Hepatol 1986;2:141–156.

240. Bernstein J, Stickler GB, Neel IV. Congenital hepatic fibrosis: Evolving morphology. Acta Pathol Microbiol Immunol Scand 1988; 4 (Suppl):17–26.

241. Perisic VN. Long-term studies on congenital hepatic fibrosis in children. Acta Paediatr 1995;84:695–696.

242. Sinaasappel M, Jansen PLM. The differential diagnosis of

243. Jansen PLM, Elferink RPJO. Hereditary hyperbilirubinemias: A molecular and mechanistic approach. Semin Liver Dis 1988;8: 168–178.

244. Welty C. Crigler-Najjar syndrome (type I) and survival. Gastroenterology 1992;102:1443.

245. Schrumpf E, Fausa O, Elgio K, et al. Hepato-biliary complications of inflammatory bowel disease. Semin Liver Dis 1988;8: 201–209.

246. Desmet VJ, Geboes K. Liver lesions in inflammatory bowel disorders. J Pathol 1987;151:247–255.

247. Darnell A, Brullet E, Campo R, et al. Liver abscesses as initial presentation of Crohn's disease. Am J Gastroenterol 1995;90: 1363–1364.

248. Sabesin SM, Fallon HJ, Andriole VT. Hepatic failure as a manifestation of cryptococcosis. Arch Intern Med 1963;111:661–669.

249. Buculvalas JC, Bove KE, Kaufman RA, et al. Cholangitis associated with *Cryptococcus neoformans.* Gastroenterology 1985;88: 1055–1059.

250. Sakaguchi N. Ultrastructural study of hepatic granulomas induced by *Cryptococcus neoformans* by quick-freezing and deep-etching method. Virchows Arch B Cell Pathol Incl Mol Pathol 1993;64:57–66.

251. Godwin TA. Cryptosporidiosis in the acquired immunodeficiency syndrome: A study of 15 autopsy cases. Hum Pathol 1991;22:1215–1224.

252. Forbes A, Blanshard C, Gazzard BG. Natural history of AIDS sclerosing cholangitis: A study of 20 cases. Gut 1993;34:116–121.

253. David JJ, Heyman MB, Ferrell L, et al. Sclerosing cholangitis associated with chronic cryptosporidiosis in a child with a congenital immunodeficiency disorder. Am J Gastroenterol 1987;82:1196–1202.

254. Wheeler DA, Edmondson HA. Cystadenoma with mesenchymal stroma (CMS) in the liver and bile ducts: A clinicopathologic study of 17 cases, 4 with malignant changes. Cancer 1985;56:1434–1445.

255. Ishak KG, Willis GW, Cummins SD, et al. Biliary cystadenoma and cystadenocarcinoma: Report of 14 cases and review of the literature. Cancer 1977;38:322–338.

256. Gabata T, Kadoya M, Matsui O, et al. Biliary cystadenoma with mesenchymal stroma of the liver. Correlation between unusual MR appearance and pathologic findings. J Magn Reson Imaging 1998;8:503–504.

257. Isenberg JN, L'Heureux PR, Warwick WJ, et al. Clinical observations on the biliary system in cystic fibrosis. Am J Gastroenterol 1976;65:134–141.

258. Vawter GF, Schwachman H. Cystic fibrosis in adults: An autopsy study. Pathol Annu 1979;14:357–382.

259. Craig JM, Haddad H, Shwachman H. The pathological changes in the liver in cystic fibrosis of the pancreas. Am J Dis Child 1957;93:357–369.

260. Oppenheimer EH, Esterly JR. Hepatic changes in young infants with cystic fibrosis: Possible relation to focal biliary cirrhosis. J Pediatr 1975;86:683–689.

261. Oppenheimer EH, Esterly JR. Pathology of cystic fibrosis: review of the literature and comparison with 146 autopsied cases. Persp Pediatr Pathol 1975;2:244–278.

262. Potter CJ, Fishbein M, Hammond S, et al. Can the histologic changes of cystic fibrosis–associated hepatobiliary disease be predicted by clinical criteria? J Pediatr Gastroenterol Nutr 1997; 25:32–36.

263. Columbo C, Apostolo M, Ferrari M, et al. Analysis of risk factors for the development of liver disease in patients with cystic fibrosis. J Pediatr 1994;124:393–399.

264. Seegmiller JE. Cystinosis. *In* Hers HA, Van Hoof F, eds. Lysosomes and storage disease. Academic Press: New York, 1973, pp 485–513.

265. Scotto JM, Stralin HG. Ultrastructure of the liver in a case of childhood cystinosis. Virchows Arch A Pathol Anat Histol 1977;377:43–48.

266. Griffiths PD. Cytomegalovirus and the liver. Semin Liver Dis 1984;4:307–313.

267. Paya CV, Hermans PE, Wiesner RH, et al. Cytomegalovirus hepatitis in liver transplantation: Prospective analysis of 93 consecutive orthotopic liver transplantations. J Infect Dis 1989; 160:752–758.

268. Clarke J, Craig RM, Saffro R, et al. Cytomegalovirus granulomatous hepatitis. Am J Med 1979;66:264–269.

269. Snover DC, Horwitz CA. Liver disease in cytomegalovirus mononucleosis: A light microscopical and immunoperoxidase study of six cases. Hepatology 1984;4:408–412.

270. Finegold MJ, Carpenter RJ. Obliterative cholangitis due to cytomegalovirus: A possible precursor of paucity of intrahepatic bile ducts. Hum Pathol 1982;13:662–665.

271. MacDonald GA, Greenson JK, DelBuono EA, et al. Mini-microabscess syndrome in liver transplant recipients. Hepatology, 1997;26:192–197.

272. Kunno A, Abe M, Yamada M, et al. Clinical and histological features of cytomegalovirus hepatitis in previously healthy adults. Liver 1997;17:129–132.

273. Kautner I, Robinson MJ, Kuhnle U. Dengue fever infection: Epidemiology, pathogenesis, clinical presentation, diagnosis, and prevention. J Pediatr 1997;131:516–524.

274. Kuo CH, Tai DI, Chang-Chien CS, et al. Liver biochemical tests and dengue fever. Am J Trop Med Hyg 1992;47:265–270.

275. Ishak KG, Walker DH, Coetzner JA, et al. Viral hemorrhagic fevers with hepatic involvement: Pathologic aspects with clinical correlations. *In* Popper H, Schaffner F, eds. Progress in Liver Diseases. Vol VII. Grune & Stratton; New York, 1982, pp 495–515.

276. Ruchelli ED, Uri A, Dimmick JE, et al. Severe perinatal liver disease and Down syndrome: An apparent relationship. Hum Pathol 1991;22:1274–1280.

277. Becroft DMO, Zwi J. Perinatal visceral fibrosis accompanying the megakaryoblastic leukemoid reaction of Down syndrome. Pediatr Pathol 1990;10:397–406.

278. Schwab M, Niemeyer C, Schwarzer U. Down syndrome, transient myeloproliferative disorder, and infantile liver fibrosis. Med Pediatr Oncol 1998;31:159–165.

279. Yagihashi N, Watanabe K, Yagihashi S. Transient abnormal myelopoiesis accompanied by hepatic fibrosis in two infants with Down syndrome. J Clin Pathol 1995;48:973–975.

280. Dubin IN, Johnson FB. Chronic idiopathic jaundice with unidentified pigment in liver cells: New clinicopathologic entity with report of 12 cases. Medicine (Baltimore) 1954;33:155–197.

281. Seymour Ca, Neale G, Peters TJ. Lysosomal changes in liver tissue from patients with the Dubin-Johnson-Sprinz syndrome. Clin Sci Mol Med 1977;52:241–248.

282. Tyagi SP, Tiwari SG, Mehdi G, et al. Dubin-Johnson syndrome. J Indian Med Assoc 1994;92:51.

283. Zuckerman AJ, Simpson DIH. Exotic virus infections of the liver. *In* Popper H, Schaffner F, eds. Progress in Liver Diseases. Vol VI. Grune & Stratton: Orlando, 1979, pp 425–438.

284. Howard CR, Ellis DS, Simpson DIH. Exotic viruses and the liver. Semin Liver Dis 1984;4:361–374.

285. Daly JJ, Baker GF. Pinworm granuloma of the liver. Am J Trop Med Hyg 1984;33:62–64.

286. Mondou EN, Gnepp DR. Hepatic granuloma resulting from *Enterobius vermicularis*. Am J Clin Pathol 1989;91:97–100.

287. Everett GD, Mitros FA. Eosinophilic gastroenteritis with hepatic eosinophilic granulomas. Am J Gastroenterol 1980;74:519–521.

288. Robert F, Omura E, Durant JR. Mucosal eosinophilic gastroenteritis with systemic involvement. Am J Med 1977;62:139–143.

289. Ishak KG, Sesterhenn IA, Goodman ZD, et al. Epithelioid hemangioendothelioma of the liver: A clinicopathologic and follow-up study of 32 cases. Hum Pathol 1984;15:839–852.

290. Dietze O, Davies SE, Williams R, et al. Malignant epithelioid hemangioendothelioma of the liver: A clinicopathological and histochemical study of 12 cases. Histopathology 1989;15:225–237.

291. Kelleher MB, Iwatsuki S, Sheahan DG. Epithelioid hemangioendothelioma of the liver. Clinicopathological correlation of 10 cases treated by orthotopic liver transplantation. Am J Surg Pathol 1989;13:999–1008.

292. Demetris AJ, Minervini M, Raikow RB, et al. Hepatic epithelioid hemangioendothelioma: Biologic questions based on pattern of recurrence in an allograft and tumor immunophenotype. Am J Surg Pathol 1997;21:263–270.

293. Walsh MM, Hytiroglou P, Thung SN, et al. Epithelioid hemangioendothelioma of the liver mimicking Budd-Chiari syndrome. Arch Pathol Lab Med 1998;122:846–848.

294. Pokharna RK, Garg PK, Gupta SD, et al. Primary epithelioid haemangioendothelioma of the liver: Case report and review of the literature. J Clin Pathol 1997;50:1029–1031.

295. White NJ, Juel-Jensun BE. Infectious mononucleosis hepatitis. Semin Liver Dis 1984;4:301–306.

296. Lloyd-Still JD, Scott JP, Crussi F. The spectrum of Epstein-Barr virus hepatitis in children. Pediatr Pathol 1986;5:337–351.

297. Purtilo DT, Sakamoto K. Epstein-Barr virus and human disease: Immune response determines the clinical and pathologic expression. Hum Pathol 1981;12:677–679.

298. Chang MY, Campbell WG. Fatal infectious mononucleosis: Association with liver necrosis and herpes-like virus particles. Arch Pathol Lab Med 1975;99:185–191.

299. Cripps DJ, Scheuer PJ. Hepatobiliary changes in erythropoietic protoporphyria. Arch Pathol 1965;80:500–508.

300. Bloomer JR, Enriquez R. Evidence that hepatic crystalline deposits in a patient with protoporphyria are composed of protoporphyrin. Gastroenterology 1982;82:569–572.

301. Klatskin G, Bloomer JR. Birefringence of hepatic pigment in erythropoietic protoporphyria. Gastroenterology 1974;67:294–302.

302. Cox TM, Alexander GJ, Sarkany RP. Protoporphyria. Semin Liver Dis 1998;18:85–93.

303. Lock G, Holstege A, Mueller AR, et al. Liver failure in erythropoietic protoporphyria associated with choledocholithiasis and severe post-transplantation polyneuropathy. Liver 1996;16:211–217.

304. Rank JM, Straka JG, Bloomer JR. Liver in disorders of porphyrin metabolism. J Gastroenterol Hepatol 1990;5:573–585.

305. Gautier M, Jehan P, Odievre M. Histologic study of biliary fibrous remnants in 48 cases of extrahepatic biliary atresia: Correlation with postoperative bile flow restoration. J Pediatr 1976;89:704–709.

306. Scotto JM, Stralin HC. Congenital extrahepatic biliary atresia. Arch Pathol Lab Med 1977;101:416–419.

307. Chandra RS, Altman RP. Ductal remnants in extrahepatic biliary atresia: A histological study with clinical correlation. J Pediatr 1978;93:196–200.

308. Gautier M, Eliot N. Extrahepatic biliary atresia: Morphological study of 98 biliary remnants. Arch Pathol Lab Med 1981;105:397–402.

309. Alagille D. Extrahepatic biliary atresia. Hepatology 1984;4 (Suppl):7S–10S.

310. Landing BH, Wells Tr, Reed GB, et al. Diseases of the bile ducts in children. *In* Gall EA, Mostofi FK, eds. The Liver. Williams & Wilkins: Baltimore, 1973, pp 480–509.

311. Landing BH, Wells TR, Reed GB, et al. Neonatal hepatitis, biliary atresia and choledochal cyst: The concept of infantile obstructive cholangiopathy. Prog Pediatr Surg 1974;6:113–119.

312. Landing BH, Wells TR, Ramicone E. Time course of the intrahepatic lesion of extrahepatic biliary atresia: A morphometric study. Pediatr Pathol 1985;4:309–319.

313. Ramm GA, Nair VG, Bridle KR, et al. Contribution of hepatic parenchymal and nonparenchymal cells to hepatic fibrogenesis in biliary atresia. Am J Pathol 1998;153:527–535.

314. Lai MW, Chang MH, Hsu SC, et al. Differential diagnosis of extrahepatic biliary atresia from neonatal hepatitis: A prospective study. J Pediatr Gastroenterol 1994;18:121–127.

315. Kasai M, Ohi R, Chiba T. Long-term survivors after surgery for biliary atresia. *In* Ohi R, ed. Biliary Atresia. Professional Postgraduate Service: Tokyo, 1987, pp. 277–281.

316. Desmet VJ. Cholestasis: Extrahepatic obstruction and secondary biliary cirrhosis. *In* MacSween RNM, Anthony PP, Scheuer PJ, et al, eds. Pathology of the Liver. 3rd ed. Churchill Livingstone: Edinburgh, 1994, pp 425–476.

317. MacSween RNM. Mechanical duct obstruction. *In* Peters RL, Craig JR, eds. Liver Pathology. Churchill Livingstone: New York, 1986, pp 161–176.

318. Afroudakis A, Kaplowitz N. Liver histopathology in chronic bile duct stenosis due to chronic alcoholic pancreatitis. Hepatology 1981;1:65–72.

319. Warshaw AL, Schapiro RH, Ferrucci JT Jr, et al. Persistent obstructive jaundice, cholangitis, and biliary cirrhosis due to common bile duct stenosis in chronic pancreatitis. Gastroenterology 1976;70:562–567.

320. Brady RO, King FM. Fabry's disease. In Dyck PJ, Thomas PK, Lambert EH, eds. Peripheral Neuropathy. Vol II. WB Saunders: New York, 1975, pp 914–927.

321. Faraggiana T, Churg J, Grishman E, et al. Light- and electron-microscopic histochemistry of Fabry's disease. Am J Pathol 1981;103:247–262.

322. Meuwissen SGM, Dingemans KP, Stryland A, et al. Ultrastructural and biochemical liver analysis in Fabry's disease. Hepatology 1982;2:263–268.

323. Bruton OC, Kanter AJ. Idiopathic familial hyperlipemia. Am J Dis Child 1951;82:153–159.

324. Roberts WC, Levy RI, Fredrickson DS. Hyperlipoproteinemia: A review of the five types with first report of necropsy findings in Type 3. Arch Pathol 1970;90:46–56.

325. Kovacs K, Lee R, Little JA. Ultrastructural changes of hepatocytes in hyperlipoproteinemia. Lancet 1972;1:752–753.

326. Moser HW, Moser AB, Chen WW, et al. Ceramidase deficiency: Farber lipogranulomatosis. In Scriver CR; Beaudet AL, Sly WS, et al, eds. The Metabolic Basis of Inherited Diseases. 6th ed McGraw-Hill: New York, 1989, pp 1645–1654.

327. Antonarakis S, Valle D, Moser HW, et al. Phenotypic variability in siblings with Farber disease. J Pediatr 1984; 104:406–409.

328. Abul-Haj SK, Martz DG, Douglas WF, et al. Farber's disease: Report of a case with observations and notes on the nature of the stored material. J Pediatr 1962;61:221–232.

329. Acosta-Ferreira W, Vercelli-Hetta J, Falconi LM. Fasciola hepatica human infection: Histopathological study of 16 cases. Virchows Arch A Pathol Anat Histopathol 1979;383:319–327.

330. Chen MG, Mott KE. Progress in assessment of morbidity due to Fasciola hepatica infection: A review of recent literature. Trop Dis Bull 1990;87(4):R1–R37.

331. Price TA, Tuazon CU, Simon GL. Fascioliasis: Case reports and review. Clin Infect Dis 1993;17:426–430.

332. Pfeifer U, Ormanns W, Klinge O. Hepatocellular fibrinogen storage in familial hypofibrinogenemia. Virchows Arch B Cell Pathol Incl Mol Pathol 1981;36:247–255.

333. Wehinger H, Klinge O, Alexandrakis E, et al. Hereditary hypofibrinogenemia with fibrinogen storage in the liver. Eur J Pediatr 1983;141:109–112.

334. Callea F, De Vos R, Tagni R, et al. Fibrinogen inclusions in liver cells: A new type of ground-glass hepatocyte. Immune light and electron microscopic characterization. Histopathology 1986;10:65–73.

335. DeCraemer D, Pipeleers-Marichal M, Vandenplas Y, et al. Peroxisome proliferation associated with fibrinogen storage in the liver. Histopathology 1996;29:171–173.

336. Brawer MK, Austin GE, Lewin KJ. Focal fatty change of the liver, a hitherto poorly recognized entity. Gastroenterology 1980;78:247–252.

337. Giorgio A, Francica G, Aloisio T, et al. Multifocal fatty infiltration of the liver mimicking metastatic disease. Gastroenterol Int 1991;4:169–172.

338. Battaglia DM, Wanless IR, Brady AP, et al. Intrahepatic sequestered segment of liver presenting as focal fatty change. Am J Gastroenterol 1995;90:2238–2239.

339. Layfield LJ. Focal fatty change of the liver. Cytologic findings in a radiographic mimic of metastases. Diagn Cytopathol 1994; 11:385–387.

340. Grove A, Vyberg B, Vyberg M. Focal fatty change of the liver: A review and a case associated with continuous ambulatory peritoneal dialysis. Virchows Arch A Pathol Anat Histopathol 1991;419:69–75.

341. Knowles DM II, Wolff M. Focal nodular hyperplasia of the liver: A clinicopathologic study and review of the literature. Hum Pathol 1976;7:533–545.

342. Wanless IR. On the pathogenesis of focal nodular hyperplasia of the liver. Hepatology 1985;5:1194–1200.

343. Kondo F, Nagao T, Sato T, et al. Etiological analysis of focal nodular hyperplasia of the liver, with emphasis on similar abnormal vasculatures to nodular regenerative hyperplasia and idiopathic portal hypertension. Pathol Res Pract 1998;194:487–495.

344. DiStasi M, Caturelli E, DeSio I, et al. Natural history of focal nodular hyperplasia of the liver: An ultrasound study. J Clin Ultrasound 1996;24:345–350.

345. Buetow PC, Pantongrag-Brown L, Buck JL, et al. Focal nodular hyperplasia of the liver: Radiologic-pathologic correlation. Radiographics 1996;16:369–388.

346. Smetana HF, Olen E. Hereditary galactose disease. Am J Clin Pathol 1962;38:3–25.

347. Appelbaum NM, Thaler MM. Reversibility of extensive liver damage in galactosemia. Gastroenterology 1975;69:496–502.

348. Suzuki H, Gilberg EF, Anido V, et al. Galactosemia: A report of two fatal cases with giant cell transformation in one. Arch Pathol 1966;82:602–609.

349. Gitzelman R. Galactosemia and other inherited disorders of galactose metabolism. In Bianchi L, Gerok W, Landmann L, et al, eds. Liver in Metabolic Diseases. MTP Press: Lancaster, 1983, pp 235–238.

350. Segal S, Blair A, Roth H. The metabolism of galactose by patients with congenital galactosemia. Am J Med 1965;38:62–70.

351. Petrelli M, Blair JD. The liver in GM gangliosidosis types 1 and 2. Arch Pathol 1975;99:111–116.

352. Volk BW, Wallace BJ. The liver in lipidosis: An electron microscopic and histochemical study. Am J Pathol 1966;49:203–225.

353. Desnick RJ, Snyder PD, Desnick SJ, et al. Sandhoff's disease: Ultrastructural and biochemical studies. In Volk RW, Aronson SM, eds. Sphingolipids, Sphingolipidoses and Allied Disorders. Plenum: New York, 1972, 351–371.

354. Hadfield MG, Mammes P, David PB. The pathology of Sandhoff's disease. J Pathol 1977;123:137–144.

355. Peters SP, Lee RE, Glen RH. Gaucher's disease: A review. Medicine (Baltimore) 1977;56:425–442.

356. Hibbs RG, Ferrans VJ, Cipriano PR, et al. A histochemical and electron microscopic study of Gaucher cells. Arch Pathol 1970; 89:137–153.

357. Brady RO, King FM. Gaucher's disease. In Hers HG, Van Hoof F, eds. Lysosomes and storage diseases. Academic Press: New York, 1973, pp 381–394.

358. Gall EA, Landing BH. Hepatic cirrhosis and hereditary disorders of metabolism. Am J Clin Pathol 1956;26:1398–1426.

359. Zimran A, Kay A, Gelbart T, et al. Gaucher disease: Clinical, laboratory, radiologic, and genetic features of 53 patients. Medicine (Baltimore) 1992;71:337–353.

360. Watson KJR, Gollan JL. Gilbert's syndrome. Baillieres Clin Gastroenterol 1989;3:337–355.

361. Barth RF, Grimley PM, Berk PD, et al. Excess lipofuscin accumulation in constitutional hepatic dysfunction (Gilbert's syndrome). Arch Pathol 1971;91:41–47.

362. McGee J O'D, Allan JG, Russell RI, et al. Liver ultrastructure in Gilbert's syndrome. Gut 1975;16:220–224.

363. McAdams AJ, Hug C, Bove KE. Glycogen storage disease, types I to X: Criteria for morphologic diagnosis. Hum Pathol 1974;5:463–487.

364. Itoh S, Ishida Y, Matsuo S. Mallory bodies in a patient with type Ia glycogen storage disease. Gastroenterology 1987;92:520–523.

365. Howell RR, Stevenson RE, Ben-Menachem Y, et al. Hepatic adenomata with type I glycogen storage disease. JAMA 1976; 236:1481–1484.

366. Reed GB, Dixon JEP, Neustein HB, et al. Type IV glycogenosis. Lab Invest 1968;19:546–557.

367. Vasquez JJ. Ground-glass hepatocytes: Light and electron microscopy. Characterization of the different types. Histol Histopathol 1990;5:379–386.

368. Lee PJ, Leonard JV. The hepatic glycogen storage diseases: Problems beyond childhood. J Inherit Metab Dis 1995;18:462–472.

369. Talenta GM, Coleman RA, Alter C, et al. Glycogen storage disease in adults. Ann Intern Med 1994;120:218–226.

370. Selby R, Starzl TE, Yunis E, et al. Liver transplantation for type I and type IV glycogen storage disease. Eur J Pediatr 1993;152 (Suppl 1):S71–S76.

371. Snover DC. Acute and chronic graft versus host disease: Histopathologic evidence for two distinct pathogenetic mechanisms. Hum Pathol 1984;15:202–205.

372. Shulman HM, Sharma P, Amos D, et al. A coded histologic study of hepatic graft-versus-host disease after human bone marrow transplantation. Hepatology 1988;8:463–470.

373. McDonald GB, Sharma P, Matthews DE, et al. Venoocclusive disease of the liver after bone marrow transplantation: Diagnosis, incidence, and predisposing factors. Hepatology 1984;4: 116–122.

374. Sloane JP, Dilly SA. Pathogenesis of graft versus host disease. Histopathology 1988;12:105–110.

375. Robert ME. Liver disease in the immunocompromised patient. Pathology 1994;3:185–206.

376. Sun NC, Smith VC. Hepatitis associated with myocarditis: Unusual manifestations of infection with coxsackie Group B, type 3. N Engl J Med 1966;274:190–193.

377. Dunn DG, Hayes P, Breen KJ, et al. The liver in congestive failure. A review. Am J Med Sci 1973;265:174–189.

378. Ware AJ. The liver when the heart fails. Gastroenterology 1978;74:627–628.

379. Lefkowitch JH, Mendez L. Morphological features of hepatic injury in cardiac disease and shock. J Hepatol 1986;2:313–327.

380. Klatt EC, Koss MN, Young TS, et al. Hepatic hyaline globules associated with passive congestion. Arch Pathol Lab Med 1988;112:510–513.

381. Fuchs S, Bogomolski-Yahalom V, Paltiel O, et al. Ischemic hepatitis: Clinical and laboratory observations of 34 patients. J Clin Gastroenterol 1998;26:183–186.

382. Cohen JA, Kaplan MM. Left-sided heart failure presenting as hepatitis. Gastroenterology 1978;74:583–587.

383. Kanel GC, Ucci AA, Kaplan MM, et al. A distinctive perivenular hepatic lesion associated with heart failure. Am J Clin Pathol 1980;73:235–239.

384. Rubel LR, Ishak KG. The liver in fatal exertional heatstroke. Liver 1983;3:249–260.

385. Biabchi L, Ohnacker H, Beck K, et al. Liver damage in heatstroke and its regression. Hum Pathol 1972;3:237–248.

386. Hassanein T, Razack A, Gavaler JS, et al. Heat stroke: Its clinical and pathological presentation, with particular attention to the liver. Am J Gastroenterol 1992;87:1382–1389.

387. Sort P, Mas A, Salmeron JM, et al. Recurrent liver involvement in heatstroke. Liver 1996;16:335–337.

388. Bacon BR, Britton RS. The pathology of hepatic iron overload: A free radical–mediated process? Hepatology 1990;11:127–137.

389. Bassett ML, Halliday JW, Powell LW. Value of hepatic iron measurements in early hemochromatosis and determination of the critical iron level associated with fibrosis. Hepatology 1986;6:24–29.

390. Conte D, Piperno A, Mandelli C, et al. Clinical biochemical and histological features of primary haemochromatosis: A report of 67 cases. Liver 1986;6:310–315.

391. Deugnier YM, Guyader D, Crantock L, et al. Primary liver cancer in genetic hemochromatosis: A clinical, pathological and pathogenetic study of 54 cases. Gastroenterology 1993; 104:228–234.

392. Bothwell TH, MacPhail AP. Hereditary hemochromatosis: Etiologic, pathologic, and clinical aspects. Semin Hematol 1998;35: 55–71.

393. Bacon BR, Sadiq SA. Hereditary hemochromatosis: Presentation and diagnosis in the 1990s. Am J Gastroenterol 1997;92: 784–789.

394. Ludwig J, Hashimoto E, Porayko MK, et al. Hemosiderosis in cirrhosis: A study of 447 native livers. Gastroenterology 1997; 112:882–888.

395. Adams PC, Kertesz AE, Valberg LS. Clinical presentation of hemochromatosis: A changing scene. Am J Med 1991;90:445–449.

396. Edwards CQ, Griffen LM, Goldgar D, et al. Prevalence of hemochromatosis among 11,065 presumably healthy blood donors. N Engl J Med 1988;318:1355–1362.

397. Silver MM, Beverley DW, Valberg LS, et al. Perinatal hemochromatosis: Clinical, morphologic, and quantitative iron studies. Am J Pathol 1987;128:538–554.

398. Blisard KS, Bartow SA. Neonatal hemochromatosis. Hum Pathol 1986;17:376–383.

399. Sigurdsson L, Reyes J, Kocoshis SA, et al. Neonatal hemochromatosis: Outcomes of pharmacologic and surgical therapies. J Pediatr Gastroenterol Nutr 1998;26:85–89.

400. Muller-Berghaus J, Knisely AS, Zaum R, et al. Neonatal haemochromatosis: Report of a patient with favourable outcome. Eur J Pediatr 1997;156:296–298.

401. Sibai BM, Ramadan MK, Usta I, et al. Maternal morbidity and mortality in 442 pregnancies with hemolysis, elevated liver enzymes, and low platelets (HELLP syndrome). Am J Obstet Gynecol 1993;169:1000–1006.

402. Martin JN Jr, Blake PG, Perry KG Jr, et al. The natural history of HELLP syndrome: Pattern of disease progression and regression. Am J Obstet Gynecol 1991;164:1500–1513.

403. Cerwenka H, Bacher H, Werkgartner G, et al. Massive liver haemorrhage and rupture caused by HELLP syndrome treated by collagen fleeces coated with fibrin glue. Eur J Surg 1998; 164:709–711.

404. Stone JH. HELLP syndrome: Hemolysis, elevated liver enzymes, and low platelets. JAMA 1998;280:559–562.

405. Saphier CJ, Repke JT. Hemolysis, elevated liver enzymes, and low platelets (HELLP) syndrome: A review of diagnosis and management. Semin Perinatol 1998;22:118–133.

406. Gurel SA, Gurel H. Early development of HELLP syndrome associated with eclampsia: A case report. Eur J Obstet Gynecol Reprod Biol 1998;76:241–243.

407. Weinstein L. Syndrome of hemolysis, elevated liver enzymes, and low platelet count: A severe consequence of hypertension in pregnancy. Am J Obstet Gynecol 1982;142:159–167.

408. Kent G, Popper H. Secondary hemochromatosis: Its association with anemia. Arch Pathol 1960;70:623–639.

409. Irving MG, Halliday JW, Powell LW. Association between alcoholism and increased hepatic iron stores. Alcoholism 1988;12: 7–13.

410. Bonkovsky HL, Banner BF, Rothman AL. Iron and chronic viral hepatitis. Hepatology 1997;25:759–768.

411. Risdon RA, Barry M, Flynn DM. Transfusional iron overload: The relationship between tissue iron concentration and hepatic fibrosis in thalassemia. J Pathol 1975;116:83–95.

412. Bothwell TH, Charlton RW. Dietary iron overload. In Kief H, ed. Iron Metabolism and Its Disorders. Excerpta Medica: Amsterdam, 1975.

413. Conn HO. Portacaval anastomosis and hepatic hemosiderin deposition: A prospective, controlled investigation. Gastroenterology 1972;62:61–72.

414. Haas JE, Muczynski KA, Krailo M, et al. Histopathology and prognosis in childhood hepatoblastoma and hepatocellular carcinoma. Cancer 1989;64:1082–1095.

415. Lack EE, Neave C, Vawter GF. Hepatoblastoma. A clinical and pathologic study of 54 cases. Am J Surg Pathol 1982;6:693–705.

416. Abenoza P, Manivel JC, Wick MR, et al. Hepatoblastoma: An immunohistochemical and ultrastructural study. Hum Pathol 1987;18:1025–1035.

417. Douglass EC. Hepatic malignancies in childhood and adolescence (hepatoblastoma, hepatocellular carcinoma, and embryonal sarcoma). Cancer Treat Res 1997;92:201–212.

418. Jain BL, Mathur DR, Vyas MC. Cytologic diagnosis of hepatoblastoma by fine needle aspiration biopsy cytology. Acta Cytol 1997;41:1858–1860.

419. Newman KD. Hepatic tumors in children. Semin Pediatr Surg 1997;6:38–41.

420. Us-Krasovec M, Pohar-Marinsek Z, Golouh R, et al. Hepatoblastoma in fine needle aspirates. Acta Cytol 1996;40:450–456.

421. Harada T, Matsuo K, Kodama S, et al. Adult hepatoblastoma: Case report and review of the literature. Aust N Z J Surg 1995; 65:686–688.

422. Stocker JT: Hepatoblastoma. Semin Diagn Pathol 1994;11:136–143.

423. Sola Perez J, Perez-Guillermo M, Bas Bernal AB, et al. Hepatoblastoma: An attempt to apply histologic classification to aspi-

rates obtained by fine needle aspiration cytology. Acta Cytol 1994;38:175–182.

424. Von Schweinitz D, Wischmeyer P, Leuschner I, et al. Clinico-pathological criteria with prognostic relevance in hepatoblas-toma. Eur J Cancer 1994;30A:1052–1058.

425. Berman MM, Libbey NP, Foster JH. Hepatocellular carcinoma of polygonal cell type with fibrous stroma—an atypical vari-ant with a favourable prognosis. Cancer 1980;46:1448–1455.

426. Hodgson HJF. Fibrolamellar cancer of the liver. J Hepatol 1987;5:241–247.

427. Berman MA, Burnham JA, Sheahan DG. Fibrolamellar carci-noma of the liver: An immunohistochemical study of nineteen cases and a review of the literature. Hum Pathol 1988;19:784–794.

428. Craig JR, Peters RL, Edmondson HA, et al. Fibrolamellar carci-noma of the liver: A tumor of adolescents and young adults with distinctive clinico-pathologic features. Cancer 1980;46:372–379.

429. Saab S, Yao F. Fibrolamellar hepatocellular carcinoma: Case reports and a review of the literature. Dig Dis Sci 1996;41:1981–1985.

430. Okuda K. Hepatocellular carcinoma: Clinicopathological as-pects. J Gastroenterol Hepatol 1997;12:S314–S318.

431. Okano A, Hajiro K, Takakuwa H, et al. Fibrolamellar carci-noma of the liver with a mixture of ordinary hepatocellular carcinoma: A case report. Am J Gastroenterol 1998;93:1144–1145.

432. Okuda K, Peters RL, Simson IW. Gross anatomic features of hepatocellular carcinoma from three disparate geographic ar-eas: Proposal of new classification. Cancer 1984;54:2165–2173.

433. Nakashima T, Okuda K, Kojiro M, et al. Pathology of hepato-cellular carcinoma in Japan: 232 consecutive cases autopsied in ten years. Cancer 1983;51:863–877.

434. Nakashima T, Kojiro M, Pathologic characteristics of hepato-cellular carcinoma. Semin Liv Dis 1986;6:259–266.

435. Kishi K, Shikata T, Hirohashi E, et al. Hepatocellular carci-noma: A clinical and pathologic analysis of 57 hepatectomy cases. Cancer 1983;51:542–548.

436. Akagi G, Furuya K, Kanamura A, et al. Liver cell dysplasia and hepatitis B surface antigen in liver cirrhosis and hepatocellular carcinoma. Cancer 1984;54:315–318.

437. LeBail B, Bernard PH, Carles J, et al. Prevalence of liver cell dysplasia and association with HCC in a series of 100 cirrhotic liver explants. J Hepatol 1997;27:835–842.

438. Bergman S, Graeme-Cook F, Pitman MB. The usefulness of the reticulin stain in the differential diagnosis of liver nodules on fine-needle aspiration biopsy cell block preparations. Mod Pathol 1997;10:1258–1264.

439. Kojiro M. Pathology of early hepatocellular carcinoma: Pro-gression from early to advanced. Hepatogastroenterology 1998;45 (Suppl 3):1203–1205.

440. Pfeifer U. Pathology of hepatocellular carcinoma. Digestion 1998;59 (Suppl 2):66–69.

441. Tsukuma H, Hiyama T, Tanaka S, et al. Risk for hepatocellular carcinoma among patients with chronic liver disease. N Engl J Med 1993;328:1797–1801.

442. Nagasue N, Yukaya H, Hamada T, et al. The natural history of hepatocellular carcinoma. Cancer 1984;54:1461–1465.

443. Zelman S. Liver fibrosis in hereditary hemorrhagic telangiecta-sia: Fibrosis of diffuse insular character. Arch Pathol 1962:74:66–72.

444. Daly JJ, Schiller AL. The liver in hemorrhagic telangiectasia (Osler-Weber-Rendu disease). Am J Med 1976;60:723–726.

445. Smith JL, Lineback ML. Hereditary hemorrhagic telangiectasia: 9 cases in one Negro family, with special reference to hepatic lesions. Am J Med 1954;17:41–49.

446. Omata M. Noncirrhotic portal hypertension. In Peters RL, Craig JR, eds. Liver Pathology. Churchill Livingstone: New York, 1986, pp 315–330.

447. Naijema T, Westermann CJ, Overtoom TT, et al. Hereditary hemorrhagic telangiectasia (Osler-Weber-Rendu disease): New insights in pathogenesis, complications, and treatment. Arch Intern Med 1996;156:714–719.

448. Phillips MJ, Little JA, Ptak TW. Subcellular pathology of hered-itary fructose intolerance. Am J Med 1968;44:910–921.

449. Hardwick DF, Dimmick JE. Metabolic cirrhosis of infancy and early childhood. Persp Pediatr Pathol 1976;3:103–144.

450. Odievre M, Gertil C, Gautier M, et al. Hereditary fructose intolerance in childhood: Diagnosis, management and course in 55 patients. Am J Dis Child 1978;132:605–608.

451. Levin B, Snodgrass GJ, Oberholzer VG, et al. Fructosaemia: Observations on seven cases. Am J Med 1968;45:826–838.

452. Long WW, Pawel B, Morrow G. Pathological case of the month: Hereditary fructose intolerance. Arch Pediatr Adolesc Med 1997;151:1165–1166.

453. Mock DM, Perman JA, Thaler MM, et al. Chronic fructose intoxication after infancy in children with hereditary fructose intolerance. N Engl J Med 1983;309:764–770.

454. Jacques SM, Qureshi F. Herpes simplex virus hepatitis in preg-nancy: A clinicopathologic study of three cases. Hum Pathol 1992;23:183–187.

455. Connor RW, Lorts G, Gilbert DN, et al. Lethal herpes simplex virus type 1 hepatitis in a normal adult. Gastroenterology 1979;76:590–594.

456. Lee JC, Fortuny IE. Adult herpes simplex hepatitis. Hum Pathol 1972;3:277–281.

457. Goodman ZD, Ishak KG, Sesterhenn IA. Herpes simplex hep-atitis in apparently immunocompetent adults. Am J Clin Pathol 1986;85:694–699.

458. Kaufman B, Gandhi SA, Louie E, et al. Herpes simplex virus hepatitis: Case report and review. Clin Infect Dis 1997;24:334–338.

459. Shanley CJ, Braun DK, Brown K, et al. Fulminant hepatic failure secondary to herpes simplex virus hepatitis: Successful outcome after orthotopic liver transplantation. Transplantation 1995;59:145–149.

460. Eshchar J, Reif L, Waron M, et al. Hepatic lesion in chicken-pox: A case report. Gastroenterology 1973;64:462–466.

461. Kasper WJ, Howe PM. Fatal varicella after a single course of corticosteroids. Pediatr Infect Dis 1990;9:729–732.

462. Goodwin RA, Shapiro JL, Thurman GH, et al. Disseminated histoplasmosis: Clinical and pathologic correlations. Medicine 1980;59:1–33.

463. Mandell W, Goldberg DM, Neu HC. Histoplasmosis in patients with the acquired immune deficiency syndrome. Am J Med 1986;81:974–978.

464. Collins MH, Jiang B, Croffie JM, et al. Hepatic granulomas in children: A clinicopathologic analysis of 23 cases including polymerase chain reaction for histoplasma. Am J Surg Pathol 1996;20:332–338.

465. Schimke RN, McKusick VA, Huang T, et al. Homocystinuria: Studies of 20 families with 38 affected members. JAMA 1963;193:711–719.

466. Gibson JB, Carson NAJ, Neill DW. Pathological findings in homocystinuria. J Clin Pathol 1964;17:427–437.

467. Carson NAJ, Dent CE, Field CMB, et al. Homocystinuria: Clini-cal and pathological review of ten cases. J Pediatr 1965;66:565–583.

468. Carson NA. Homocystinuria. Proc R Soc Med 1970;63:41–43.

469. Wilkins MJ, Lindley R, Dourakis SP, et al. Surgical pathology of the liver in HIV infection. Histopathology 1991;18:459–464.

470. Lebovics E, Thung SN, Schaffner F, et al. The liver in the acquired immunodeficiency syndrome: A clinical and histo-logic study. Hepatology 1985;5:293–298.

471. Glasgow BJ, Anders K, Layfield LJ, et al. Clinical and patho-logic findings of the liver in the acquired immune deficiency syndrome (AIDS). Am J Clin Pathol 1985;83:582–588.

472. Kahn E, Greco A, Daum F, et al. Hepatic pathology in pediat-ric acquired immunodeficiency syndrome. Hum Pathol 1991;22:1111–1119.

473. Nakanuma Y, Liew CT, Peters RL, et al. Pathologic features of the liver in acquired immune deficiency syndrome (AIDS). Liver 1986;6:158–166.

474. Lefkowitz JH. The liver in AIDS. Semin Liv Dis 1997;17:335–344.

475. Poles MA. HIV-related hepatic disease: When and why to biopsy. Gastrointest Endosc Clin North Am 1998;8:939–962.

476. Kennedy M, O'Reilly M, Bergin CJ, et al. Liver biopsy pathol-ogy in human immunodeficiency virus infection. Eur J Gas-troenterol Hepatol 1998;10:255–258.

477. Poles MA, Dieterich DT, Schwarz ED, et al. Liver biopsy findings in 501 patients infected with human immunodeficiency virus (HIV). J Acquir Immune Defic Syndr Hum Retrovirol 1996;11:170–177.

478. Viteri AL, Greene JF. Bile duct abnormalities in the acquired immune deficiency syndrome. Gastroenterology 1987;92:2014–2018.

479. Forbes A, Blanshard C, Gazzard BG. Natural history of AIDS sclerosing cholangitis: A study of 20 cases. Gut 1993;34:116–121.

480. Van Steenbergen W, Fevery J, Broeckaert L, et al. Hepatic echinococcosis ruptured into the biliary tree: Clinical, radiological and therapeutic features during five episodes of spontaneous biliary rupture in three patients with hepatic hydatidosis. J Hepatol 1987;4:133–139.

481. Hira PR, Lindberg LG, Francis I, et al. Diagnosis of cystic hydatid disease: Role of aspiration cytology. Lancet 1988;2:655–657.

482. Akinoglu A, Demiryurek H, Guzel C. Alveolar hydatid disease of the liver: A report on thirty-nine surgical cases in eastern Anatolia. Am J Trop Med Hyg 1991;45:182–189.

483. Khuroo MS, Wani NA, Javid G, et al. Percutaneous drainage compared with surgery for hepatic hydatid cysts. N Engl J Med 1997;337:881–887.

484. Ciftcioglu MA, Yildirgan MI, Akcay MN, et al. Fine needle aspiration biopsy in hepatic *Echinococcus multilocularis*. Acta Cytol 1997;41:649–652.

485. DiMatteo G, Bove A, Chiarini S, et al. Hepatic echinococcus disease: Our experience over 22 years. Hepatogastroenterology 1996;43:1562–1565.

486. Klein S, Nealon WH. Hepatobiliary abnormalities associated with total parenteral nutrition. Semin Liv Dis 1988;8:237–246.

487. Cohen C, Olsen MM. Paediatric total parenteral nutrition. Arch Pathol Lab Med 1981;105:152–156.

488. Body JJ, Bleiberg H, Bron D, et al. Total parenteral nutrition–induced cholestasis mimicking large bile duct obstruction. Histopathology 1982;6:787–792.

489. Benjamin D. Hepatobiliary dysfunction in infants and children associated with long-term total parenteral nutrition: A clinicopathologic study. Am J Clin Pathol 1981;76:276–283.

490. Wolfe BM, Walker BK, Shaul DB, et al. Effect of total parenteral nutrition on hepatic histology. Arch Surg 1988;123:1084–1090.

491. Goplerud JM. Hyperalimentation associated hepatotoxicity in the newborn. Ann Clin Lab Sci 1992;22:79–84.

492. Croffy B, Kopelman R, Kaplan M. Hypereosinophilic syndrome: Association with chronic active hepatitis. Dig Dis Sci 1988;33:233–239.

493. Foong A, Scholes JV, Gleich GJ, et al. Eosinophil-induced chronic active hepatitis in the idiopathic hypereosinophilic syndrome. Hepatology 1991;13:1090–1094.

494. Fauci AS, Harley JB, Roberts WC, et al. The idiopathic hypereosinophilic syndrome: Clinical, pathophysiologic and therapeutic considerations. Ann Intern Med 1982;97:78–92.

495. Cha SH, Park CM, Cha IH, et al. Hepatic involvement in hypereosinophilic syndrome: Value of portal venous phase imaging. Abdom Imaging 1998;23:154–157.

496. Gore I, Isaacson NH. Pathology of hyperpyrexia: Observations at autopsy in 17 cases of fever therapy. Am J Pathol 1949;25:1029–1046.

497. Movitt ER, Gerstl B, Davis AE. Needle liver biopsy in thyrotoxicosis. Arch Intern Med 1953;91:729–739.

498. Piper J, Poulsen E. Liver biopsy in thyrotoxicosis. Acta Med Scand 1947;127:439–447.

499. Sola J, Pardo-Mindan FJ, Zozaya J, et al. Liver changes in patients with hyperthyroidism. Liver 1991;11:193–197.

500. Huang MJ, Liaw YF. Clinical associations between thyroid and liver disease. J Gastroenterol Hepatol 1995;10:344–350.

501. Fong TL, McHutchison JG, Reynolds TB. Hyperthyroidism and hepatic dysfunction: A case series analysis. J Clin Gastroenterol 1992;14:240–244.

502. Baker A, Kaplan M, Wolfe H. Central congestive fibrosis of the liver in myxoedema ascites. Ann Intern Med 1972;77:927–929.

503. Clancy RL, Mackay IR. Myxoedematous ascites. Med J Aust 1970;2:415–416.

504. Ludwig J, Wiesner RH, LaRusso NF. Idiopathic adulthood ductopenia: A cause of chronic cholestatic liver disease and biliary cirrhosis. J Hepatol 1988;7:193–199.

505. Zafrani ES, Metreau J-M, Douvin C, et al. Idiopathic biliary ductopenia in adults: A report of five cases. Gastroenterology 1990;99:1823–1828.

506. Desmet VJ. Histopathology of chronic cholestasis and adult ductopenic syndrome. Clin Liver Dis 1998;2:249–264.

507. Ludwig J. Idiopathic adulthood ductopenia: An update. Mayo Clin Proc 1998;73:285–291.

508. Klatskin G. Hepatic granulomata: Problems in interpretation. Mt Sinai J Med 1977;44:798–812.

509. Ishak KG. Granulomas of the liver. In Ioachim HL, ed. Pathology of Granulomas. Raven Press: New York, 1983, pp 307–369.

510. Nakhleh RE, Glock M, Snover DC. Hepatic pathology of chronic granulomatous disease of childhood. Arch Pathol Lab Med 1992;116:71–75.

511. Simon HB, Wolff SM. Granulomatous hepatitis and prolonged fever of unknown origin: A study of 13 patients. Medicine 1973;52:1–21.

512. Sartin JS, Walker RC. Granulomatous hepatitis: A retrospective review of 88 cases at the Mayo Clinic. Mayo Clin Proc 1991;66:914–918.

513. Zoutman DE, Ralph ED, Frei JV. Granulomatous hepatitis and fever of unknown origin: An 11-year experience of 23 cases with three years' follow-up. J Clin Gastroenterol 1991;13:69–75.

514. Mikkelsen WP, Edmondson HA, Peters RL, et al. Extra- and intrahepatic portal hypertension without cirrhosis (hepatoportal sclerosis). Ann Surg 1965;162:602–620.

515. Okuda K, Kono K, Ohnishi K, et al. Clinical study of eighty-six cases of idiopathic portal hypertension and comparison with cirrhosis with splenomegaly. Gastroenterology 1984;86:600–610.

516. Peters RL. Idiopathic portal hypertension: Pathologic changes. In Okuda K, Omata M, eds. Idiopathic Portal Hypertension: Proceedings of the International Symposium on Idiopathic Portal Hypertension. University of Tokyo Press: Tokyo, 1983, pp 85–97.

517. Okuda K, Nakashima T, Okudaira M, et al. Liver pathology of idiopathic portal hypertension: Comparison with noncirrhotic portal fibrosis of India. Liver 1982;2:176–192.

518. Almoudarres M, Vega KJ, Trotman BW. Noncirrhotic portal hypertension in the adult: Case report and review of the literature. J Assoc Acad Minor Phys 1998;9:53–55.

519. Oikawa H, Masuda T, Sato S, et al. Changes in lymph vessels and portal veins in the portal tract of patients with idiopathic portal hypertension: A morphometric study. Hepatology 1998;27:1607–1610.

520. Nakanuma Y, Hoso M, Sasaki M, et al. Histopathology of the liver in non-cirrhotic portal hypertension of unknown aetiology. Histopathology 1996;28:195–204.

521. Joshi VV. Indian childhood cirrhosis. Perspect Pediatr Pathol 1987;11:175–192.

522. Lefkowitch JH, Honig CL, King ME, et al. Hepatic copper overload and features of Indian childhood cirrhosis. N Engl J Med 1982;307:271–277.

523. Tanner MS, Portmann B. Indian childhood cirrhosis. Arch Dis Child 1981;56:4–6.

524. Pandit A, Bhave S. Present interpretation of the role of copper in Indian childhood cirrhosis. Am J Clin Nutr 1996;63:830S–835S.

525. Bhusnurmath SR, Walia BN, Singh S, et al. Sequential histopathologic alterations in Indian childhood cirrhosis treated with D-penicillamine. Hum Pathol 1991;22:653–658.

526. Lathrop DB. Cystic disease of the liver and kidney. Pediatrics 1959;24:215–224.

527. Lieberman E, Salinas-Madrigal L, Gwinn JL, et al. Infantile polycystic disease of the kidneys and liver. Medicine 1971;50:227–318.

528. Landing BH, Walls TR, Claireaux AE. Morphometric analysis of liver lesions in cystic diseases of childhood. Hum Pathol 1980;11:549–560.

529. Desmet VJ. Congenital diseases of intrahepatic bile ducts: Var-

iations on the theme "ductal plate malformation." Hepatology 1992;16:1069–1083.

530. Gang DL, Herrin JT. Infantile polycystic disease of the liver and kidneys. Clin Nephrol 1986;25:28–36.

531. Dachman AH, Lichtenstein JE, Friedman AC, et al. Infantile hemangioendothelioma of the liver: Radiologic pathologic–clinical correlation. Am J Radiol 1983;140:1091–1096.

532. Stanley P, Geer GD, Miller JH, et al. Infantile hepatic hemangiomas. Cancer 1989;64:936–949.

533. Fok TF, Chan MS, Metreweli C, et al. Hepatic haemangioendothelioma presenting with early heart failure in a newborn: Treatment with hepatic artery embolization and interferon. Acta Paediatr 1996;85:1373–1375.

534. Han SJ, Tsai CC, Tsai HM, et al. Infantile hemangioendothelioma with a highly elevated serum alpha-fetoprotein level. Hepatogastroenterology 1998;45:459–461.

535. Someren A. "Inflammatory pseudotumor" of liver with occlusive phlebitis: Report of a case in a child and review of the literature. Am J Clin Pathol 1978;69:176–181.

536. Kessler E, Turani H, Kayser S, et al. Inflammatory pseudotumor of the liver. Liver 1988;8:17–23.

537. Horiuchi R, Uchida T, Kojima T, et al. Inflammatory pseudotumor of the liver: Clinicopathologic study and review of the literature. Cancer 1990;65:1583–1590.

538. Zamir D, Jarchowsky J, Singer C, et al. Inflammatory pseudotumor of the liver—a rare entity and a diagnostic challenge. Am J Gastroenterol 1998;93:1538–1540.

539. Selves J, Meggetto F, Brousset P, et al. Inflammatory pseudotumor of the liver: Evidence for follicular dendritic reticulum cell proliferation associated with clonal Epstein-Barr virus. Am J Surg Pathol 1996;20:747–753.

540. Passalides A, Keramidas D, Mavrides G. Inflammatory pseudotumor of the liver in children: A case report and review of the literature. Eur J Pediatr Surg 1996;6:35–37.

541. Lai HS, Duh YC, Chen WJ. Inspissated bile syndrome followed by choledochal cyst formation. Surgery 1998;126:706–708.

542. Brown DM. Bile plug syndrome: Successful management with a mucolytic agent. J Pediatr Surg 1990;25:351–352.

543. Amano S, Hazama F, Kubagawa H, et al. General pathology of Kawasaki disease. Acta Pathol Jpn 1980;30:681–694.

544. Ohshio G, Furukawa F, Fujiwara H, et al. Hepatomegaly and splenomegaly in Kawasaki disease. Pediatr Pathol 1985;4:257–264.

545. Bader-Meunier B, Hadchouel M, Fabre M, et al. Intrahepatic bile duct damage in children with Kawasaki disease. J Pediatr 1992;120:750–752.

546. Gear JH, Meyers KE, Steele M. Kawasaki disease manifesting with acute cholangitis: A case report. S Afr Med J 1992;81:31–33.

547. Ohshio G, Furukawa F, Fujiwara H, et al. Hepatomegaly and splenomegaly in Kawasaki disease. Pediatr Pathol 1985;4:257–264.

548. Webber BL, Freiman I. The liver in kwashiorkor: A clinical and electron microscopic study. Arch Pathol 1974;98:400–408.

549. Praharaj KC, Choudhury U. The liver in kwashiorkor: A clinicohistopathological study. J Indian Med Assoc 1977;69:77–80.

550. Doherty JF, Adam EJ, Griffin GE, et al. Ultrasonographic assessment of the extent of hepatic steatosis in severe malnutrition. Arch Dis Child 1992;67:1348–1352.

551. Tai da Rocha-Afodu J. The liver in kwashiorkor. Scand J Gastroenterol Suppl 1986;124:9–24.

552. Grundy P, Ellis R. Histiocytosis X: A review of the etiology, pathology, staging and therapy. Med Pediatr Oncol 1986;14:664–671.

553. Heyn RM, Hamoudi A, Newton WA Jr. Pretreatment liver biopsy in 20 children with histiocytosis X: A clinicopathologic correlation. Med Pediatr Oncol 1990;18:110–118.

554. Favara BE. The pathology of "histiocytosis." Am J Pediatr Hematol Oncol 1981;3:45–56.

555. Favara BE, McCarthy RC, Meirau GW. Histiocytosis X. Hum Pathol 1983;14:663–676.

556. Baumgartner I, von Hochstetter A, Baumert B, et al. Langerhans'-cell histiocytosis in adults. Med Pediatr Oncol 1997;28:9–14.

557. The French Langerhans' Cell Histiocytosis Study Group. A multicentre retrospective survey of Langerhans' cell histiocytosis: 348 cases observed between 1983 and 1993. Arch Dis Child 1996;75:17–24.

558. Favara BE. Histopathology of the liver in histiocytosis syndromes. Pediatr Pathol Lab Med 1996;16:413–433.

559. Concepcion W, Esquivel CO, Terry A, et al. Liver transplantation in Langerhans' cell histiocytosis (histiocytosis X). Semin Oncol 1991;18:24–28.

560. Walker DH, McCormick JB, Johnson KM, et al. Pathologic and virologic study of fatal Lassa fever in man. Am J Pathol 1982;107:349–356.

561. Edington GM, White HA. The pathology of Lassa fever. Trans R Soc Trop Med Hyg 1972;66:381–389.

562. Peters CJ, Liu CT, Anderson GW Jr, et al. Pathogenesis of viral hemorrhagic fevers: Rift Valley fever and Lassa fever contrasted. Rev Infect Dis 1989;11 (Suppl 4):S743–S749.

563. McCormick JB, Walker DH, King IJ, et al. Lassa fever hepatitis: A study of fatal Lassa fever in humans. Am J Trop Med Hyg 1986;35:401–407.

564. Moreno A, Marazuela M, Yebra M, et al. Hepatic fibrin-ring granuloma in visceral leishmaniasis. Gastroenterology 1988;95:1123–1126.

565. Duarte MIS, Mariano ON, Corbett CEP. Liver parenchymal cell parasitism in human visceral leishmaniasis. Virchows Arch A Pathol Anat Histopathol 1989;415:1–6.

566. Duarte MIS, Corbett CEP. Histopathological patterns of the liver involvement in visceral leishmaniasis. Rev Inst Med Trop São Paulo 1987;29:131–136.

567. Daneshbod K. Visceral leishmaniasis (kala-azar) in Iran: A pathologic and electron microscopic study. Am J Clin Pathol 1972;57:156–166.

568. El Hag IA, Hashim FA, el Toum IA, et al. Liver morphology and function in visceral leishmaniasis (kala-azar). J Clin Pathol 1994;47:547–551.

569. Karat ABA, Job CK, Rao PSS. Liver in leprosy: Histological and biochemical findings. BMJ 1971;1:307–310.

570. Powell CS, Swan LL. Leprosy: Pathologic changes observed in fifty consecutive necropsies. Am J Pathol 1955;31:1131–1147.

571. Desikan KV, Job CK. A review of postmortem findings in 37 cases of leprosy. Int J Leprosy 1968;36:32–44.

572. Chen TSN, Drutz DJ, Whelan GR. Hepatic granulomas in leprosy: Their relation to bacteremia. Arch Pathol Lab Med 1976;100:182–185.

573. Taneja K, Khanna NV, Shiv VK, et al. Hepatic ultrasonography in patients with lepromatous leprosy. Indian J Lepr 1990;62:443–447.

574. Patnaik JK, Saha PK, Satpathy SK, et al. Hepatic morphology in reactional states of leprosy. Int J Lepr Other Mycobact Dis 1989;57:499–505.

575. Ferreira VA, Vianna MR, Yasuda PH, et al. Detection of leptospiral antigen in the human liver and kidney using an immunoperoxidase staining procedure. J Pathol 1987;151:125–131.

576. Ciceroni L, Pinto A, Benedetti E, et al. Human leptospirosis in Italy, 1986–1993. Eur J Epidemiol 1995;11:707–710.

577. Den Haan PJ, van Vliet AC, Hazenberg BP. Weil's disease as a cause of jaundice. Neth J Med 1993;42:171–174.

578. Zafrani ES, Degos F, Guigui B, et al. The hepatic sinusoid in hairy cell leukemia: An ultrastructural study of 12 cases. Hum Pathol 1987;18:801–807.

579. Roquet ML, Zafrani ES, Farcet JP, et al. Histopathological lesions of the liver in hairy cell leukemia: A report of 14 cases. Hepatology 1985;5:496–500.

580. Locasiulli A, Vergani GM, Uderzo C, et al. Chronic liver disease in children with leukemia in long-term remission. Cancer 1983;52:1080–1087.

581. Yamada Y, Kamihira S, Murata K, et al. Frequent hepatic involvement in adult T cell leukemia: Comparison with non-Hodgkin's lymphoma. Leuk Lymphoma 1997;26:327–335.

582. Scheimberg IB, Pollock DJ, Collins PW, et al. Pathology of the liver in leukemia and lymphoma: A study of 110 autopsies. Histopathology 1995;26:311–321.

583. Droz D, Noel LH, Carnot F, et al. Liver involvement in non-amyloid light chain deposits disease. Lab Invest 1984;50:683–689.

584. Bedossa P, Febre M, Paraf F, et al. Light chain deposition

disease with liver dysfunction. Hum Pathol 1988;19:1008–1014.

585. Pelletier G, Fabre M, Attali P, et al. Light chain deposition disease presenting with hepatomegaly: An association with amyloid-like fibrils. Postgrad Med J 1988;64:804–808.

586. Faa G, Van Eyken P, De Vos R, et al. Light chain deposition disease of the liver associated with AL-type amyloidosis and severe cholestasis. J Hepatol 1991;12:75–82.

587. Bedossa P, Fabre M, Paraf F, et al. Light chain deposition disease with liver dysfunction. Hum Pathol 1988;19:1008–1014.

588. Westin J, Eyrich R, Falsen E, et al. Gamma heavy chain disease: Reports of three patients. Acta Med Scand 1972;192:281–292.

589. Yu VL, Miller WP, Wing EJ, et al. Disseminated listeriosis presenting as acute hepatitis. Am J Med 1982;73:773–777.

590. Lindgren P, Pla JC, Hogberg U, et al. *Listeria monocytogenes*–induced liver abscess in pregnancy. Acta Obstet Gynecol Scand 1997;76:486–488.

591. Marino P, Maggioni M, Preatoni A, et al. Liver abscesses due to *Listeria monocytogenes*. Liver 1996;16:67–69.

592. Manian FA. Liver abscess due to *Listeria monocytogenes*. Clin Infect Dis 1994;18:841–842.

593. Tremm WR, Witzelben CA, Piccoli DA, et al. Medium-chain and long-chain acyl-CoA dehydrogenase deficiency: Clinical, pathologic and ultrastructural differentiation from Reye syndrome. Hepatology 1986;6:1270–1278.

594. Losty HC, Lee P, Alfaham M, et al. Fatty infiltration in the liver in medium chain acyl-CoA dehydrogenase deficiency. Arch Dis Child 1991;66:727–728.

595. Allison F, Bennett MJ, Pollitt RJ, et al. Acquired deficiency of long-chain acyl-CoA dehydrogenase in liver: A cautionary tale. J Inherit Metab Dis 1990;13:333–336.

596. Goellner MH, Agger WA, Burgess JH, et al. Hepatitis due to recurrent Lyme disease. Ann Intern Med 1988;108:707–708.

597. Duray PH. Clinical pathologic correlations of Lyme disease. Rev Infect Dis 1989;11 (Suppl 6):S1487–S1493.

598. Horowitz HW, Dworkin B, Forseter G, et al. Liver function in early Lyme disease. Hepatology 1996;23:1412–1417.

599. Kazakoff MA, Sinusas K, Macchia C. Liver function test abnormalities in early Lyme disease. Arch Fam Med 1993;2:409–413.

600. Duray PH. Histopathology of clinical phases of human Lyme disease. Rheum Dis Clin North Am 1989;15:691–710.

601. Van Steenbergen W, Joosten E, Marchall G, et al. Hepatic lymphangiomatosis. Gastroenterology 1985;88:1968–1972.

602. Haratake J, Koide O, Takeshita H. Hepatic lymphangiomatosis: Report of two cases with an immunohistochemical study. Am J Gastroenterol 1992;87:906–909.

603. Stavropoulos M, Vagianos C, Scopa CD, et al. Solitary hepatic lymphangioma. A rare benign tumor: A case report. HPB Surg 1994;8:33–36.

604. Haratake J, Koide O, Takeshita H. Hepatic lymphangiomatosis: Report of two cases, with an immunohistochemical study. Am J Gastroenterol 1992;87:906–909.

605. Abt AB, Kirschner RH, Belliveau RE, et al. Hepatic pathology associated with Hodgkin's disease. Cancer 1974;33:1564–1571.

606. Belliveau RE, Wiernik PH, Abt AB. Liver enzymes and pathology in Hodgkin's disease. Cancer 1974;34:300–305.

607. Dich NH, Goodman ZD, Klein MA. Hepatic involvement in Hodgkin's disease: Clues to histologic diagnosis. Cancer 1989;64:2121–2126.

608. Bruguera M, Caballero T, Carreras E, et al. Hepatic sinusoidal dilatation in Hodgkin's disease. Liver 1987;7:76–80.

609. Sans M, Andreu V, Bordas JM, et al. Usefulness of laparoscopy with liver biopsy in the assessment of liver involvement at diagnosis of Hodgkin's and non-Hodgkin's lymphoma. Gastrointest Endosc 1998;47:391–395.

610. Kadin ME, Donaldson SS, Dorfman RF. Isolated granulomas in Hodgkin's disease. N Engl J Med 1970;283:859–861.

611. Osborne BM, Butler JJ, Guarda LA. Primary lymphoma of the liver: Ten cases and a review of the literature. Cancer 1985;56:2902–2910.

612. DeMent SH, Mann RB, Staal SP, et al. Primary lymphomas of the liver: Report of six cases and review of the literature. Am J Clin Pathol 1987;88:255–263.

613. Ryan J, Straus DJ, Lange C, et al. Primary lymphoma of the liver. Cancer 1988;61:370–375.

614. Lei KI. Primary non-Hodgkin's lymphoma of the liver. Leuk Lymphoma 1998;29:293–299.

615. Al-Fadda M, Fashir BM. Primary large cell lymphoma presenting as hilar mass and obstructive jaundice. Am J Gastroenterol 1998;93:274–275.

616. Maes M, Depardieu C, Dargent JL, et al. Primary low-grade B-cell lymphoma of MALT-type occurring in the liver. A study of two cases. J Hepatol 1997;27:922–927.

617. Mohler M, Gutzler F, Kallinowski B, et al. Primary hepatic high-grade non-Hodgkin's lymphoma and chronic hepatitis C infection. Dig Dis Sci 1997;42:2241–2245.

618. Joshi YK, Tandon BN, Acharya SK, et al. Acute hepatic failure due to *Plasmodium falciparum* liver injury. Liver 1986;6:357–360.

619. Ramachandran S, Perera MVF. Jaundice and hepatomegaly in primary malaria. J Trop Med Hyg 1976;79:207–210.

620. Crane GG. Hyperreactive malarious splenomegaly (tropical splenomegaly syndrome). Parasitology Today 1986;2:4–9.

621. De Brito T, Barone AA, Faria RM. Human liver biopsy in *P. falciparum* and *P. vivax* malaria: A light and electron microscopy study. Virchows Arch A Pathol Anat Histopathol 1969;348:220–229.

622. Hollingdale MR. Malaria and the liver. Hepatology 1985;5:327–335.

623. Ravichandiran K, Sumitha K, Selvam R. Liver function tests in recurrent *P. vivax* malaria. J Commun Dis 1996;28:231–240.

624. Davies MP, Borrk GM, Weir WR, et al. Liver function tests in adults with *Plasmodium falciparum* infection. Eur J Gastroenterol Hepatol 1996;8:873–875.

625. Mishra SK, Mohanty S, Das BS, et al. Hepatic changes in *P. falciparum* malaria. Indian J Malariol 1992;29:167–171.

626. Anand AC, Ramji S, Narula AS, et al. Malarial hepatitis: A heterogeneous syndrome? Natl Med J India 1992;5:59–62.

627. Petushkova NA. First-trimester diagnosis of an unusual case of β-mannosidosis. Prenat Diagn 1991;11:279–283.

628. Gordon BA, Carson R, Haust MD. Unusual clinical and ultrastructural features in a boy with biochemically typical mannosidosis. Acta Paediatr Scand 1980;69:787–792.

629. Monus Z, Konyar E, Szabo L. Histomorphologic and histochemical investigations in mannosidosis: A light and electron microscopic study. Virchows Arch B Cell Pathol Incl Mol Pathol 1977;26:159–173.

630. Simon DM, Krause R, Galambos JT. Peliosis hepatis in a patient with marasmus. Gastroenterology 1988;95:805–809.

631. Martini GA. Marburg virus disease. Postgrad Med J 1973;49:542–546.

632. Piggot JA, Hochholzer L. Human melioidosis: A histopathologic study of acute and chronic melioidosis. Arch Pathol Lab Med 1970;90:101–111.

633. Sheehy TW, Deller JJ Jr, Weber DR. Melioidosis. Ann Intern Med 1967;67:897–900.

634. Stocker JT, Ishak KG. Mesenchymal hamartoma of the liver. Pediatr Pathol 1983;1:245–267.

635. DeMaioribus CA, Lally KP, Sim K, et al. Mesenchymal hamartoma of the liver. Arch Surg 1990;125:598–600.

636. Tzen CY, Chen BF, Chang PY, et al. Mesenchymal hamartoma of the liver. A case report. Chung Hua I Hsueh Tsa Chih 1998;61:427–431.

637. Alwaidh MH, Woodhall CR, Carty HT. Mesenchymal hamartoma of the liver: A case report. Pediatr Radiol 1997;27:247–249.

638. Ros PR, Goodman ZD, Ishak KG, et al. Mesenchymal hamartoma of the liver. Radiologic-pathologic correlation. Radiology 1986;158:619–624.

639. Hagberg B, Sourander P, Svennerholm L. Sulfatide lipidosis in childhood. Am J Dis Child 1962;104:644–656.

640. Wolfe HJ, Pietra GG. The visceral lesions of metachromatic leukodystrophy. Am J Pathol 1964;44:921–930.

641. Cole G, Proctor NS. Adult metachromatic leucodystrophy. S Afr Med J 1974;48:1371–1374.

642. Pol S, Romana C, Richard S, et al. *Enterocytozoon bieneusi* infection in acquired immunodeficiency syndrome–related sclerosing cholangitis. Gastroenterology 1992;102:1778–1781.

643. Pol S, Romana C, Richard S, et al. Microsporidia infection in patients with the human immunodeficiency virus and unexplained cholangitis. N Engl J Med 1993;328:95–99.

644. Terada S, Reddy KR, Jeffers LJ, et al. Microsporidian hepatitis in the acquired immunodeficiency syndrome. Ann Intern Med 1987;107:61–62.

645. Cowley GP, Miller RF, Papadaki L, et al. Disseminated microsporidiosis in a patient with acquired immunodeficiency syndrome. Histopathology 1997;30:386–389.

646. Spranger J. Mucolipidosis I. In Bergsma D, ed. Disorders of connective tissue. Stratton Intercontinental: New York, 1975, pp 279–282.

647. Riches WG, Smuckler EA. A severe infantile mucolipidosis: Clinical, biochemical and pathologic features. Arch Pathol Lab Med 1983;107:147–152.

648. Kenyon KR, Sensenbrenner JA, Wyllie RG. Hepatic ultrastructure and histochemistry in mucolipidosis II (I-cell disease). Pediatr Res 1973;7:560–568.

649. Neufeld EF, Muenzer J. The mucopolysaccharidoses. In Scriver CR, Beaudet AL, Sly WS, et al, eds. The Metabolic Basis of Inherited Disease. 6th ed. McGraw-Hill: New York, 1989, pp 1565–1587.

650. Van Hoof F. Mucopolysaccharidoses. In Hers HA, Van Hoof F, eds. Lysosomes and Storage Disease. Academic Press: New York, 1973, pp 217–259.

651. Parfrey NA, Hutchins GM. Hepatic fibrosis in the mucopolysaccharidoses. Am J Med 1986;81:825–829.

652. Resnick JM, Whitley CB, Leonard AS, et al. Light and electron microscopic features of the liver in mucopolysaccharidosis. Hum Pathol 1994;25:276–286.

653. Resnick JM, Krivit W, Snover DC, et al. Pathology of the liver in mucopolysaccharidosis: Light and electron microscopic assessment before and after bone marrow transplantation. Bone Marrow Transplant 1992;10:273–280.

654. Parfrey NA, Hutchins GM. Hepatic fibrosis in the mucopolysaccharidoses. Am J Med 1986;81:825–829.

655. Thiruvengadam R, Penetranti R, Grolsky HJ, et al. Multiple myeloma presenting as space-occupying lesions of the liver. Cancer 1990;65:2784–2786.

656. Thomas FB, Clausen KP, Greenberger NJ. Liver disease in multiple myeloma. Arch Intern Med 1973;132:195–202.

657. Yoon YS, Min YH, Chou CY, et al. Liver involvement in multiple myeloma proven by peritoneoscopy—a case report. Yonsei Med J 1993;34:90–97.

658. Greene JB, Gurdip SS, Lewin S, et al. Mycobacterium avium-intracellulare: A cause of disseminated life-threatening infection in homosexuals and drug abusers. Ann Intern Med 1982; 97:539–546.

659. Maasenkeil G, Opravil M, Salfinger M, et al. Disseminated coinfection with Mycobacterium avium complex and Mycobacterium kanasii in a patient with AIDS and liver abscess. Clin Infect Dis 1992;14:618–619.

660. Wallace JM, Hannah JB. Mycobacterium avium complex infection in patients with the acquired immunodeficiency syndrome: A clinicopathologic study. Chest 1988;93:926–932.

661. Nightingale SD, Byrd LT, Southern PM, et al. Incidence of Mycobacterium avium-intracellulare complex bacteremia in human immunodeficiency virus–positive patients. J Infect Dis 1992;165:1082–1085.

662. Torriani FJ, McCutchan JA, Bozzette SA, et al. Autopsy findings in AIDS patients with Mycobacterium avium complex bacteremia. J Infect Dis 1994;170:1601–1605.

663. Hopewell PC. Tuberculous and nontuberculous mycobacterial infections. In Stein JH, ed. Internal Medicine. 2nd ed. Little, Brown: Boston, 1987, pp 1746–1748.

664. Dubois A, Dauzat M, Pignodel C, et al. Portal hypertension in lymphoproliferative and myeloproliferative disorders: Hemodynamic and histological correlations. Hepatology 1993;17: 246–250.

665. Pereira A, Bruguera M, Cervantes F, et al. Liver involvement at diagnosis of primary myelofibrosis: A clinicopathological study of twenty-two cases. Eur J Haematol 1988;40:355–361.

666. Nishimura RN, Ishak KG, Reddick R, et al. Lafora disease: Diagnosis by liver biopsy. Ann Neurol 1979;8:409–415.

667. Collins GH, Cowden RR, Nevis AH. Myoclonus epilepsy with Lafora bodies. Arch Pathol 1968;86:239–254.

668. Ishihara T, Yokota T, Yamashita Y, et al. Comparative study of the intracytoplasmic inclusions in Lafora disease and type IV glycogenesis by electron microscopy. Acta Pathol Jpn 1987;37: 1591–1601.

669. Footitt DR, Quinn N, Kocen RS, et al. Familial Lafora body disease of late onset: Report of four cases in one family and a review of the literature. J Neurol 1997;244:40–44.

670. Elliott EJ, Talbot IC, Pye IF, et al. Lafora disease: A progressive myoclonus epilepsy. J Paediatr Child Health 1992;28:455–458.

671. Montgomery CK, Ruebner BH. Neonatal hepatocellular giant cell transformation: A review. In Rosenberg HS, Bolande RP, eds. Perspectives in Pediatric Pathology. Year Book Medical Publishers: Chicago, 1976, pp 85–101.

672. Ruebner B, Thaler MM. Giant cell transformation in infantile liver disease. In Javitt NB, ed. Neonatal Hepatitis and Biliary Atresia. US Government Printing Press: Washington, DC, 1976, pp 299–311.

673. Oledzka-Slotwinska H, Desmet V. Morphologic study on neonatal liver "giant" cell transformation. Exp Mol Biol 1969;10: 162–175.

674. Shet TM, Kandalkar BM, Vora IM. Neonatal hepatitis—an autopsy study of 14 cases. Indian J Pathol Microbiol 1998;41:77–84.

675. Dick MC, Mowat AP. Hepatitis syndrome in infancy—an epidemiological survey with 10-year follow-up. Arch Dis Child 1985;60:512–516.

676. Elleder M, Smid F, Hymova H. Liver findings in Niemann-Pick disease type C. Histochem J 1984;16:1147–1170.

677. Ashkenazi A, Yarom R, Gutman A, et al. Niemann-Pick disease and giant cell transformation of the liver. Acta Paediatr Scand 1971;60:285–294.

678. Tamaru J, Iwasaki I, Horie H, et al. Niemann-Pick disease associated with liver disorders. Acta Pathol Jpn 1985;35:1267–1272.

679. Takahashi T, Akiyama K, Tomihara M, et al. Heterogeneity of liver disorder in type B Niemann-Pick disease. Hum Pathol 1997;28:385–388.

680. Buchino JJ. Niemann-Pick type C. Pediatr Pathol 1993;13:841–845.

681. Mishra S, Hiranandani M, Yachha SK, et al. Niemann-Pick disease presenting as hepatic disorder. Indian J Gastroenterol 1992;11:39–40.

682. Tassoni JP Jr, Fawaz KA, Johnston DE. Cirrhosis and portal hypertension in a patient with adult Niemann-Pick disease. Gastroenterology 1991;100:567–569.

683. Kim J, Minamoto GY, Grieco MH. Nocardial infection as a complication of AIDS: Report of six cases and review. Rev Infect Dis 1991;13:624–629.

684. Ramseyer LT, Nguyen DL. Nocardia brasiliensis liver abscesses in an AIDS patient: Imaging findings. Am J Roentgenol 1993;160:898–899.

685. Raby N, Forbes G, Williams R. Nocardia infection in patients with liver transplants or chronic liver disease: Radiologic findings. Radiology 1990;174:713–716.

686. Forbes GM, Harvey FA, Philpott-Howard JN, et al. Nocardiosis in liver transplantation: Variation in presentation, diagnosis and therapy. J Infect 1990;20:11–19.

687. Stromeyer FW, Ishak KG. Nodular transformation (nodular "regenerative" hyperplasia) of the liver. Hum Pathol 1981;12:60–71.

688. Mones JM, Saldana MJ, Albores-Saavedra J. Nodular regenerative hyperplasia of the liver. Arch Pathol Lab Med 1984;108: 741–743.

689. Voinchet O, Degott C, Scoazec JY, et al. Peliosis hepatis, nodular regenerative hyperplasia of the liver, and light-chain deposition in a patient with Waldenström's macroglobulinemia. Gastroenterology 1988;95:482–486.

690. Goritsas CP, Repanti M, Papadaki E, et al. Intrahepatic bile duct injury and nodular regenerative hyperplasia of the liver in a patient with polyarteritis nodosa. J Hepatol 1997;26:727–730.

691. Kanel GC. Hepatic lesions resembling alcoholic liver disease. In Ferrell LD, ed. Diagnostic problems in liver pathology. Hanley & Belfus: Philadelphia, 1994, pp 77–104.

692. Ludwig J, Viggiano TR, McGill DB, et al. Nonalcoholic steatohepatitis: Mayo Clinic experiences with a hitherto unnamed disease. Mayo Clin Proc 1980;55:434–438.

693. Itoh S, Yougel T, Kawagoe K. Comparison between nonalcoholic steatohepatitis and alcoholic hepatitis. Am J Gastroenterol 1987;82:650–654.

694. Powell EE, Cooksley WGE, Hanson R, et al. The natural history of nonalcoholic steatohepatitis: A follow-up study of forty-two patients for up to 21 years. Hepatology 1990;11:74–80.

695. Lee RG. Nonalcoholic steatohepatitis: A study of 49 patients. Hum Pathol 1989;20:594–598.

696. Bacon BR, Farahvash MJ, Janney CG, et al. Nonalcoholic steatohepatitis. An expanded clinical entity. Gastroenterology 1994;107:1103–1109.

697. O'Connor BJ, Kathamna B, Tavill AS. Nonalcoholic fatty liver (NASH syndrome). Gastroenterologist 1997;5:316–329.

698. Ludwig J, McGill DB, Lindor KD. Review: Nonalcoholic steatohepatitis. J Gastroenterol Hepatol 1997;12:398–403.

699. Diehl AM, Goodman Z, Ishak KG. Alcohol-like liver disease in nonalcoholics: A clinical and histologic comparison with alcohol-induced liver injury. Gastroenterology 1988;95:1056–1062.

700. Popper H, Schaffner F. Liver: Structure and Function. McGraw-Hill: New York, 1957, pp 404–407.

701. Evans H, Bourgeois CH, Comer DS, et al. Biliary tract changes in opisthorchiasis. Am J Trop Med Hyg 1971;20:667–671.

702. Elkins DB, Haswell-Elkins MR, Mairiang E, et al. A high frequency of hepatobiliary disease and suspected cholangiocarcinoma associated with heavy *Opisthorchis viverrini* infection in a small community in north-east Thailand. Trans R Soc Trop Med Hyg 1990;84:715–719.

703. Riganti M, Pungpak S, Punpoowong B, et al. Human pathology of *Opisthorchis viverrini* infection: A comparison of adults and children. Southeast Asian J Trop Med Public Health 1989;20:95–100.

704. Teixeira F, Gayotto LCDC, de Brito T. Morphological patterns of the liver in South American blastomycosis. Histopathology 1978;2:231–237.

705. Wanless IR, Lentz JS, Roberts EA. Partial nodular transformation of the liver in an adult with persistent ductus venosus. Arch Pathol Lab Med 1985;109:427–432.

706. Sherlock S, Feldman CA, Moran B, et al. Partial nodular transformation of the liver. Am J Pathol 1959;35:943–953.

707. Terayama N, Terada T, Hoso M, et al. Partial nodular transformation of the liver with portal vein thrombosis: A report of two autopsy cases. J Clin Gastroenterol 1995;20:71–76.

708. Tsui WM, So KT. Partial nodular transformation of liver in a child. Histopathology 1993;22:594–596.

709. Kahn E, Daum F, Markowitz J, et al. Nonsyndromatic paucity of interlobular bile ducts: Light and electron microscopic evaluation of sequential liver biopsies in early childhood. Hepatology 1986;6:890–901.

710. Alagille D, Estrada A, Hadchouel M, et al. Syndromatic paucity of interlobular bile ducts (Alagille syndrome or arteriohepatic dysplasia): Review of 80 cases. J Pediatr 1987;110:195–200.

711. Kahn El, Daum F, Markowitz J, et al. Arteriohepatic dysplasia. II. Hepatobiliary morphology. Hepatology 1983;3:77–84.

712. Kahn E. Paucity of interlobular bile ducts: Arteriohepatic dysplasia and nonsyndromatic duct paucity. *In* Abramowsky CR, Bernstein J, Rosenberg HS, eds. Perspectives in Pediatric Pathology. Transplantation Pathology–Hepatic Morphogenesis. Karger: Basel, 1991, pp 168–215.

713. Hashida Y, Junis EJ. Syndromatic paucity of interlobular bile ducts: Hepatic histopathology of the early and endstage liver. Pediatr Pathol 1988;8:1–15.

714. Dahms BB, Petrelli M, Wyllie R, et al. Arteriohepatic dysplasia in infancy and childhood: A longitudinal study of six patients. Hepatology 1982;2:350–358.

715. Kocak N, Gurakan F, Yuce A, et al. Nonsyndromatic paucity of interlobular bile ducts: Clinical and laboratory findings of 10 cases. J Pediatr Gastroenterol Nutr 1997;24:44–48.

716. Bosman C, Renda F, Boldrini R, et al. Intrahepatic cholestasis by paucity of interlobular bile ducts in infancy. Recent Prog Med 1994;85:375–383.

717. Hadchouel M. Paucity of interlobular bile ducts. Semin Diagn Pathol 1992;9:24–30.

718. Yanoff M, Rawson AJ. Peliosis hepatis: An anatomic study with demonstration of two varieties. Arch Pathol 1964;77:159–165.

719. Radin DR, Kanel GC. Peliosis hepatis in a patient with human immunodeficiency virus infection. AJR 1991;156:91–92.

720. Zak FG. Peliosis hepatis. Am J Pathol 1950;26:1–15.

721. Ahsan N, Holman MJ, Riley TR, et al. Peliosis hepatis due to *Bartonella henselae* in transplantation: A hemato-hepato-renal syndrome. Transplantation 1998;65:1000–1003.

722. Alkan S, Orenstein JM. Bacillary peliosis hepatis. N Engl J Med 1991;324:1513–1514.

723. Jayanetra P, Nitiyanant P, Ajello L, et al. Penicilliosis marneffei in Thailand: A report of five human cases. Am J Trop Med Hyg 1984;33:637–644.

724. Kantipong P, Panich V, Pongsurachet V, et al. Hepatic penicilliosis in patients without skin lesions. Clin Infect Dis 1998;26:1215–1217.

725. Heath TC, Patel A, Fisher D, et al. Disseminated penicillium marneffei: Presenting illness of advanced HIV infection; a clinicopathological review, illustrated by a case report. Pathology 1995;27:101–105.

726. Self JT, Hopps HC, Williams AO. Pentastomiasis in Africans. Trop Geogr Med 1975;27:1–13.

727. Prathap K, Lau KS, Bolton JM. Pentastomiasis: A common finding at autopsy in Malaysian aborigines. Am J Trop Med Hyg 1969;18:20–27.

728. Guardia SN, Sepp H, Scholten T, et al. Pentastomiasis in Canada. Arch Pathol Lab Med 1991;115:515–517.

729. Nakano M, Worner TM, Lieber CS. Perivenular fibrosis in alcoholic liver injury: Ultrastructure and histologic progression. Gastroenterology 1982;83:777–785.

730. Poblete RB, Rodriguez K, Foust RT, et al. *Pneumocystis carinii* hepatitis in the acquired immunodeficiency syndrome (AIDS). Ann Intern Med 1989;110:737–738.

731. Northfelt DW, Clement MJ, Safrin S. Extrapulmonary pneumocystosis: Clinical features in human immunodeficiency virus infection. Medicine 1990;69:392–398.

732. Sarmento e Castro R, Vasconcelos O, Carneiro F, et al. Hepatic pneumocytosis without concomitant PCP in a patient with AIDS. J Infect 1997;34:257–259.

733. Boldorini R, Guzzetti S, Meroni L, et al. Acute hepatic and renal failure caused by *Pneumocystit carinii* in patients with AIDS. J Clin Pathol 1995;48:975–978.

734. Colombo JL, Sammut PH, Langnas AN, et al. The spectrum of *Pneumocystis carinii* infection after liver transplantation in children. Transplantation 1992;54:621–624.

735. Merkel IS, Good CB, Nalesnik M, et al. Chronic *Pneumocystis carinii* infection of the liver: A case report and review of the literature. J Clin Gastroenterol 1992;15:55–58.

736. Mowrey FH, Lundbergh EA. The clinical manifestations of essential polyangitis (periarteritis nodosa) with emphasis on the hepatic manifestations. Ann Intern Med 1954;40:1145–1164.

737. Rousselet MC, Kettani S, Rohmer V, et al. A case of temporal arteritis with intrahepatic arterial involvement. Pathol Res Pract 1989;185:329–331.

738. Mouthon L, Deblois P, Sauvaget F, et al. Hepatitis B virus–related polyarteritis nodosa and membranous nephropathy. Am J Nephrol 1995;15:266–269.

739. Ahmed HA, Arulambalam KJ, Nickols CD. Polyarteritis nodosa of the liver—a case report and review of the literature. Mater Med Pol 1986;18:231–234.

740. Von Knorring J, Wasastjerna C. Liver involvement in polymyalgia rheumatica. Scand J Rheumatol 1976;5:179–204.

741. Thompson K, Roberts PF. Chronic hepatitis in polymyalgia rheumatica. Postgrad Med J 1976;52:236–238.

742. Long R, James O. Polymyalgia rheumatica and liver disease. Lancet 1972;1:77–79.

743. Kyle V. Laboratory investigations including liver in polymyalgia rheumatica/giant cell arteritis. Baillieres Clin Rheumatol 1991;5:475–484.

744. Burke M, Sasson E, Baratz M, et al. Hepatic granuloma in polymyalgia rheumatica. J Am Geriatr Soc 1984;32:472–473.

745. Cortes JM, Oliva H, Paradinas FJ, et al. The pathology of the

liver in porphyria cutanea tarda. Histopathology 1980;4:471–485.

746. Lefkowitch JH, Grossman ME. Hepatic pathology in porphyria cutanea tarda. Liver 1983;3:19–29.

747. Campo E, Bruguera M, Rodes J. Are there diagnostic histologic features of porphyria cutanea tarda in liver biopsy specimens? Liver 1990;10:185–190.

748. Tsukazaki N, Watanabe M, Irifune H. Porphyria cutanea tarda and hepatitis C virus infection. Br J Dermatol 1998;138:1015–1017.

749. Elder GH. Porphyria cutanea tarda. Semin Liver Dis 1998;18:67–75.

750. Siersema PD, Rademakers LH, Cleton MI, et al. The difference in liver pathology between sporadic and familial forms of porphyria cutanea tarda: The role of iron. J Hepatol 1995;23:259–267.

751. Nakanuma Y, Tsuneyama K, Gershwin ME, et al. Pathology and immunopathology of primary biliary cirrhosis with emphasis on bile duct lesions: Recent progress. Semin Liver Dis 1995;15:313–328.

752. Portmann B, Popper H, Neuberger J, et al. Sequential and diagnostic features in primary biliary cirrhosis based on serial histologic study in 209 patients. Gastroenterology 1985;88:1777–1790.

753. Kaplan MM. Primary biliary cirrhosis. N Engl J Med 1987;316:521–528.

754. Kloppel G, Kirchhof M, Berg PA. Natural course of primary biliary cirrhosis. I. A morphological, clinical and serological analysis of 103 cases. Liver 1982;2:141–151.

755. Scheuer PJ. Ludwig symposium on biliary disorders. II. Pathologic features and evolution of primary biliary cirrhosis and primary sclerosing cholangitis. Mayo Clin Proc 1998;73:179–183.

756. Laurin JM, Lindor KD. Primary biliary cirrhosis. Dig Dis 1994;12:331–350.

757. Roll J, Boyer JL, Barry D, et al. The prognostic importance of clinical and histologic features in asymptomatic and symptomatic primary biliary cirrhosis. N Engl J Med 1983;308:1–7.

758. Chapman RW. Primary sclerosing cholangitis. J Hepatol 1985;1:179–186.

759. Nakanuma Y, Hiraf N, Kono N, et al. Histological and ultrastructural examination of the intrahepatic biliary tree in primary sclerosing cholangitis. Liver 1986;6:317–325.

760. Ludwig J, LaRusso NF, Wiesner RH. Primary sclerosing cholangitis. *In* Peters RL, Craig JR, eds. Liver Pathology. Churchill Livingstone: New York, 1986, pp 193–214.

761. Debray D, Pariente D, Urvoas E, et al. Sclerosing cholangitis in children. J Pediatr 1994;124:49–56.

762. Casali AM, Carbone G, Cavalli G. Intrahepatic bile duct loss in primary sclerosing cholangitis: A quantitative study. Histopathology 1998;32:449–453.

763. Ponsioen CI, Tytgat GN. Primary sclerosing cholangitis: A clinical review. Am J Gastroenterol 1998;93:515–523.

764. Ludwig J. Small-duct primary sclerosing cholangitis. Semin Liver Dis 1991;11:11–17.

765. Ludwig J, Barham SS, LaRusso NF, et al. Morphologic features of chronic hepatitis associated with primary sclerosing cholangitis or chronic ulcerative colitis. Hepatology 1981;1:632–640.

766. Weisner RH, Grambsch PSC, Dickinson ER, et al. Primary sclerosing cholangitis: Natural history, prognostic factors, and survival analysis. Hepatology 1989;10:430–436.

767. De Vos R, De Wolf-Peeters C, Desmet VJ, et al. Progressive intrahepatic cholestasis (Byler's disease): Case report. Gut 1975;16:943–950.

768. Whitington PF, Freese DK, Alonso EM, et al. Clinical and biochemical findings in progressive familial intrahepatic cholestasis. J Pediatr Gastroenterol Nutr 1994;18:134–141.

769. Whitington PF, Freese DK, Alonso EM, et al. Progressive familial intrahepatic cholestasis (Byler's disease). *In* Lentze M, Reichen J, eds. Paediatric cholestasis: Novel approaches to treatment. Kluwer Academic Publishers: Dordrecht, 1992, pp 165–183.

770. Jansen PL, Muller MM. Progressive familial intrahepatic cholestasis types 1, 2, and 3. Gut 1998;42:766–767.

771. Alonso EM, Snover DC, Montag A, et al. Histologic pathology of the liver in progressive familial intrahepatic cholestasis. J Pediatr Gastroenterol Nutr 1994;18:128–133.

772. Riely CA. Familial intrahepatic cholestatic syndromes. Semin Liver Dis 1987;7:119–133.

773. Reynolds TB, Kanel GC. Alcoholic liver disease. *In* Stein JH, ed. Internal Medicine. 4th ed. Mosby: St. Louis, 1994, pp 611–618.

774. Wanless IR. Vascular disorders. *In* MacSween RNM, Anthony PP, Scheuer PJ, et al, eds. Pathology of the Liver. Churchill Livingstone: Edinburgh, 1994, pp 535–562.

775. Lin CS. Suppurative pylephlebitis and liver abscess complicating colonic diverticulitis: Report of two cases and review of literature. Mt Sinai J Med 1973;40:48–55.

776. Slovis TL, Haller JO, Cohen HL, et al. Complicated appendiceal inflammatory disease in children: Pylephlebitis and liver abscess. Radiology 1989;171:823–825.

777. Saxena R, Adolph M, Ziegler JR, et al. Pylephlebitis: A case report and review of outcome in the antibiotic era. Am J Gastroenterol 1996;91:1251–1253.

778. Greenstein AJ, Lowenthal BA, Hammer GFS, et al. Continuing patterns of disease in pyogenic liver abscess: A study of 38 cases. Am J Gastroenterol 1984;79:217–226.

779. Perera MR, Kirk A, Noone P, et al. Presentation, diagnosis and management of liver abscess. Lancet 1980;2:629–632.

780. Stain S, Yellin AE, Donovan AJ, et al. Pyogenic liver abscess: Modern treatment. Arch Surg 1991;126:991–996.

781. Williams CN. Hepatic abscess. Can J Gastroenterol 1998;12:249–250.

782. Hansen PS, Schonheyder HC. Pyogenic hepatic abscess: A 10-year population-based retrospective study. APMIS 1998;106:396–402.

783. Bernstein M, Edmondson HA, Barbour BH. The liver lesion in Q fever: Clinical and pathologic features. Arch Intern Med 1965;116:491–498.

784. Murphy E, Griffiths MR, Hunter JA, et al. Fibrin-ring granulomas: A non-specific reaction to liver injury? Histopathology 1991;19:91–93.

785. Pellegrin M, Delsol G, Auvergant JC, et al. Granulomatous hepatitis in Q fever. Hum Pathol 1980;11:51–57.

786. Travis LB, Travis WD, Li C-Y, et al. Q fever: A clinicopathologic study of five cases. Arch Pathol Lab Med 1986;110:1017–1020.

787. Marazuela M, Moreno A, Yebra M, et al. Hepatic fibrin-ring granulomas: A clinicopathologic study of 23 patients. Hum Pathol 1991;22:607–613.

788. Ruiz-Contreras J, Gonzalez Montero R, Ramos Amador JT, et al. Q fever in children. Am J Dis Child 1993;147:300–302.

789. Aagenaes O, Van der Hagen CB, Refsum S. Hereditary recurrent intrahepatic cholestasis from birth. Arch Dis Child 1968;43:646–657.

790. Shiraki K, Okaniwa M, Landing BH. Cholestatic syndromes of infancy and childhood. *In* Zakim D, Boyer TD, eds. Hepatology: A Textbook of Liver Diseases. WB Saunders: Philadelphia, 1982, pp 1176–1192.

791. Haemmerli UP, Wyss HI. Recurrent intrahepatic cholestasis of pregnancy: A report of six cases, and review of the literature. Medicine 1967;46:299–321.

792. Reyes H. The spectrum of liver and gastrointestinal disease seen in cholestasis of pregnancy. Gastroenterol Clin North Am 1992;21:905–921.

793. Holland RL. Recurrent intrahepatic cholestasis of pregnancy. S D J Med 1987;40:9–12.

794. Rioseco AJ, Ivankovic MB, Manzur A, et al. Intrahepatic cholestasis of pregnancy: A retrospective case-control study of perinatal outcome. Am J Obstet Gynecol 1994;170:890–895.

795. Chou S-T, Chan CW. Recurrent pyogenic cholangitis: A necropsy study. Pathology 1980;12:415–428.

796. Kashi H, Lam F, Giles GR. Recurrent pyogenic cholangiohepatitis. Ann R Coll Surg Engl 1989;71:387–389.

797. Craig JR. Recurrent pyogenic cholangiohepatitis. *In* Peters RL, Craig JR, eds. Liver Pathology. Churchill Livingstone: New York, 1986, pp 215–219.

798. Sperling RM, Koch J, Sandhu JS, et al. Recurrent pyogenic cholangitis in Asian immigrants to the United States: Natural history and role of therapeutic ERCP. Dig Dis Sci 1997;42:865–871.

799. Wilson MK, Stephen MS, Mather M, et al. Recurrent pyogenic cholangitis or "oriental cholangiohepatitis" in occidentals: Case reports of four patients. Aust N Z J Surg 1996;66:649–652.

800. Reye RDK, Morgan G, Baral J. Encephalopathy and fatty degeneration of the viscera: A disease entity in childhood. Lancet 1963;2:749–752.

801. Chang C-H, Uchwat F, Masalskis F, et al. Morphologic grading of hepatic mitochondrial alterations in Reye's syndrome: Potential prognostic implication. Pediatr Pathol 1985;4:265–275.

802. Heubi JE, Partin JC, Partin JS, et al. Reye's syndrome: Current concepts. Hepatology 1987;7:155–164

803. Bove KE, McAdams AJ, Partin JC, et al. The hepatic lesion in Reye's syndrome. Gastroenterology 1975;69:685–697.

804. Brown RE, Ishak KG. Hepatic zonal degeneration and necrosis in Reye syndrome. Arch Pathol Lab Med 1976;100:123–126.

805. Partin JC, Schubert WK, Partin JS. Mitochondrial ultrastructure in Reye's syndrome (encephalopathy and fatty degeneration of the viscera). N Engl J Med 1971;285:1339–1343.

806. Kimura S, Kobayashi T, Tanaka Y, et al. Liver histopathology in clinical Reye syndrome. Brain Dev 1991;13:95–100.

807. Rau R, Pfenninger K, Boni A. Liver function tests and liver biopsies in patients with rheumatoid arthritis. Ann Rheum Dis 1975;34:198–199.

808. Dietrichson O, From A, Christofferson P, et al. Morphological changes in liver biopsies from patients with rheumatoid arthritis. Scand J Rheumatol 1976;5:65–69.

809. Rau R, Karger T, Herborn G, et al. Liver biopsy findings in patients with rheumatoid arthritis undergoing longterm treatment with methotrexate. J Rheumatol 1989;16:489–493.

810. Laffon A, Moreno A, Gutierrez-Bucero A, et al. Hepatic sinusoidal dilatation in rheumatoid arthritis. J Clin Gastroenterol 1989;11:653–657.

811. Kremer JM, Lee RG, Tolman KG. Liver histology in rheumatoid arthritis patients receiving long-term methotrexate therapy. Arthritis Rheum 1989;32:121–129.

812. Heathcote J, Deodhar KP, Scheuer PJ, et al. Intrahepatic cholestasis in childhood. N Engl J Med 1976;295:801–805.

813. Rey-Conde TF, Badrick TC, Robson JM. Rubella and the liver. Med J Aust 1996;165:238.

814. Arai M, Wada N, Maruyama K, et al. Acute hepatitis in an adult with acquired rubella infection. J Gastroenterol 1995;30: 539–542.

815. Sugaya N, Nirasawa M, Mitamura K, et al. Hepatitis in acquired rubella in children. Am J Dis Child 1988;142:817–818.

816. McLellan RK, Gleiner JA. Acute hepatitis in an adult with rubeola. JAMA 1982;247:2000–2001.

817. Williams AO. Autopsy study of measles in Ibadan, Nigeria. Ghana Med J 1970;9:23–27.

818. De Brito T, Vieira WT, Dias M. Jaundice in typhoid hepatitis: A light and electron microscopy study based on liver biopsies. Acta Hepatogastroenterol 1977;24:426–433.

819. Pramoolsinsap C, Viranuvatti V. Salmonella hepatitis. J Gastroenterol Hepatol 1998;13:745–750.

820. Ramachandran S, Godfrey JJ, Perera MNP. Typhoid hepatitis. JAMA 1974;230:236–240.

821. Hornick RB, Greisman SE, Woodward TE, et al. Typhoid fever. Pathogenesis and immunological control. N Engl J Med 1970;283:686–691.

822. El-Newihi HM, Alamy ME, Reynolds TB. Salmonella hepatitis: Analysis of 27 cases and comparison with acute viral hepatitis. Hepatology 1996;24:516–519.

823. Khosla SN, Singh R, Singh GP, et al. The spectrum of hepatic injury in enteric fever. Am J Gastroenterol 1988;83:413–416.

824. Alexander JF, Galambos JT. Granulomatous hepatitis. The usefulness of liver biopsy in the diagnosis of tuberculosis and sarcoidosis. Am J Gastroenterol 1973;59:23–30.

825. Ishak KG. Sarcoidosis of the liver and bile ducts. Mayo Clin Proc 1998;73:467–472

826. Hercules HC, Bethlem NM. Value of liver biopsy in sarcoidosis. Arch Pathol Lab Med 1984;108:831–834.

827. Pereira-Lima J, Schaffner F. Chronic cholestasis in hepatic sarcoidosis with clinical features resembling primary biliary cirrhosis. Am J Med 1987;83:144–148.

828. Devaney K, Goodman ZD, Epstein MS, et al. Hepatic sarcoidosis: Clinicopathological features in 100 patients. Am J Surg Pathol 1993; 17:1272–1280.

829. Dunn MA, Kamel R. Hepatic schistosomiasis. Hepatology 1981;1:653–661.

830. Warren KS, Domingo EO, Cowan RBT. Granuloma formation around schistosome eggs as a manifestation of delayed hypersensitivity. Am J Pathol 1967:51:735–756.

831. Andrade ZA, Peixoto E, Guerret S, et al. Hepatic connective tissue changes in hepatosplenic schistosomiasis. Hum Pathol 1992;23:566–573.

832. Warren KS. The kinetics of hepatosplenic schistosomiasis. Semin Liver Dis 1984;4:293–300.

833. Bhagwandeen SB. The histopathology of early schistosomiasis. Afr J Med Sci 1976;5:125–130.

834. Tsui WM, Chow LT. Advanced schistosomiasis as a cause of hepar lobatum. Histopathology 1993;23:495–497.

835. Camacho-Lobato K, Borges DR. Early liver dysfunction in schistosomiasis. J Hepatol 1998;29:233– 240.

836. Elliott DE, Schistosomiasis: Pathophysiology, diagnosis, and treatment. Gastroenterol Clin North Am 1996;25:599–625.

837. Mills LR, Mwakyusa D, Milner PF. Histopathologic features of liver biopsy specimens in sickle cell disease. Arch Pathol Lab Med 1988;112:290–294.

838. Schubert TT. Hepatobiliary system in sickle cell disease. Gastroenterology 1986;90:2013–2021.

839. Bauer TW, Moore GW, Hutchins GM. The liver in sickle cell disease. A clinicopathologic study of 70 patients. Am J Med 1980;69:833–837.

840. Kraus JS, Freant LJ, Lee JR. Gastrointestinal pathology in sickle cell disease. Ann Clin Lab Sci 1998;28:19–23.

841. Johnson CS, Omata M, Tong MJ, et al. Liver involvement in sickle cell disease. Medicine 1985;64:349–356.

842. Omata M, Johnson CS, Tong M, et al. Pathological spectrum of liver diseases in sickle cell disease. Dig Dis Sci 1986;31:247–256.

843. Geist DC. Solitary nonparasitic cyst of the liver. Arch Surg 1955;71:867–880.

844. Flagg RS, Robinson DW. Solitary nonparasitic hepatic cysts. Arch Surg 1967;95:964–973.

845. Koperna T, Vogl S, Satzinger U, et al. Nonparasitic cysts of the liver. Results and options of surgical treatment. World J Surg 1997;21:850–854.

846. Donovan MJ, Kozakewich H, Perez-Atayde A. Solitary nonparasitic cysts of the liver. The Boston Children's Hospital experience. Pediatr Pathol Lab Med 1995; 15:419–428.

847. Keller SM, Goldfarb AB, Zisbrod Z. Solitary nonparasitic liver cysts. N Y State J Med 1985;85:95–96.

848. Neerhoff MG, Zelman W, Sullivan T. Hepatic rupture in pregnancy: A review. Obstet Gynecol Surv 1989;44:407–409.

849. Smith LG, Moise KJ, Dildy GA, et al. Spontaneous rupture of liver during pregnancy. Current therapy. Obstet Gynecol 1991; 77:171–175.

850. Wijesinghe PS, Gunasekera PC, Sirisena J. Spontaneous hepatic rupture in pregnancy. Ceylon Med J 1998;43:109–111.

851. Genta RM. Global prevalence of strongyloidiasis: Critical review and epidemiologic insights into the prevention of disseminated disease. Rev Infect Dis 1989;11:755–767.

852. Poltera AA, Katsimbura N. Granulomatous hepatitis due to *Strongyloides stercoralis*. J Pathol 1974;113:241–246.

853. Christoffersen P, Poulsen H, Skeie E. Focal liver cell necroses accompanied by infiltration of granulocytes arising during operation. Acta Hepatosplenologica 1970;17:240–245.

854. McDonald GSA, Courtney MG. Operation-associated neutrophils in a percutaneous liver biopsy: Effect of prior transjugular procedure. Histopathology 1986;10:217–222.

855. Brooks SEH, Audretsch JJ. Hepatic ultrastructure in congenital syphilis. Arch Pathol Lab Med 1978;102:502–505.

856. Sobel HJ, Wolf EH. Liver involvement in early syphilis. Arch Pathol Lab Med 1972;93:565–568.

857. Feher J, Somogyi T, Timmer M, et al. Early syphilitic hepatitis. Lancet 1975;2:896–899.

858. Lee RV, Thornton GF, Conn HO. Liver disease associated with secondary syphilis. N Engl J Med 1971;284:1423–1425.

859. Romen J, Rybak B, Dave P, et al. Spirochetal vasculitis and bile ductular damage in early hepatic syphilis. Am J Gastroenterol 1980;74:352–354.

860. Maincent G, Labadie H, Fabre M, et al. Tertiary hepatic syphilis. A treatable cause of multinodular liver. Dig Dis Sci 1997; 42:447–450.

861. Relvas S, Carreira F, Castro B. Liver involvement in secondary syphilis. Am J Gastroenterol 1992;87:1528.

862. Young MF, Sanowski RA, Manne RA. Syphilitic hepatitis. J Clin Gastroenterol 1992;15:174–176.

863. Karpati G, Carpenter S, Engel AG, et al. The syndrome of systemic carnitine deficiency: Clinical, morphologic, biochemical and pathophysiologic features. Neurology 1975;25:16–24.

864. Treem WR, Stanley CA, Finegold DN, et al. Primary carnitine deficiency due to failure of carnitine transport in kidney, muscle and fibroblasts. N Engl J Med 1988;319:1331–1336.

865. Bremmer J. Carnitine metabolism and functions. Physiol Rev 1983;63:1420–1480.

866. Haworth JC, Demaugre F, Booth FA, et al. Atypical features of the hepatic form of carnitine palmitoyltransferase deficiency in a Hutterite family. J Pediatr 1992;121:553–557.

867. Dubois EL, Wierzchowiecki M, Cox MB, et al. Duration and death in systemic lupus erythematosus: An analysis of 249 cases. JAMA 1974;227:1399–1402.

868. Runyon BA, LeBrecqui DR, Anuras S. The spectrum of liver disease in systemic lupus erythematosus: Report of 33 histologically-proved cases and review of the literature. Am J Med 1980;69:187–194.

869. Miller MH, Urowitz MB, Gladman DD, et al. The liver in systemic lupus erythematosus. Q J Med 1984;211:401–409.

870. Matsumoto T, Yoshimine T, Shimouchi K, et al. The liver in systemic lupus erythematosus: Pathologic analysis of 52 cases and review of Japanese autopsy registry data. Hum Pathol 1992;23:1151–1158.

871. Van Hoek B. The spectrum of liver disease in systemic lupus erythematosus. Neth J Med 1996;48:244–253.

872. Bale PM, Clifton-Bligh P, Benjamin BNP, et al. Pathology of Tangier disease. J Clin Pathol 1971;24:609–616.

873. Ferrans VJ, Fredrickson DS. The pathology of Tangier disease. Am J Pathol 1975;78:101–136.

874. Dechelotte P, Kantelip B, de Laguillamie BV. Tangier disease: A histological and ultrastructural study. Pathol Res Pract 1985; 180:424–430.

875. Rolfes DB, Ishak KG. Liver disease in toxemia of pregnancy. Am J Gastroenterol 1986;81:1138–1144.

876. Manas KJ, Welsh JD, Rankin RA, et al. Hepatic hemorrhage without rupture in preeclampsia. N Engl J Med 1985;312:424–426.

877. Karadia S, Walford C, McSwiney M, et al. Hepatic rupture complicating eclampsia in pregnancy. Br J Anaesth 1996;77: 792–794.

878. Ralston SJ, Schwaitzberg SD. Liver hematoma and rupture in pregnancy. Semin Perinatol 1998;22:141–148.

879. Howard EW 3rd, Jones HL. Massive hepatic necrosis in toxemia of pregnancy. Tex Med 1993;89:74–80.

880. Kronthal AJ, Fishman EK, Kuhlman JE, et al. Hepatic infarction in preeclampsia. Radiology 1990;177:726–728.

881. Alexander J, Cuellar RE, Van Thiel DH. Toxemia of pregnancy and the liver. Semin Liver Dis 1987;7:55–58.

882. Gourley GR, Chesney PJ, Davis JP, et al. Acute cholestasis in patients with toxic shock syndrome. Gastroenterology 1981;81: 928–931.

883. Ishak KG, Rogers WA. Cryptogenic acute cholangitis: Association with toxic shock syndrome. Am J Clin Pathol 1981;76: 619–626.

884. Weitberg AB, Alper JC, Diamond I, et al. Acute granulomatous hepatitis in the course of acquired toxoplasmosis. N Engl J Med 1979;300:1093–1096.

885. Bonacini M, Alamy M, Kanel G. Duodenal and hepatic toxoplasmosis in a patient with HIV infection: Review of the literature. Am J Gastroenterol 1996;91:1838–1840.

886. Tiwari I, Rolland CF, Popple AW. Cholestatic jaundice due to toxoplasma hepatitis. Postgrad Med J 1982;58:299–300.

887. Feldman HA. Toxoplasmosis. N Engl J Med 1968;279:1370, 1431.

888. Mastroianni A, Coronado O, Scarani P, et al. Liver toxoplasmosis and acquired immunodeficiency syndrome. Recent Prog Med 1996;87:353–355.

889. Alvarez SZ, Carpio R. Hepatobiliary tuberculosis. Dig Dis Sci 1983;28:193–200.

890. Hunt JS, Silverstein MJ, Sparks FC, et al. Granulomatous hepatitis. A complication of BCG immunotherapy. Lancet 1973;2: 820–821.

891. Brmbolic BJ, Boricic I, Salemovic DR, et al. Focal tuberculosis of the liver with local hemorrhage in a patient with acquired immunodeficiency syndrome. Liver 1996;16:218–220.

892. Prive L. Pathological findings in patients with tyrosinemia. Can Med Assoc J 1967;97:1054–1056.

893. Dehner LP, Snover DC, Sharp HL, et al. Hereditary tyrosinemia type I (chronic form): Pathologic findings in the liver. Hum Pathol 1989;20:149–159.

894. Day DL, Letourneau JG, Allan BT, et al. Hepatic regenerating nodules in hereditary tyrosinemia. Am J Roentgenol 1987;149: 391–393.

895. Esquivel CO, Gutierrez C, Cox KL, et al. Hepatocellular carcinoma and liver cell dysplasia in children with chronic liver disease. J Pediatr Surg 1994;29:1465–1469.

896. Manowski Z, Silver MM, Roberts EA, et al. Liver cell dysplasia and early liver transplantation in hereditary tyrosinemia. Mod Pathol 1990;3:694–701.

897. Kvittingen EA. Hereditary tyrosinemia type I—an overview. Scand J Clin Lab Invest 1986;46 (Suppl 184):27–34.

898. Mistilis SP. Pericholangitis and ulcerative colitis. I. Pathology, etiology and pathogenesis. Ann Intern Med 1965;63:1–16.

899. Chalasani N, Smallwood G. Idiopathic ulcerative colitis in patients with primary sclerosing colitis undergoing orthotopic liver transplantation. Am J Gastroenterol 1998;93:481–482.

900. Shulman HM, Fisher LB, Schoch HG, et al. Venoocclusive disease of the liver after marrow transplantation: Histological correlates of clinical signs and symptoms. Hepatology 1994; 1171–1181.

901. Rollins BJ. Hepatic veno-occlusive disease. Am J Med 1986;81: 297–306.

902. McDonald GB, Sharma P, Matthews DE, et al. Venocclusive disease of the liver after bone marrow transplantation. Diagnosis, incidence, and predisposing factors. Hepatology 1984;4: 116–122.

903. Jeffries MA, McDonnell WM, Tworek JA, et al. Venoocclusive disease of the liver following renal transplantation. Dig Dis Sci 1998;43:229–234.

904. Buckley JA, Hutchins GM. Association of hepatic veno-occlusive disease with the acquired immunodeficiency syndrome. Mod Pathol 1995;8:398–401.

905. Uchida T, Kronborg I, Peters RL. Acute viral hepatitis: Morphologic and functional correlations in human livers. Hum Pathol 1984;15:267–277.

906. Peters RL. Viral hepatitis: A pathologic spectrum. Am J Med Sci 1975;270:17–31.

907. Ishak KG. Viral hepatitis: The morphologic spectrum. In Gall EA, Mostofi FK, eds. The Liver. Williams & Wilkins: Baltimore, 1973, pp 218–268.

908. Phillips MJ, Poucell S. Modern aspects of the morphology of viral hepatitis. Hum Pathol 1981;12:1060–1084.

909. Seeff LB. Acute viral hepatitis. In Kaplowitz N, ed. Liver and biliary diseases. 2nd ed. Williams & Wilkins: Baltimore, 1996, pp 289–316.

910. Seeff LB, Beebe GW, Hoofnagle JW, et al. A serologic followup of the 1942 epidemic of postvaccination hepatitis in the U.S. Army. N Engl J Med 1987;316:965–970.

911. Sciot R, Van Damme B, Desmet VJ. Cholestatic features in hepatitis A. J Hepatol 1986;3:172–181.

912. Okuno T, Sano A, Deguchi T, et al. Pathology of acute hepatitis A in humans: Comparison with acute hepatitis B. Am J Clin Pathol 1984;81:162–169.

913. Teixeira MR, Weller IVD, Murray A, et al. The pathology of hepatitis A in man. Liver 1982;2:53–60.

914. Shapiro CN, Coleman PJ, McQuillan GM, et al. Epidemiology of hepatitis A: Seroepidemiology and risk groups in the US. Vaccine 1992;10 (Suppl 1):S59–S62.

915. Glikson M, Galun E, Oren R, et al. Relapsing hepatitis A: Review of 14 cases and literature survey. Medicine 1992;71: 14–23.

916. Lednar WM, Lemon SM, Kirkpatrick JW, et al. Frequency of

illness associated with epidemic hepatitis A virus infection in adults. Am J Epidemiol 1985;122:226–233.

917. Mohite BJ, Rath S, Vineeta B, et al. Mechanisms of liver cell damage in acute hepatitis B. J Med Virol 1987;22:199–210.

918. Koff RS. Natural history of acute hepatitis B in adults reexamined. Gastroenterology 1987;92:2035–2036.

919. McMahon BJ, Alward WLM, Hall DB, et al. Acute hepatitis B virus infection: Relation of age to the clinical expression of disease and subsequent development of the carrier state. J Infect Dis 1985;151:599–603.

920. Craig JR, Govindarajan S, De Cock KM. Delta viral hepatitis: Histopathology and course. Pathol Annu 1986;21:1–21.

921. Govindarajan S, De Cock KM, Redeker AG. Natural history of delta superinfection in chronic hepatitis B virus–infected patients: Histopathologic study with multiple liver biopsies. Hepatology 1986;6:640–644.

922. Lefkowitch JH, Goldstein H, Yatto R, et al. Cytopathic liver injury in acute delta virus hepatitis. Gastroenterology 1987;92:1262–1266.

923. Alter MJ, Margolis HS, Krawczynski K, et al. The natural history of community-acquired hepatitis C in the United States. N Engl J Med 1992;327:1899–1905.

924. Ohno T. The "gold-standard," accuracy, and the current concepts: Hepatitis C virus genotype and viremia. Hepatology 1996;24:1312–1315.

925. Sharara AI, Hunt CM, Hamilton JD. Hepatitis C. Ann Intern Med 1996;125:658–668.

926. Scheuer PJ, Ashrafzadeh P, Sherlock S, et al. The pathology of hepatitis C. Hepatology 1992;15:567–571.

927. Gerber MA. Histopathology of HCV infection. In Davis GL, ed. Hepatitis C. WB Saunders: Philadelphia, 1997, pp 529–541.

928. Goodman ZD, Ishak KG. Histopathology of hepatitis C virus infection. Semin Liver Dis 1995;15:70–81.

929. Ramalingaswami V, Purcell RH. Waterborne non-A, non-B hepatitis. Lancet 1988;1:571–573.

930. De Cock KM, Bradley DW, Sandford NL, et al. Epidemic non-A, non-B hepatitis in patients from Pakistan. Ann Intern Med 1987;106:227–230.

931. Khuroo MS. Study of an epidemic of non-A, non-B hepatitis. Am J Med 1980;68:818–824.

932. Khuroo MS, Teli MR, Skidmore S, et al. Incidence and severity of viral hepatitis in pregnancy. Am J Med 1981;70:252–255.

933. Bansal J, He J, Yarbough PO et al. Hepatitis E virus infection in eastern India. Am J Trop Med Hyg 1998;59:258–260.

934. Alter HJ, Nakatsuji Y, Melpolder J, et al. The incidence of transfusion-associated hepatitis G virus infection and its relation to liver disease. N Engl J Med 1997;336:747–754.

935. Miyakawa Y, Mayumi M. Hepatitis G virus—a true hepatitis virus or an accidental tourist. N Engl J Med 1997;336:795–796.

936. Alter MJ, Gallagher M, Morris TT, et al. Acute non-A-E hepatitis in the United States and the role of hepatitis G virus infection. N Engl J Med 1997;336:741–746.

937. Masuko K, Mitsui T, Iwano K, et al. Infection with hepatitis GB virus C in patients on maintenance hemodialysis. N Engl J Med 1996;334:1485–1490.

938. Karayiannis P, Pickering J, Zampino R, et al. Natural history and molecular biology of hepatitis G virus/GB virus C. Clin Diagn Virol 1998;10:103–111.

939. Phillips MJ, Blendis LM, Poucell S, et al. Syncytial giant-cell hepatitis: Sporadic hepatitis with distinctive pathological features, a severe clinical course, and paramyxoviral features. N Engl J Med 1991;324:455–460.

940. Devaney K, Goodman ZD, Ishak KG, et al. Postinfantile giant-cell transformation in hepatitis. Hepatology 1992;16:327–333.

941. Lau JYN, Koukoulis G, Mieli-Verbani G, et al. Syncytial giant-cell hepatitis—a specific disease entity? J Hepatol 1992;15:216–219.

942. Arankalle VA, Chadha MS, Tsarey SA, et al. Seroepidemiology of water-borne hepatitis in India and evidence for a third enterically-transmitted hepatitis agent. Proc Natl Acad Sci USA 1994;91:3428–3432.

943. Boyer JL, Klatskin G. Patterns of necrosis in acute viral hepatitis: Prognostic value of bridging (subacute hepatic) necrosis. N Engl J Med 1970;283:1063–1071.

944. Nisman RM, Ganderson AP, Vlahcevic ZR, et al. Acute viral hepatitis with bridging hepatic necrosis: An overview. Arch Intern Med 1979;139:1289–1291.

945. Schmid M, Cueni B. Portal lesions in viral hepatitis with submassive hepatic necrosis. Hum Pathol 1972;3:209–216.

946. Milandri M, Gaub J, Ranek L. Evidence for liver cell proliferation during fatal acute liver failure. Gut 1980;21:423–427.

947. Smedile A, Farci P, Verme G, et al. Influence of delta infection on severity of hepatitis B. Lancet 1982;2:945–947.

948. Horney JT, Galambos JT. The liver during and after fulminant hepatitis. Gastroenterology 1977;73:639–645.

949. Peters RL. Viral inflammatory disease. In Peters RL, Craig JR, eds. Liver Pathology. Churchill Livingstone: New York, 1986, pp 73–123.

950. Edmondson HA, Peters RL. Liver. In Kissane JM, Anderson WAD, eds. Pathology. 8th ed. CV Mosby: St. Louis, 1985, pp 1096–1212.

951. Desmet VJ, Gerber MA, Hoofnagle JH, et al. Classification of chronic hepatitis: Diagnosis, grading and staging. Hepatology 1994;19:1513–1520.

952. Barnaba V, Balsano F. Immunologic and molecular basis of viral persistence: The hepatitis B virus model. J Hepatol 1992;14:391–400.

953. Huang SN, Neurath AR. Immunohistologic demonstration of hepatitis B viral antigens in liver with reference to its significance in liver injury. Lab Invest 1979;40:1–17.

954. Anthony PP, Vogel CL, Barker LF. Liver cell dysplasia: A premalignant condition. J Clin Pathol 1973;26:217–223.

955. Liaw YF, Lin DY, Chen TJ, et al. Natural course after the development of cirrhosis in patients with chronic type B hepatitis: A prospective study. Liver 1989;9:235–241.

956. Korenman J, Baker B, Waggoner J, et al. Long-term remission of chronic hepatitis B after alpha-interferon therapy. Ann Intern Med 1991;114:629–634.

957. Govindarajan S, Kanel GC, Peters RL. Incidence of delta antibody among chronic hepatitis B virus infected patients in the Los Angeles area: Its correlation with the liver biopsy diagnosis. Gastroenterology 1983;85:160–162.

958. Kanel GC, Govindarajan S, Peters RL. Chronic delta infection and liver biopsy changes in chronic active hepatitis B. Ann Intern Med 1984;101:51–54.

959. Rizetto M, Verme G, Gerin JL, et al. Hepatitis delta virus disease. Prog Liver Dis 1986;8:417–431.

960. Seeff LB. The natural history of chronic hepatitis C virus infection. In Davis GL, ed. Hepatitis C. WB Saunders: Philadelphia; 1997, pp 587–602.

961. Kage M, Shimatu K, Nakashima E, et al. Long term evolution of fibrosis from chronic hepatitis to cirrhosis in patients with hepatitis C: Morphometric analysis of repeated biopsies. Hepatology 1997;25:1028–1031.

962. DiBisceglie AM, Martin P, Kassianides C, et al. Recombinant interferon alpha therapy for chronic hepatitis C—a randomized, double-blind, placebo-controlled trial. N Engl J Med 1989;321:1506–1510.

963. Diamantis ID, Kouroumalis E, Koulentaki M, et al. Influence of hepatitis G virus infection on liver disease. Eur J Clin Microbiol Infect Dis 1997;16:916–919.

964. Taylor MRH, Keane CT, O'Connor P, et al. The expanded spectrum of toxocaral disease. Lancet 1988;1:692–695.

965. Schantz PM. Toxocara larva migrans now. Am J Trop Med Hyg 1989;41 (Suppl):S21–S34.

966. Ishibashi H, Shimamura R, Hirata Y, et al. Hepatic granuloma in toxocaral infection: Role of ultrasonography in hypereosinophilia. J Clin Ultrasound 1992;20:204–210.

967. Hegde S, Maiya PP, Dandekar C, et al. Visceral larva migrans. Indian Pediatr 1995;32:1245–1246.

968. Jain R, Sawhney S, Bhargava DK, et al. Hepatic granulomas due to visceral larva migrans in adults: Appearance on US and MRI. Abdom Imaging 1994;19:253–256.

969. Ljungstrom I, van Knapen F. An epidemiological and serological study of toxocara infection in Sweden. Scand J Infect Dis 1989;21:87–93.

970. Brooks AP. Portal hypertension in Waldenström's macroglobulinemia. BMJ 1976;1:689–690.

971. Gertz MA, Kyle RA, Noel P. Primary systemic amyloidosis: A rare complication of immunoglobulin M monoclonal gammo-

pathies and Waldenström's macroglobulinemia. J Clin Oncol 1993;11:914–920.

972. Jensen DM, Papadakis M, Payne JA. Chronic liver disease manifesting as Waldenström's macroglobulinemia. Arch Intern Med 1982;142:2318–2319.

973. Oram S, Cochrane GM. Weber-Christian disease with visceral involvement: An example with hepatic enlargement. BMJ 1958;2:281–284.

974. Kimura H, Kayo M, Iyo K, et al. Alcoholic hyaline (Mallory bodies) in a case of Weber-Christian disease: Electron microscopic observations of liver involvement. Gastroenterology 1986;78:807–812.

975. Edge J, Dunger DB, Dillon MJ. Weber-Christian panniculitis and chronic active hepatitis. Eur J Pediatr 1986;145:227–229.

976. Sieracki C, Fine G. Whipple's disease. Observations on systemic involvement. II. Gross and histologic observations. Arch Pathol 1959;67:81–93.

977. Cho C, Linscheer WG, Hirschkorn MA, et al. Sarcoid-like granulomas as an early manifestation of Whipple's disease. Gastroenterology 1984;87:941–947.

978. Saint-Marc Girardin M-F, Zafrani ES, Chaumette MT, et al. Hepatic granulomas in Whipple's disease. Gastroenterology 1984;86:753–756.

979. Feldman M. Whipple's disease. Am J Med Sci 1986;291:56–67.

980. Cho C, Linscheer WG, Hirschkorn MA, et al. Sarcoidlike granulomas as an early manifestation of Whipple's disease. Gastroenterology 1984;87:941–947.

981. Scheinberg IH, Sternlieb I. Wilson's disease. WB Saunders: Philadelphia, 1984.

982. Stromeyer FW, Ishak KG. Histology of the liver in Wilson's disease: A study of 34 cases. Am J Clin Pathol 1980;73:12–24.

983. Goldfischer S, Sternlieb I. Changes in the distribution of hepatic copper in relation to the progression of Wilson's disease (hepatolenticular degeneration). Am J Pathol 1968;53:883–901.

984. Archer GJ, Morrie RD. Wilson's disease and chronic active hepatitis. Lancet 1977;1:486–487.

985. Sumithran E, Looi LM. Copper-binding protein in liver cells. Hum Pathol 1985;16:677–682.

986. Rector WG, Uchida T, Kanel GC, et al. Fulminant hepatic and renal failure complicating Wilson's disease. Liver 1984;4:341–347.

987. Baban NK, Hubbs DT, Roy TM. Wilson's disease. South Med J 1997;90:535–538.

988. Steindl P, Ferenci P, Dienes HP, et al. Wilson's disease in patients presenting with liver disease: A diagnostic challenge. Gastroenterology 1997;113:212–218.

989. McCullough AJ, Fleming CR, Thistle JL, et al. Diagnosis of Wilson's disease presenting as fulminant hepatic failure. Gastroenterology 1983;84:161–167.

990. Tankanow RM. Pathophysiology and treatment of Wilson's disease. Clin Pharm 1991;10:839–849.

991. Saito T. Presenting symptoms and natural history of Wilson's disease. Eur J Pediatr 1987;146:261–265.

992. Lough J, Fawcett J, Wiegensberg B. Wolman's disease: An electron microscopic, histochemical and biochemical study. Arch Pathol 1970;89:103–110.

993. Bona G, Bracco G, Gallina MR, et al. Wolman's disease: Clinical and biochemical findings of a new case. J Inherit Metab Dis 1988;11:423–424.

994. Wolman M. Wolman disease and its treatment. Clin Pediatr 1995;34:207–212.

995. Uno Y, Taniguchi A, Tanaka E. Histochemical studies in Wolman's disease—report of an autopsy case accompanied with a large amount of milky ascites. Acta Pathol Jpn 1973;23:779–790.

996. Roytta M, Fagerlund AS, Toikkanen S, et al. Wolman disease: Morphological, clinical and genetic studies on the first Scandinavian cases. Clin Genet 1992;42:1–7.

997. Francis TI, Moore DL, Edington GM, et al. A clinicopathological study of human yellow fever. Bull WHO 1972;46:659–667.

998. Vieira W, Gayotto LC, De Kima CP, et al. Histopathology of the human liver in yellow fever with special emphasis on the diagnostic role of the Councilman body. Histopathology 1983;7:195–208.

999. DeBrito T, Siqueira SA, Santos RT, et al. Human fatal yellow fever: Immunohistochemical detection of viral antigens in the liver, kidney and heart. Pathol Res Pract 1992;188:177–181.

1000. Setchell KDR, Street JM. Inborn errors of bile acid metabolism. Semin Liver Dis 1987;7:85–99.

1001. Danks DM, Tippett P, Adams C, et al. Cerebro-hepato-renal syndrome of Zellweger: A report of eight cases with comments upon the incidence, the liver lesion, and a fault of pipecolic acid metabolism. J Pediatr 1975;86:382–387.

1002. Powers JM, Moser HW, Moser AB, et al. Fetal cerebrohepatorenal (Zellweger's) syndrome: Dysmorphic, radiologic, biochemical, and pathologic findings in four affected fetuses. Hum Pathol 1985;16:610–620.

1003. Roels F, Cornelis A, Poll-The BT, et al. Hepatic peroxisomes are deficient in infantile Refsum disease: A cytochemical study of four cases. Am J Med Genet 1986;25:257–271.

1004. Peuschel SM, Oyer CE. Cerebrohepatorenal (Zellweger) syndrome: Clinical, neuropathological, and biochemical findings. Childs Nerv Syst 1995;11:639–642.

1005. Raafat F, Smith K, Halloran EA, et al. Zellweger syndrome: A histochemical diagnosis of two cases. Pediatr Pathol 1991;11:413–420.

1006. Benbow EW, Delamore IW, Stoddart RW, et al. Disseminated zygomycosis associated with erythroleukaemia: Confirmation by lectin stains. J Clin Pathol 1985;38:1039–1044.

1007. Neyer RD, Rosen P, Armstrong D. Phycomycosis complicating leukaemia and lymphoma. Ann Intern Med 1972;77:871–879.

1008. Pagano L, Ricci P, Tonso A, et al. Mucormycosis in patients with haematological malignancies: A retrospective clinical study of 37 cases. GIMEMA Infection Program (Gruppo Italiano Malattie Ematologiche Maligne dell' Adulto). Br J Haematol 1997;99:331–336.

1009. Erdem G, Caglar M, Ceyhan M, et al. Hepatic mucormycosis in a child with fulminant hepatic failure. Turk J Pediatr 1996;38:511–514.

1010. Al-Asiri RH, Van Dijken PJ, Mahmood MA, et al. Isolated hepatic mucormycosis in an immunocompetent child. Am J Gastroenterol 1996;91:606–607.

1011. Zimmerman HJ, Ishak KG. Hepatic injury due to drugs and toxins. In MacSween RNM, Anthony PP, Scheuer PJ, et al, eds. Pathology of the Liver. Churchill Livingstone: Edinburgh, 1994, pp 563–633.

1012. Black M. Drug-induced liver disease. Clin Liver Dis 1998;2:457–642.

1013. Kaplowitz N. Drug metabolism and hepatotoxicity. In Kaplowitz N, ed. Liver and Biliary Diseases. 2nd ed. Williams & Wilkins: Baltimore, 1996, pp 103–120.

1014. Zimmerman HJ. Drug-induced liver disease. In Schiff ER, Sorrell MF, Maddrey WC, eds. Schiff's Diseases of the Liver. 8th ed. Lippincott-Raven: Philadelphia, 1999, pp 973–1064.

1015. Davis GL. Hepatitis C. In Schiff ER, Sorrell MF, Maddrey WC, eds. Schiff's Diseases of the Liver. 8th ed. Lippincott-Raven: Philadelphia, 1999, pp 793–836.

1016. Sjogren MH. Hepatitis A. In Schiff ER, Sorrell MF, Maddrey WC, eds. Schiff's Diseases of the Liver. 8th ed. Lippincott-Raven: Philadelphia, 1999, pp 745–756.

1017. Chan HL, Ghany MG, Lok ASF. Hepatitis B. In Schiff ER, Sorrell MF, Maddrey WC, eds. Schiff's Diseases of the Liver. 8th ed. Lippincott-Raven: Philadelphia, 1999, pp 757–790.

1018. Rizetto M, Smedile A: Hepatitis D. In Schiff ER, Sorrell MF, Maddrey WC, eds. Schiff's Diseases of the Liver. 8th ed. Lippincott-Raven: Philadelphia, 1999, pp 837–847.

1019. Krawczynski K, Aggarwal R. Hepatitis E. In Schiff ER, Sorrell MF, Maddrey WC, eds. Schiff's Diseases of the Liver. 8th ed. Lippincott-Raven: Philadelphia, 1999, pp 849–860.

1020. Schiff ER, de Medina MD. Hepatitis G. In Schiff ER, Sorrell MF, Maddrey WC, eds. Schiff's Diseases of the Liver. 8th ed. Lippincott-Raven: Philadelphia, 1999, pp 861–867.

INDEX

Note: Page numbers in *italics* refer to illustrations; page numbers followed by t refer to tables.

Abetalipoproteinemia, histology and clinical/laboratory findings in, 116t

Abscess, characteristics of, 8
 formation of, 8, 8t, 9–10
  assessment of, 4
 in amebiasis, 128t
 pyogenic, histologic and clinical/laboratory features of, 191t
 in bacterial sepsis, 133t

Acetaminophen, ischemic necrosis with minimal inflammation and, 63

Acidic alpha-mannosidase A and B deficiency, histologic and clinical/laboratory features of, 177t

Acidophil bodies, formation of, 3
 in hepatitis A, 204t
 in viral hepatitis, 59

Acquired immunodeficiency syndrome, peliotic lesions with, *101,* 185t
 Pneumocystis carinii infection in, 187t

Actinomyces israelii, infection with, histology and clinical/laboratory findings in, 116t

Actinomycosis, histology and clinical/laboratory findings in, 116t

Acyl-CoA dehydrogenase deficiency, long- and medium-chain, histologic and clinical/laboratory features of, 174t

Adenoma, bile duct, benign mass lesion of, *70*
 histology and clinical/laboratory findings in, 118t
 liver cell, benign mass lesion of, *70*
  drugs/toxins causing, 222t
  extramedullary hematopoiesis in, *105*
  granulomas in, *44*
  histology and clinical/laboratory findings in, 118t
  Mallory bodies and, *66*

Adenomatosis, multiple hepatocellular, 118t

Adenomatous hyperplasia, ductular, in clonorchiasis, 140t
 histology and clinical/laboratory findings in, 119t

Adenovirus infection, histology and clinical/laboratory findings in, 119t

Adult polycystic disease, cyst in, *28*
 histology and clinical/laboratory findings in, 120t

Afibrinogenemia, histologic and clinical/laboratory findings in, 151t

AIDS, peliotic lesions with, *101,* 185t
 Pneumocystis carinii infection in, 187t

Alagille's syndrome, 94
 bile duct paucity and, *21*
 histologic and clinical/laboratory features of, 185t

Alcoholic cirrhosis, histology and clinical/laboratory findings in, 120t
 regenerative nodules in, 89
 sinusoidal collagen deposits in, in active drinker, *95*
 vascular thrombosis and occlusion in, *111*

Alcoholic fatty liver, granulomas in, *44*
 histology and clinical/laboratory findings in, 116t, 121t
 inclusions in, *50*
 of pregnancy, 117t

Alcoholic foamy degeneration, histology and clinical/laboratory findings in, *39,* 121t

Alcoholic hepatitis, 2, 8
 acute, histology and clinical/laboratory findings in, 117t
 lobular necrosis with inflammation in, *55*
 portal neutrophils and, *83*
 sinusoidal circulating neutrophils in, *104*
 sinusoidal collagen deposits in, *94*

Alcoholism, fatty change in, *39, 78*

Allograft(s), acute failure of, histology and clinical/laboratory findings in, *62,* 123t
 fibrosing cholestatic hepatitis of, histology and clinical/laboratory findings in, 124t
 harvesting injury of, cholestasis and, *25,* 25t
  histology and clinical/laboratory findings in, 124t
  ischemic necrosis with minimal inflammation in, *62*
  red blood cell extravasation and, *102*
  sinusoidal hemorrhage with, *99*
 ischemic necrosis of, secondary to hepatic artery thrombosis, *62,* 125t
 lymphoproliferative disorder of, post transplant, histology and clinical findings in, 125t
 primary nonfunction of, 123t
 rejection of, acute (cellular), histology and clinical/laboratory findings in, *12, 109,* 122t
  portal eosinophils in, 87
  chronic (ductopenic), bile duct paucity and, 19, *20,* 20t
   histology and clinical/laboratory findings in, 123t
  hyperacute (humoral), histology and clinical/laboratory findings in, 124t
  lobular necrosis with, 61
  vascular, histology and clinical/laboratory findings in, *109,* 126t
 vanishing bile duct syndrome of, 123t

Alpers' disease, histology and clinical/laboratory findings in, 126t

Alpha$_1$-antichymotrypsin deficiency, histology and clinical/laboratory findings in, 126t

Alpha$_1$-antitrypsin deficiency, diagnostic features of, *29,* 30t
 cirrhosis with, portal fibrosis and, 89
 histology and clinical/laboratory findings in, 127t
 inclusions in, vs. inclusions in alcoholic fatty liver, *50*

Alpha-fetoprotein, in hepatoblastoma, 159t
 in hepatocellular carcinoma, 161t

Alpha-galactosidase deficiency, Fabry's disease with, 150t

Amebiasis, histology and clinical/laboratory findings in, 128t

Amiodarone, Mallory bodies and, *67*
 sinusoidal collagen deposits in, *96*

Amyloid, 129t
 sinusoidal and globular, *31*

Amyloidosis, diagnostic features of, 5, 30t
 extracellular (non-collagen) deposits in, *36*
 histology and clinical/laboratory findings in, *31,* 129t

Androgens, liver cell adenoma and, 118t

Angiomatosis, bacillary, histology and clinical/laboratory findings in, 132t
 peliotic lesions with, *100*

Angiomyolipoma, benign mass lesion of, *70*
 diagnostic features of, 30t
 histology and clinical/laboratory findings in, 129t

Angiosarcoma, diagnostic features of, 30t
 drugs/toxins causing, 222t
 epithelioid hemangioendothelioma and, 146t
 histology and clinical/laboratory findings in, *32,* 130t
 thorium dioxide pigment in, 77
 vascular channels on, *72*

Antigen(s), factor VIII–associated, in angiosarcoma, *32*
 hepatitis B surface, *35*
  immunoperoxidase stains for, 124t
 major histocompatibility complex, bile duct paucity and, 19

Antigen(s) *(Continued)*
    in acute allograft rejection, 122t
Apoptosis, in hepatitis A, 204t
    in liver cell injury, 3
Armillifer armillatus, infection with, histologic and clinical/laboratory features of, 186t
Arteries, hepatic, foam cell arteriopathy of, in vascular allograft rejection, 126t
        inflammation of, 4, 108, 108t, *109–110*
    small, assessment of, 2
Arteriohepatic dysplasia, histologic and clinical/laboratory features of, 185t
Arterioles, hepatic, 2, 11
        inflammation of, 108, 108t, *109–110*
Arylsulfatase A, deficiency of, 179t
Ascariasis, histology and clinical/laboratory findings in, 130t
Aspergillosis, histology and clinical/laboratory findings in, 131t
Autoimmune hepatitis. See *Hepatitis, autoimmune.*

Babesiosis, histology and clinical/laboratory findings in, 132t
Bacillary angiomatosis, histology and clinical/laboratory findings in, 132t
    peliotic lesions with, *100*
Bacterial sepsis, abscess formation and, *9,* 191t
    fatty change in, *39*
    histology and clinical/laboratory findings in, 133t
    increased neutrophils in, *12, 84, 104*
    vasculitis in, *109*
Bartonella infection, histology and clinical/laboratory findings in, 132t
Beta-galactosidase, deficiency of, in gangliosidosis, 153t
Bile, assessment of, 3–4
    in cholestasis, 3
    inspissated, 15
    staining characteristics of, 4t
Bile duct(s), adenoma of, benign mass lesion of, *70*
        histology and clinical/laboratory findings in, 118t
    assessment of, 2
    epithelium of, benign mass lesions of, conditions causing, 69t
        bile duct paucity and, *19*
        hemosiderin in, in hemochromatosis, *75–76*
        in cytomegalovirus infection, 144t
        malignant mass lesions of, 71t
        malignant transformation of, in cystadenoma, *33*
        periductal fibrosis of, 18, 18t, *18–19*
    fibrosis of, in primary sclerosing cholangitis, 189t
    in clonorchiasis, 140t
    in extrahepatic biliary atresia, 147t
    interlobular, in acute cholangitis, 11
        in allograft ischemia secondary to hepatic artery thrombosis, 125t
        in primary biliary cirrhosis, 188t
        lymphocytic inflammation of, 13, 13t, *14–15*
            drugs/toxins causing, 220t
        paucity of, 19, 20t, *20–21*
            extramedullary hematopoiesis and, *106*
            histologic and clinical/laboratory features of, 185t
            in cirrhosis, *89, 92*
            syndromatic, *94*
        reduplication and ectasia of, 15, 15t, *16–17*
        vs. cholangioles, 2
    intrahepatic, clonorchiasis in, *32*
        histologic and clinical/laboratory features of, 185t
        paucity of, syncytial giant cells in, *108*
        syndromatic, 20t, *21*
    loss of, in chronic (ductopenic) allograft rejection, 123t
    metaplastic, in acute cholangiolitis, 11
    neutrophilic inflammation of, 11, 11t, *12–13.* See also *Cholangitis, acute.*
        drugs/toxins causing, 219t
    periductal fibrosis of, 18, 18t, *18–19*
        drugs/toxins causing, 220t
    proliferation of, in extrahepatic biliary obstruction, 149t
    vanishing, in allografts, 123t

Bile infarcts, in extrahepatic biliary obstruction, *57,* 149t
Bile lakes, in extrahepatic biliary obstruction, 149t
Bile plugs, 25, 25t, *26–27.* See also *Cholestasis.*
Biliary atresia, bile duct proliferation and ectasia and, *17*
    extrahepatic, histology and clinical/laboratory findings in, 147t
        portal fibrosis leading to cirrhosis with, *91*
        syncytial giant cells in, *107*
    intrahepatic, histologic and clinical/laboratory features of, 185t
Biliary cirrhosis, 88, *89–90*
    in extrahepatic biliary obstruction, 149t
    nonsuppurative cholangitis and, 13
    primary, 4
        bile duct paucity and, 19, 20t, *21*
        bile duct proliferation and, *17*
        copper-binding protein in, *76*
        granulomas in, *46*
        histologic and clinical/laboratory features of, 188t
        lymphocytic inflammation of bile ducts and, *14*
        Mallory bodies and, *68*
        periportal inflammation with, *81*
        plasma cells with, *85*
        portal eosinophils with, *87*
        regenerating nodules with, *92*
Biliary concretions, 15, 15t
    periductal fibrosis of bile ducts and, 18, 18t, *19*
Biliary fibrosis, in congenital hepatic fibrosis, 141t
    in cystic fibrosis, 143t
    in extrahepatic biliary obstruction, 149t
Biliary hamartoma, bile duct proliferation and ectasia and, *16*
    diagnostic features of, 30t
    histology and clinical/laboratory findings in, 134t
Biliary obstruction, acute cholangitis and, 11
    extrahepatic, bile duct paucity and, 19, *20,* 20t
        bile duct proliferation and, *17*
        cholestasis and, 25t, *26*
        histologic and clinical/laboratory findings in, 148t, 149t
        Mallory bodies and, *67*
        necroinflammatory change with, *57*
        neutrophilic inflammation of bile ducts and, 11t, *12–13*
        periductal fibrosis of bile ducts and, 18, *18,* 18t
        portal fibrosis leading to cirrhosis with, *91*
Blastomyces dermatitidis infection, histology and clinical/laboratory findings in, 134t
Blastomycosis, North American, histology and clinical/laboratory features of, 134t
    South American, histology and clinical/laboratory features of, 184t
Blood flow, arterial, red blood cell extravasation and, 102
Blood transfusions, hemosiderosis and, 158t
Bone marrow transplantation, graft-versus-host disease and, 154t
Borrelia infection, histology and clinical/laboratory findings in, 134t, 175t
Borreliosis, histology and clinical/laboratory findings in, 134t
Boutonneuse fever, histology and clinical/laboratory findings in, 135t
Brucella infection, histology and clinical/laboratory findings in, 135t
Brucellosis, granulomas in, *44*
    histology and clinical/laboratory findings in, 135t
Budd-Chiari syndrome, drugs/toxins causing, 221t
    histology and clinical/laboratory findings in, 136t
    red blood cell extravasation and, *102*
    vascular thrombosis and occlusion with, *112*
Byler's syndrome (progressive familial intrahepatic cholestasis), 25, *27*
    bile duct paucity and, 20t, *21*
    cirrhosis with, *92*
    histologic and clinical/laboratory features of, 190t

Calcification, 22, 22t, *22–24*
    assessment of, 4
    dystrophic, 22
    in hydatid cyst, *34*
    metastatic, 22
Candida albicans, 136t
Candidiasis, abscess formation and, *9*
    histology and clinical/laboratory findings in, 136t

Capillaria hepatica infection, histology and clinical/laboratory findings in, 137t

Capillariasis, histology and clinical/laboratory findings in, 137t

Cardiac cirrhosis, 111
in Budd-Chiari syndrome, 136t
in right-sided heart failure, 156t
in veno-occlusive disease, 203t

Carnitine, systemic deficiency of, histologic and clinical/laboratory features of, 199t

Caroli's disease, bile duct proliferation and ectasia and, *16*
histology and clinical/laboratory findings in, 137t

Cat-scratch disease, histology and clinical/laboratory findings in, 137t

Cavernous hemangioma, calcification and, *22,* 22t
diagnostic features of, 30t
histology and clinical/laboratory findings in, *32,* 138t

Ceramidase deficiency, histologic and clinical/laboratory findings in, 150t

Cerebroside deficiency, in Gaucher's disease, 153t

Chlorothiazide, neutrophilic inflammation of bile ducts and, *12*

Chlorpromazine, necroinflammatory change with, *57*

Cholangiocarcinoma, drugs/toxins causing, 222t
histology and clinical/laboratory findings in, 138t
malignant duct epithelium in, *72*
sinusoidal collagen deposits in, *95*

Cholangiohepatitis, recurrent pyogenic, abscess formation and, *10*
histologic and clinical/laboratory features of, 192t
neutrophilic inflammation of bile ducts and, *13*
periductal fibrosis of bile ducts and, 18, 18t, *19*
portal neutrophils and, *84*

Cholangioles, biliary concretions of, 15, 15t
in acute cholangiolitis, 11
proliferation of, in cystic fibrosis, 143t
reduplication and ectasia of, 15, 15t, *16–17*
vs. interlobular bile ducts, 2

Cholangiolitis, acute, in acute viral hepatitis, 208t
in extrahepatic biliary obstruction, 148t
vs. acute cholangitis, 11

Cholangiopathy, HIV infection–associated, histologic and clinical/laboratory findings in, 164t
lymphocytic inflammation of bile ducts and, *14*

Cholangitis, abscess formation and, *9*
acute, 11, 11t, *12–13*
extrahepatic biliary obstruction and, 148t
portal neutrophils and, 83, *83–84*
ischemic, in allograft ischemia secondary to hepatic artery thrombosis, 125t
nonsuppurative, 13, 13t, *14–15*
in acute cellular allograft rejection, 122t
primary sclerosing, 4
bile duct paucity and, 19, 20t, *21*
cirrhosis with, *92*
copper-binding protein in, *76*
histologic and clinical/laboratory features of, 189t
Mallory bodies and, *68*
periductal fibrosis of bile ducts and, 18, 18t, *19*

Choledochal cyst, histology and clinical/laboratory findings in, 139t

Choledocholithiasis, in extrahepatic biliary obstruction, 148t

Cholestasis, adjacent to space-occupying lesions, 119t
assessment of, 3
benign, histology and clinical/laboratory findings in, 133t
categories of, 25
chronic, Mallory bodies and, 66, *68*
extrahepatic, 25
functional, 124t
in bacterial sepsis, 133t
in cystic fibrosis, 143t
in extrahepatic biliary obstruction, 148t, 149t
in fibrosing cholestatic hepatitis of allograft, 124t
in hyperalimentation, 166t
in lobular necrosis with inflammation, 55, *56*
in primary sclerosing cholangitis, 189t
intrahepatic, 25
benign postoperative, 133t
benign recurrent, 25t, *26,* 133t

Cholestasis *(Continued)*
progressive familial, 25, *27*
bile duct paucity and, 20t, *21*
cirrhosis with, *92*
histologic and clinical/laboratory features of, 190t
lobular, in extrahepatic biliary obstruction, 149t
Norwegian, histologic and clinical/laboratory features of, 192t
recurrent, intrahepatic, of pregnancy, histologic and clinical/laboratory features of, 192t
with lymphedema, histologic and clinical/laboratory features of, 192t
simple, 25, 25t, *25–27*
drugs/toxins causing, 219t
with inflammation, drugs/toxins causing, 219t

Cholesterol ester storage disease, histology and clinical/laboratory findings in, 139t

Circulatory failure, acute, histologic and clinical/laboratory findings in, 155t

Cirrhosis, alcoholic, histology and clinical/laboratory findings in, 120t
regenerative nodules in, *89*
sinusoidal deposits in, *95*
vascular thrombosis and occlusion with, *111*
cardiac, 111
in Budd-Chiari syndrome, 136t
in right-sided heart failure, 156t
in veno-occlusive disease, 203t
causes of, 89t
in classic chronic viral hepatitis, 209t
Indian childhood, *67, 76*
histology and clinical/laboratory features of, 168t
portal fibrosis progressing to, 88, 89t, *89–93*
primary biliary. See *Biliary cirrhosis, primary.*
signs of, 2

Clonorchiasis, diagnostic features of, 30t
histology and clinical/laboratory findings in, *32,* 140t

Clonorchis sinensis, infection with, histology and clinical/laboratory findings in, 15, *32,* 140t

Cocaine, fatty change with, *40*

Coccidioidomycosis, diagnostic features of, 30t
histologic features of, *32*

Collagen deposits, in acute sclerosing hyaline necrosis, 117t
in alcoholic cirrhosis, 120t
in nonalcoholic steatohepatitis, 183t
sinusoidal, 94, *94,* 95t, *95–97*
assessment of, 2, 3
in Budd-Chiari syndrome, *112*
in progressive perivenular alcoholic cirrhosis, *112*
in veno-occlusive disease, *113*

Copper, 73, 74t
bile duct paucity and, 19
diseases producing, 74t
in cystic fibrosis, 143t
in Wilson's disease, 77

Copper-binding protein, 73
bile duct paucity and, 19
diseases producing, 74t, *76–77*
in cystic fibrosis, 143t
in Wilson's disease, 77

Councilman (acidophil) bodies, formation of, 3
in hepatitis A, 204t
in viral hepatitis, *59*

Coxiella burnetii, infection with, histologic and clinical/laboratory features of, 191t

Coxsackievirus infection, group B, histologic and clinical/laboratory findings in, 155t

Crigler-Najjar syndrome, histology and clinical/laboratory findings in, 141t

Crohn's disease, fatty change in, *40*
granulomas in, *44*
histology and clinical/laboratory findings in, 141t

Cryptococcosis, histology and clinical/laboratory findings in, 142t

Cryptococcus neoformans, infection with, histology and clinical/laboratory findings in, 142t

Cryptosporidiosis, histology and clinical/laboratory findings in, 142t

Cryptosporidium parvum, infection with, histology and clinical/laboratory findings in, 142t

Cyst(s), assessment of, 4
  choledochal, histology and clinical/laboratory findings in, 139t
  ciliated hepatic foregut, histology and clinical/laboratory findings in, 140t
  hepatic, 27, 27t, *28*
    lining of, 27
  hydatid. See *Hydatid cysts.*
  in adult polycystic disease, *28*, 120t
  in amebiasis, 128t
  in cystadenoma, with or without mesenchymal stroma, 142t
  in infantile microcystic disease, 169t
  nonparasitic, *28*
    calcification and, 22t, *24*
    histologic and clinical/laboratory features of, 197t
Cystadenoma, calcification and, *22*, 22t
  malignant transformation of, 27
  with or without mesenchymal stroma, histology and clinical findings in, 30t, *33*, 142t
Cystathionine beta-synthase deficiency, histologic and clinical/laboratory findings in, 163t
Cystic fibrosis, bile duct paucity and, *20*, 20t
  bile duct proliferation and ectasia and, *16*
  histology and clinical/laboratory findings in, 143t
  portal fibrosis leading to cirrhosis with, *90*
Cystinosis, diagnostic features of, 30t
  histology and clinical/laboratory findings in, 143t
Cytomegalovirus infection, abscess formation and, *10*
  diagnostic features of, 30t
  histology and clinical/laboratory findings in, 144t
  inclusions in, *48, 53*
  lobular necrosis with inflammation in, *55*

Dengue fever, histology and clinical/laboratory findings in, 144t
Diagnostic lesions, 29, *29*, 30t, *31–35*
Down syndrome, histology and clinical/laboratory findings in, 145t
Drugs/toxins, bile duct damage with, *12*, 219t–220t
  cholestasis and, 25t, *26*, 219t
  fatty change and, *40*, 220t
  granulomas and, *45*, 221t
  hepatic venous outflow obstruction and, 221t
  inclusions and, 222t
  ischemic necrosis with minimal inflammation and, *63*
  liver cell injury and, 217–224
  lobular necrosis and, *65*, 218t, 219t
  lobular necrosis with inflammation and, *57*
  Mallory bodies and, *67*, 223t
  neoplasms and, 222t
  periportal inflammation and, *81*
  pigments due to, 223t
  portal eosinophils and, *87*
  portal fibrosis and, *90*, 220t
  sinusoidal damage and, *96*, 221t
  vasculitis and, 221t
  veno-occlusive disease and, 221t
Dubin-Johnson syndrome, histology and clinical/laboratory findings in, 145t
  lipochrome in, *73, 77*
Ductopenia, 19, 20t, *20–21*
  idiopathic adulthood, histologic and clinical/laboratory features of, 167t
Dysfibrinogenemia, histologic and clinical/laboratory findings in, 151t

Ebola virus infection, histology and clinical/laboratory findings in, 145t
Echinococcus granulosus, infection with, histologic and clinical/laboratory findings in, 165t
Echinococcus hydatid cyst. See *Hydatid cyst.*
Echinococcus multilocularis, infection with, histologic and clinical/laboratory findings in, 165t
Eclampsia, histologic and clinical/laboratory features of, 200t
Encephalitozoon infection, histologic and clinical/laboratory features of, 179t

Endophlebitis, in acute sclerosing hyaline necrosis, 117t
Endophthalmitis, in schistosomiasis, 196t
Endoscopic retrograde cholangiopancreatography, for extrahepatic biliary obstruction, 148t
Endothelial damage, necrotizing, in hyperacute (humoral) allograft rejection, 124t
Endothelialitis, in acute cellular allograft rejection, 122t
Entamoeba histolytica, 128t
Enterobiasis, histology and clinical/laboratory findings in, 145t
Enterobius vermicularis infection, histology and clinical/laboratory findings in, 145t
Enterocytozoon infection, histologic and clinical/laboratory features of, 179t
Eosinophilic gastroenteritis, histology and clinical/laboratory findings in, 146t
Eosinophilic globules, diPAS, in alpha$_1$-antitrypsin deficiency, 127t
Eosinophils, portal, 86, 86t, *87–88*
Epilepsy, myoclonus, histologic and clinical/laboratory features of, 181t
  inclusions in, *51*
Epithelioid cells, 106
Epithelium, bile duct. See *Bile ducts, epithelium of.*
  biliary, as cyst lining, 27t, *28*
Epstein-Barr virus infection, histology and clinical/laboratory findings in, 146t
  increased sinusoidal circulating lymphocytes in, *104*
  lymphocytic inflammation of bile ducts and, *14*
  necroinflammatory change with, *57*
  post transplant lymphoproliferative disorder and, 125t
  vasculitis in, *110*
Erythropoietic protoporphyria, diagnostic features of, 30t
  histology and clinical/laboratory findings in, 147t
  protoporphyrin in, *78*
Extracellular deposits (not collagen), 36, 36t, *36–37*
  vs. sinusoidal collagen deposits, 3

Fabry's disease, histologic and clinical/laboratory findings in, 150t
Factor VIII–related antigen, epithelioid hemangioendothelioma and, 146t
Familial hyperlipoproteinemia, histologic and clinical/laboratory findings in, 150t
Familial intrahepatic cholestasis, progressive, 25, *27*
  bile duct paucity and, 20t, *21*
  cirrhosis with, *92*
  histologic and clinical/laboratory features of, 190t
Farber's lipogranulomatosis, histologic and clinical/laboratory findings in, 150t
Fasciola hepatica, infection with, histologic and clinical/laboratory findings in, 151t
Fascioliasis, histologic and clinical/laboratory findings in, 151t
Fat, type of, 3
Fatty change, alcoholic, 2, *39, 78*
  assessment of, 3
  disorders associated with, 37, 38t, *39–42*
  drugs/toxins causing, *40*, 220t
  focal, histologic and clinical/laboratory findings in, 151t
  in cystic fibrosis, 143t
  in hyperalimentation, 166t
  in nonalcoholic steatohepatitis, 183t
  in primary sclerosing cholangitis, 189t
  microvesicular or macrovesicular, 37, 38t
Fatty liver, acute, of pregnancy, histology and clinical/laboratory findings in, 117t
  alcoholic, acute, histology and clinical/laboratory findings in, 116t
  histology and clinical/laboratory findings in, 121t
  inclusions in, *50*
Ferrous sulfate, ischemic necrosis with minimal inflammation due to, *63*
Fibrinogen storage disease, diagnostic features of, 30t
  histologic and clinical/laboratory findings in, 151t
Fibrosis, assessment of, 2–3
  biliary, in congenital hepatic fibrosis, 141t
    in cystic fibrosis, 143t
    in extrahepatic biliary obstruction, 149t

Fibrosis *(Continued)*
  bridging, assessment of, 2
    in alcoholic cirrhosis, 120t
    in chronic hepatic venous outflow obstruction, 111
    in hepatic venules, in Budd-Chiari syndrome, 136t
    in primary biliary cirrhosis, 188t
    in primary sclerosing cholangitis, 189t
    in right-sided heart failure, 156t
    in veno-occlusive disease, 203t
  congenital hepatic, bile duct proliferation and ectasia and, *16*
    histology and clinical/laboratory features of, 141t
    portal fibrosis without progression to cirrhosis and, *93*
  cystic. See *Cystic fibrosis.*
  diffuse interstitial, in alcoholic cirrhosis, 120t
  in acute sclerosing hyaline necrosis, 117t
  in classic chronic viral hepatitis, 209t
  periductal, of bile ducts, 18, 18t, *18–19*
    drugs/toxins causing, 220t
  perivenular alcoholic, histology and clinical/laboratory features of, 186t
  portal. See *Portal fibrosis.*
  progressive perivenular alcoholic, histologic and clinical/laboratory features of, 190t
    vascular thrombosis and occlusion with, *112*
  sinusoidal, 94, *94*, 95t, *95–97*
    in progressive perivenular alcoholic fibrosis, 190t
  true, vs. lobular collapse, 2
Fibrous bands, assessment of, 2
Foam cells, arteriopathy of, in vascular allograft rejection, 126
Foamy degeneration, 37
  alcoholic, *39*
    histology and clinical/laboratory findings in, 121t
Focal fatty change, histologic and clinical/laboratory findings in, 151t
Focal nodular hyperplasia, cholestasis and, 25t, *26*
  diagnostic features of, 30t
  drugs/toxins causing, 222t
  histology and clinical/laboratory features of, 152t
  of hepatocytes, benign, *70*
Formalin pigment, 78
Fructose intolerance, hereditary, histologic and clinical/laboratory findings in, 162t

Galactosemia, histologic and clinical/laboratory findings in, 152t
Gangliosidosis, histologic and clinical/laboratory findings in, 153t
Gastroenteritis, eosinophilic, histology and clinical/laboratory findings in, 146t
Gaucher's disease, histologic and clinical/laboratory findings in, 153t
  Kupffer cell inclusions in, *53*
Gilbert's syndrome, histologic and clinical/laboratory findings in, 153t
Glucocerebrosidase deficiency, histologic and clinical/laboratory findings in, 153t
Glycogen storage disease, cirrhosis with, *91*
  histologic and clinical/laboratory findings in, 154t
Glycosphingolipidosis, histologic and clinical/laboratory findings in, 150t
Graft-versus-host disease, histologic and clinical/laboratory findings in, 154t
Granuloma(s), 43, 43t, *44–47*
  assessment of, 3
  drugs/toxins causing, 221t
  epithelioid, 43
    in primary biliary cirrhosis, *85,* 188t
    in sarcoidosis, 195t
  in chronic granulomatous disease of childhood, 139t
  in Farber's lipogranulomatosis, 150t
  in idiopathic granulomatous hepatitis, 168t
  in leishmaniasis, 172t
  in leprosy, 172t
  in Q fever, *42,* 191t
  in schistosomiasis, *34*
  inflammatory, 43
  lobular necrosis and inflammation and, *55*
  ring, 191t

Granulomatous disease of childhood, chronic, histology and clinical/laboratory findings in, 139t
Granulomatous hepatitis, idiopathic, histologic and clinical/laboratory features of, 168t
Ground-glass appearance, assessment of, 3
  in hepatitis B, 30t, *35, 51, 60*
    vs. hepatocellular carcinoma inclusions, *50*
  of hepatocyte inclusions, 48

Halothane, hypersensitivity to, portal eosinophils with, *87*
  lobular confluent necrosis due to, *65*
Hamartoma, biliary, bile duct proliferation and ectasia and, *16*
  histology and clinical/laboratory features of, 134t
  mesenchymal, histologic and clinical/laboratory features of, 179t
Hansen's disease (leprosy), granulomas in, *45*
  histologic and clinical/laboratory features of, 172t
Heart failure, extracellular (non-collagen) deposits in, *37*
  left-sided, with and without hypotension, *103*
    histologic and clinical/laboratory findings in, 155t
  right-sided, histologic and clinical/laboratory findings in, 156t
    sinusoidal collagen deposits in, *96*
    sinusoidal dilatation and congestion and, *99*
Heat stroke, histologic and clinical/laboratory findings in, 156t
HELLP syndrome, histologic findings in, 158t
  in pregnancy, 197t
Hemangioendothelioma, epithelioid, histology and clinical/laboratory findings in, 146t
  infantile, histologic and clinical/laboratory features of, 169t
  malignant, histology and clinical/laboratory findings in, 130t
Hemangioepithelioma, epithelioid, diagnostic features of, 30t
Hemangioma, cavernous, calcification and, *22,* 22t
  diagnostic features of, 30t
  histology and clinical/laboratory findings in, *32,* 138t
Hematopoiesis, extramedullary, sinusoidal, 4, 105, 105t, *105–106*
Hematopoietic lesions, malignant, 71t
Hematoxylin-eosin stain, extracellular (non-collagen) deposits on, 36, 36t, *36–37*
Hemicirrhosis, in primary sclerosing cholangitis, 189t
Hemochromatosis, hemosiderin in, *75*
  histologic and clinical/laboratory findings in, 157t
  neonatal, histologic and clinical/laboratory findings in, 157t
  regenerative nodules with, *91*
  vs. hemosiderosis secondary to iron overload, *75–76*
Hemolysis, elevated liver enzymes, low platelets (HELLP syndrome), histologic findings in, 158t
  in pregnancy, 197t
Hemorrhage, acute, in right-sided heart failure, 156t
  sinusoidal, 4, 98, 98t, *99*
    drugs/toxins causing, 221t
Hemorrhagic telangiectasia, hereditary, histologic and clinical/laboratory findings in, 162t
Hemosiderin deposits, 73
  assessment of, 3–4
  diseases producing, 73t
  drugs/toxins causing, 223t
  in alcoholic cirrhosis, 120t
  in cystic fibrosis, 143t
  in hemochromatosis, *91,* 157t
    vs. secondary iron overload, *75–76*
  in Hodgkin's lymphoma, 175t
  in leukemia, 173t
  in malaria, 177t
  in neonatal hepatitis, *107*
  in non-Hodgkin's lymphoma, 176t
  staining characteristics of, 4t
Hemosiderosis, histologic and clinical/laboratory findings in, 158t
  secondary to iron overload, vs. hemochromatosis, *75–76*
Hemozoin, in malaria, *79,* 177t
Hepar lobatum, 143t
  in chronic granulomatous disease of childhood, 139t
  in syphilis, 199t
Hepatic arteries, foam cell arteriopathy of, in vascular allograft rejection, 126
  inflammation of, 4, 108, 108t, *109–110*

Hepatic arteries (Continued)
  small, assessment of, 2
  thrombosis of, allograft ischemia with, 125t
Hepatic arterioles, assessment of, 2
Hepatic cord-sinusoid pattern, in parenchymal architectural structure, 3
Hepatic fibrosis, congenital, bile duct proliferation and ectasia and, 16
  cirrhosis and, absence of, in portal fibrosis, 93
  histology and clinical/laboratory findings in, 141t
Hepatic injury, secondary, with nonsinusoidal vascular thrombosis and occlusion, 111, 111t, 111–113
Hepatic veins, occlusion of, in Budd-Chiari syndrome, 136t
  in veno-occlusive disease, 203t
  portal, 2, 4
  thrombosis and occlusion of, hepatic injury with, 111, 111t, 111–113
  vasculitis of, 108, 108t, 109–110
Hepatic venous outflow obstruction. See Venous outflow obstruction.
Hepatitis, alcoholic. See Alcoholic hepatitis.
  autoimmune, histology and clinical/laboratory findings in, 131t
    portal neutrophils and, 83
    syncytial giant cells in, 107
    untreated, lobular necrosis with, 55, 64
      periportal inflammation with, 81
      plasma cells with, 84, 84t, 85
  fibrosing cholestatic, of allograft, 124t
  granulomatous, idiopathic, histologic and clinical/laboratory features of, 168t
  neonatal, histologic and clinical/laboratory features of, 182t
    multinucleated giant cells in, 107
    vs. cystic fibrosis, 143t
  nonspecific reactive, histologic and clinical/laboratory features of, 184t
  peliotic lesions with, 101
  surgical, abscess formation and, 10
    characteristics of, 8
    histologic and clinical/laboratory features of, 198t
  viral. See Viral hepatitis.
Hepatitis B surface antigen, 35
  immunoperoxidase stains for, 124t
Hepatoblastoma, calcification and, 22t, 23
  diagnostic features of, 30t
  histologic and clinical/laboratory findings in, 159t
  melanin in, 78
Hepatocellular carcinoma, 5
  acinar type of, histologic and clinical/laboratory findings in, 161t
  alcoholic cirrhosis and, 120t
  diagnostic features of, 30t
  drugs/toxins causing, 222t
  ductular type of, histologic and clinical/laboratory findings in, 161t
  fatty change with, 41
  fibrolamellar type of, histologic and clinical/laboratory findings in, 160t
    inclusions in, 51
    peliotic lesions with, 100
    sinusoidal collagen deposits in, 96
  findings in, 71
  in chronic viral hepatitis C, 209t
  Mallory bodies and, 67
  trabecular type of, 72
    calcification and, 22t, 23
    cholestasis and, 27
    histologic and clinical/laboratory findings in, 161t
    inclusions in, 51
    syncytial giant cells in, 107
Hepatocytes, adenoma of. See Adenoma, liver cell.
  assessment of, 3
  ballooning of, 3, 62–63, 124t
  dropout of, 3
    in acute viral hepatitis with bridging necrosis, 208t
    in harvesting injury of allograft, 124t
    in hepatitis A, 204t
    in left-sided heart failure, 155t
    in lobular confluent necrosis, 64, 64–65
    in lobular necrosis with minimal inflammation, 62
    red blood cell extravasation and, 102, 102–103
    sinusoidal hemorrhage and, 98

Hepatocytes (Continued)
  drug-induced injury of, 63, 217–224
  focal nodular hyperplasia of, benign, 70
  giant cell transformation of, 3
  in extrahepatic biliary obstruction, 149t
  in nodular regenerative hyperplasia, 71
  inclusions in, 48, 48, 49t, 50–52
    drugs/toxins causing, 222t
  ischemic necrosis of, with minimal inflammation, 61, 62–63
  malignant mass lesions of, 71t
  trapped, in classic chronic viral hepatitis, 209t
Hepatolenticular degeneration (Wilson's disease). See Wilson's disease.
Hepatomegaly, in leishmaniasis, 172t
Hepatorenal syndrome, in acute sclerosing hyaline necrosis, 117t
  in progressive perivenular alcoholic fibrosis, 190t
Hepatotoxicity. See Drugs/toxins.
Herpes simplex virus infection, diagnostic features of, 30t
  histologic and clinical/laboratory findings in, 162t
  inclusions in, 48
Herpes zoster infection, histologic and clinical/laboratory findings in, 163t
Histiocytosis, Langerhans' cell, histologic and clinical/laboratory features of, 171t
Histoplasma capsulatum, infection with, 163t
Histoplasmosis, granulomas in, 45
  histologic and clinical/laboratory findings in, 163t
  Kupffer cell inclusions in, 53
Hodgkin's lymphoma, diagnostic features of, 30t
  histologic and clinical/laboratory features of, 175t
  portal eosinophils in, 87
Homocystinuria, histologic and clinical/laboratory findings in, 163t
Human immunodeficiency virus infection, cholangiopathy associated with, 14, 164t
  histologic and clinical/laboratory findings in, 164t
Hunter's syndrome, histologic and clinical/laboratory features of, 180t
Hurler's syndrome, histologic and clinical/laboratory features of, 180t
Hyaline necrosis, acute sclerosing, 2, 4–5, 8, 117t
Hydatid cysts, calcification and, 22t, 24
  diagnostic features of, 30t
  histologic and clinical/laboratory findings in, 165t
  histologic features of, 34
  plasma cells with, 85
  sinusoidal dilatation and congestion and, 98
Hyperalimentation, histologic and clinical/laboratory features of, 166t
  in infants, sinusoidal collagen deposits in, 96
Hypereosinophilic syndrome, histologic and clinical/laboratory features of, 166t
Hyperimmune reaction, 177t
Hyperlipoproteinemia, familial, histologic and clinical/laboratory findings in, 150t
Hyperplasia, focal nodular. See Focal nodular hyperplasia.
  nodular regenerative. See Nodular regenerative hyperplasia.
Hyperpyrexia, histologic and clinical/laboratory features of, 167t
Hypersensitivity reaction. See Drugs/toxins.
Hypertension, idiopathic portal, 94
  histologic and clinical/laboratory features of, 168t
  pregnancy-induced, spontaneous rupture in pregnancy and, 197t
Hyperthyroidism, histologic and clinical/laboratory features of, 167t
Hypofibrinogenemia, histologic and clinical/laboratory findings in, 151t
Hypotension, absence of, in left-sided heart failure, red blood cell extravasation and, 102, 103
Hypothyroidism, histologic and clinical/laboratory features of, 167t
  vascular thrombosis and occlusion with, 112

I-cell disease, histologic and clinical/laboratory features of, 180t
Immunocompromise, cytomegalovirus infection and, 144t
  granulomas in, 46
  herpes simplex virus infection and, 162t
Inclusions, amyloid, 31
  assessment of, 3
  drugs/toxins causing, 222t

Inclusions (*Continued*)
hepatitis B surface antigen, in viral hepatitis type B, *35*
hepatocyte, herpes simplex virus infection and, 162t
in alpha₁-antitrypsin deficiency, *29*
nuclear and cytoplasmic, 48, *48,* 49t, *50–52*
in Kupffer cells, 53, *53,* 54t
in portal macrophages, 53, *54,* 54t
viral, in cytomegalovirus infection, *10,* 144t
Indian childhood cirrhosis, copper-binding protein in, *76*
histologic and clinical/laboratory features of, 168t
Mallory bodies and, *67*
Infantile hemangioendothelioma, histologic and clinical/laboratory features of, 169t
Infantile microcystic disease, histologic and clinical/laboratory features of, 169t
Inflammation, lobular, assessment of, 3
lymphocytic, of bile ducts, 13, 13t, *14–15*
drugs/toxins causing, 220t
minimal to absent, with lobular necrosis, 61, 61t, *62–63*
neutrophilic, of bile ducts, 11, 11t, *12–13.* See also *Cholangitis, acute.*
drugs/toxins causing, 219t
of nonsinusoidal vessels, 108, 108t, *109–110*
periportal, portal lymphocytes with, 80, 80t, *81–82*
with lobular confluent necrosis, 64, *64–65*
with lobular necrosis, 55, *55,* 56t, *57–60*
drugs/toxins causing, 218t
Inflammatory bowel disease, fatty change in, *40*
Inflammatory infiltrates, assessment of, 2
benign mass lesions of, conditions causing, 69t
in hepatitis A, 204t
in Hodgkin's lymphoma, 175t
in non-Hodgkin's lymphoma, 176t
mixed portal, in acute cellular allograft rejection, 122t
with lobular confluent necrosis, 64, *64–65*
Inflammatory pseudotumor, histologic and clinical/laboratory features of, 170t
Inspissated bile syndrome, histologic and clinical/laboratory features of, 170t
Iron deposits, in hemochromatosis, 157t
in hemosiderosis, 158t
Iron overload, hemosiderosis secondary to, vs. hemochromatosis, *75–76*
secondary, histologic and clinical/laboratory findings in, 158t
Isoniazid, 5
necroinflammatory change with, *57*

Jejunoileal bypass, nonalcoholic steatohepatitis and, granulomas with, *46*

Kala azar, histologic and clinical/laboratory features of, 172t
Kasai procedure, 147t
Kawasaki disease, histologic and clinical/laboratory features of, 170t
Klatskin tumor, 138t
Kupffer cells, 3
in cryptococcosis, 142t
in gangliosidosis, 153t
in Gaucher's disease, 153t
in hepatitis A, 204t
in Niemann-Pick disease, histologic and clinical/laboratory features of, 182t
inclusions in, 53, *53,* 54t
drugs/toxins causing, 222t
pigments in, 73
Kwashiorkor, histologic and clinical/laboratory features of, 171t

Laboratory tests, histologic correlation with, 29
Lafora bodies, 3
Lafora's disease, histologic and clinical/laboratory features of, 181t
inclusions in, *51*

Langerhans' cell histiocytosis, histologic and clinical/laboratory features of, 171t
Larva migrans, visceral, histologic and clinical/laboratory features of, 212t
portal eosinophils with, *88*
Lassa fever, histologic and clinical/laboratory features of, 171t
ischemic necrosis with minimal inflammation and, *63*
Leishmania donovani, infection with, histologic and clinical/laboratory features of, 172t
Leishmaniasis, granulomas in, *45*
histologic and clinical/laboratory features of, 172t
Leprosy, granulomas in, *45*
histologic and clinical/laboratory features of, 172t
Leptospira icterohaemorrhagica, infection with, histologic and clinical/laboratory features of, 173t
Leptospirosis, histologic and clinical/laboratory features of, 173t
Leukemia, acute lymphocytic, 173t
acute myelogenous, 173t
chronic lymphocytic, *104,* 173t
chronic myelogenous, *105,* 173t
hairy cell, 173t
histologic and clinical/laboratory features of, 173t
types of, 173t
Leukodystrophy, metachromatic, histologic and clinical/laboratory features of, 179t
Light chain disease, histologic and clinical/laboratory features of, 174t
Lipidosis, sphingomyelin-cholesterol, histologic and clinical/laboratory features of, 182t
sulfatide, histologic and clinical/laboratory features of, 179t
Lipochrome, 73, 74t
assessment of, 3–4
drugs/toxins causing, 223t
in Dubin-Johnson syndrome, 73, *77*
in Gilbert's disease, 153t
staining characteristics of, 4t
Lipogranulomas, in alcoholic fatty liver, *44,* 121t
Lipogranulomatosis, Farber's, histologic and clinical/laboratory findings in, 150t
Listeria monocytogenes, infection with, histologic and clinical/laboratory features of, 174t
Listeriosis, histologic and clinical/laboratory features of, 174t
Liver biopsy, assessment of, 2–4
clinical-pathologic correlation with, 4–5
differential diagnosis of, 5
Liver cells. See also *Hepatocytes.*
adenoma of, benign mass lesion of, *70*
drugs/toxins causing, 222t
extramedullary hematopoiesis in, *105*
granulomas in, *44*
histology and clinical/laboratory findings in, 118t
Mallory bodies and, *66*
injury to, from drugs and toxins, 217–224
Liver fluke infection, histology and clinical/laboratory findings in, *32,* 140t
Liver transplantation. See also *Allograft(s).*
lobular necrosis with minimal to absent inflammation in, 61
Long-chain acyl-CoA dehydrogenase deficiency, histologic and clinical/laboratory features of, 174t
Lupus erythematosus, systemic, histologic and clinical/laboratory features of, 200t
Lyme disease, histologic and clinical/laboratory features of, 175t
Lymphangioma, histologic and clinical/laboratory features of, 175t
Lymphocytes, circulating, in sinusoids, 103, 103t, *104*
in primary biliary cirrhosis, 188t
in vasculitis, *109*
near inflamed bile ducts, 2
portal, minimal to absent periportal activity and, 79, 79t, *80*
periportal activity and, 80, 80t, *81–82*
Lymphocytic inflammation, of bile ducts, 13, 13t, *14–15*
Lymphoma, Hodgkin's. See *Hodgkin's lymphoma.*
non-Hodgkin's, histologic and clinical/laboratory features of, 176t
portal lymphocytic infiltrates with, *80*
types of, 176t
Lymphoproliferative disease, post transplant, 125t
Epstein-Barr virus infection and, 146t

Macrophages, portal, inclusions in, 53, *54,* 54t
  drugs/toxins causing, 222t
Major histocompatibility complex antigens, bile duct paucity and, 19
  in acute cellular allograft rejection, 122t
Malaria, diagnostic features of, 30t
  hemozoin in, *79*
  histologic and clinical/laboratory features of, 177t
Mallory bodies, 48, 66, 66t, *66–68*
  assessment of, 3
  drug-induced, *96.* 223t
  in acute sclerosing hyaline necrosis, *55, 94,* 117t
  in alcoholic hepatitis, 2
  in extracellular locations, 36, *36t*
Mannosidosis, histologic and clinical/laboratory features of, 177t
Marasmus, histologic and clinical/laboratory features of, 178t
Marburg virus infection, histologic and clinical/laboratory features of, 178t
Maroteaux-Lamy syndrome, histologic and clinical/laboratory features of, 180t
Mass lesions, benign, 69, 69t, *70–71*
  malignant, primary, 71, 71t, *72*
Mediterranean spotted fever, 135t
Medium-chain acyl-CoA dehydrogenase deficiency, histologic and clinical/laboratory features of, 174t
Medullary sponge kidney, 137t
Megamitochondria, 3
  in alcoholic fatty liver, *50*
  in alcoholic foamy degeneration, 121t
Melanin, in hepatoblastoma, *78*
Melioidosis, histologic and clinical/laboratory features of, 178t
Mesenchymal stroma, in cystadenoma, diagnostic features of, 30t
  histologic and clinical/laboratory features of, *33,* 142t
Methimazole, cholestasis and, 26
Methotrexate, periportal inflammation with, *81*
  portal fibrosis progressing to cirrhosis with, *90*
Microabscess(es), characteristics of, 8, *9*
Microcystic disease, infantile, histologic and clinical/laboratory features of, 169t
Microsporidiosis, histologic and clinical/laboratory features of, 179t
Morquio syndrome, histologic and clinical/laboratory features of, 180t
Mucocutaneous lymph node syndrome, 170t
Mucolipidoses, histologic and clinical/laboratory features of, 180t
Mucopolysaccharidoses, histologic and clinical/laboratory features of, 180t
Multiple myeloma, histologic and clinical/laboratory features of, 180t
  plasma cells with, *85*
Multiple sulfatase deficiency, 179t
Mycobacterium avium-intracellulare infection, granulomas in, *46*
  histologic and clinical/laboratory features of, 181t
Mycobacterium leprae infection, histologic and clinical/laboratory features of, 172t
Mycobacterium tuberculosis infection, histologic and clinical/laboratory features of, 201t
Myelofibrosis, extramedullary hematopoiesis in, *106*
Myeloproliferative disorders, histologic and clinical/laboratory features of, 181t
Myoclonus epilepsy, histologic and clinical/laboratory features of, 181t
  inclusions in, *51*

Necrosis, acute sclerosing hyaline. See *Sclerosing hyaline necrosis, acute.*
  chronic sclerosing hyaline, histologic and clinical/laboratory features of, 190t
  ischemic, in hyperacute (humoral) allograft rejection, 124t
    neutrophilic infiltration and, 61
    sinusoidal hemorrhage and, 98
    with minimal inflammation, 61, *63*
  liver cell, in left-sided heart failure, 155t
  lobular, confluent, 64, 64t, *64–65*
    drugs/toxins causing, 219t
    with inflammation, 55, *55,* 56t, *57–60*

Necrosis *(Continued)*
    drugs/toxins causing, 218t
    with minimal/absent inflammation, 61, 61t, *62–63*
      drugs/toxins causing, 218t
  lytic, in acute sclerosing hyaline necrosis, 117t
    in extrahepatic biliary obstruction, 149t
  massive hepatic, in acute viral hepatitis, 208t
  panacinar, in acute viral hepatitis, *65,* 208t
  piecemeal, in classic chronic viral hepatitis, 209t
    in primary biliary cirrhosis, 188t
    in primary sclerosing cholangitis, 189t
    periportal activity with, 80, 80t, *81–82*
  submassive hepatic, in acute viral hepatitis, 208t
  zonal, *63, 64, 65*
Neonates, cytomegalovirus infection in, 144t
  extrahepatic biliary atresia in, 147t
  galactosemia in, 152t
  hemochromatosis in, histologic and clinical/laboratory findings in, 157t
  hepatitis in, histologic and clinical/laboratory features of, 182t
    multinucleated giant cells in, *107*
    vs. cystic fibrosis, 143t
Neoplasms, drugs/toxins causing, 222t
  obstruction by, extrahepatic biliary obstruction and, 148t
  primary hepatic, cholestasis and, 25
Neutrophils, adjacent to space-occupying lesions, 119t
  circulating, in sinusoids, 103, 103t, *104*
  clusters of, characteristics of, 8
    in surgical hepatitis, *10*
    in acute sclerosing hyaline necrosis, *94*
  in bacterial sepsis, *9,* 133t
  in nonalcoholic steatohepatitis, 183t
  in portal tracts, without bile duct orientation, 83, 83t, *83–84*
  infiltration of, in extrahepatic biliary obstruction, 148t
    in primary biliary cirrhosis, 188t
    ischemic necrosis and, 61
    of bile ducts, 11, 11t, *12–13.* See also *Cholangitis, acute.*
  Mallory bodies and, 66, *66–68*
  near inflamed bile ducts, 2
Niacin, lobular confluent necrosis due to, *65*
Niemann-Pick disease, histologic and clinical/laboratory features of, 182t
Nocardiosis, histologic and clinical/laboratory features of, 182t
Nodular hyperplasia, focal. See *Focal nodular hyperplasia.*
Nodular regenerative hyperplasia, benign, *71*
  drugs/toxins causing, 222t
  histologic and clinical/laboratory features of, 183t
Nodular transformation, partial, histologic and clinical/laboratory features of, 184t
Nodules, in cirrhosis, types of, 88
  in partial nodular transformation, 184t
  macroregenerative, histology and clinical/laboratory findings in, 119t
  regenerative, in alcoholic cirrhosis, 120t
    in hemochromatosis, *91*
Non-Hodgkin's lymphoma, histologic and clinical/laboratory features of, 176t
  portal lymphocytic infiltrates with, *80*
  types of, 176t
North American blastomycosis, histology and clinical/laboratory findings in, 134t
Norwegian cholestasis, histologic and clinical/laboratory features of, 192t

Oral contraceptives, liver cell adenoma and, 118t
Orcein stain, 73
  bile duct paucity and, 19
  for copper-binding protein in liver diseases, *76–77*
  for HBsAg particles, 48
Osler-Rendu-Weber disease, histologic and clinical/laboratory findings in, 162t
Ossification, 22, 22t, *22–24*
  assessment of, 4
Oxyphenisatin, portal fibrosis progressing to cirrhosis with, *90*

Pale bodies, in hepatocellular carcinoma, *51, 100*

Paracoccidioides brasiliensis infection, histologic and clinical/laboratory features of, 184t

Paracoccidioidomycosis, histologic and clinical/laboratory features of, 184t

Parenchyma, architectural structure of, 3
assessment of, 3–4

Partial nodular transformation, histologic and clinical/laboratory features of, 184t

PAS stain, after diastase digestion, for necroinflammatory change, 55
for glycogenated nuclei, 48
in alpha₁-antitrypsin deficiency, *29*

Paucity of intrahepatic duct. See *Bile duct(s), intrahepatic, paucity of.*

Peliosis, in sinusoids, 4

Peliosis hepatis, histologic and clinical/laboratory features of, 185t

Peliotic lesions, drugs/toxins causing, 221t
in bacillary angiomatosis, 132t
in liver cell adenoma, 118t
of sinusoids, 100, 100t, *100–101*

Penicilliosis, histologic and clinical/laboratory features of, 186t

Penicillium marneffei infection, histologic and clinical/laboratory features of, 186t

Pentastomiasis, histologic and clinical/laboratory features of, 186t

Periodic acid–Schiff stain, after diastase digestion, for necroinflammatory change, 55
for glycogenated nuclei, 48
in alpha₁-antitrypsin deficiency, *29*

Periportal activity, minimal to absent, portal lymphocytes and, 79, 79t, *80*
portal lymphocytes and, 80, 80t, *81–82*

Perivenular alcoholic fibrosis, progressive, histologic and clinical/laboratory features of, 190t
vascular thrombosis and occlusion with, *112*

Perivenular fibrosis, alcoholic etiology, histologic and clinical/laboratory features of, 186t

Perls's stain, in hemochromatosis, 75

Pigments, 73, 73t–74t, *75–79.* See also names of specific pigments (e.g., *Hemosiderin deposits*).
assessment of, 3–4
drugs/toxins causing, 223t

Plasma cells, in portal tracts, 84, 84t, *85–86*

Plasmodium falciparum infection (malaria), diagnostic features of, 30t
hemozoin in, 79
histologic and clinical/laboratory features of, 177t

Pneumocystis carinii infection, diagnostic features of, 30t
histologic and clinical/laboratory features of, 187t

Polyarteritis nodosa, histologic and clinical/laboratory features of, 187t
vasculitis in, *110*

Polyclonal disease, 125t

Polymyalgia rheumatica, histologic and clinical/laboratory features of, 187t

Porphyria cutanea tarda, diagnostic features of, 30t
histologic and clinical/laboratory features of, 188t

Portal fibrosis, bile duct paucity and, 19
drugs/toxins causing, 220t
in extrahepatic biliary obstruction, 149t
in primary sclerosing cholangitis, 189t
in schistosomiasis, 196t
noncirrhotic, 168t
progressing to cirrhosis, 88, 89t, *89–93*
with paucity of interlobular bile ducts and no cirrhosis, *94*
without progression to cirrhosis, 93, *93–94*
diseases causing, 89t

Portal hypertension, idiopathic, *94*
histologic and clinical/laboratory features of, 168t

Portal macrophages, inclusions in, 53, *54,* 54t
drugs/toxins causing, 222t

Portal tracts, assessment of, 2
cyst near, *28*
eosinophils in, 86, 86t, *87–88*
granulomas in, 43
in Hodgkin's lymphoma, 175t
in primary sclerosing cholangitis, 189t

Portal tracts *(Continued)*
lymphocytes in, 80, 80t, *81–82*
neutrophils in, without bile duct orientation, 83, 83t, *83–84*
plasma cells in, 84, 84t, *85–86*

Portal veins, assessment of, 2
inflammation of, 4
thrombophlebitis of, 190t

Preeclampsia, 200t

Pregnancy, acute fatty liver of, histology and clinical/laboratory findings in, 117t
recurrent intrahepatic cholestasis of, histologic and clinical/laboratory features of, 192t
spontaneous [liver] rupture in, histologic and clinical/laboratory features of, 197t
toxemia of, extracellular (non-collagen) deposits in, *37*
histologic and clinical/laboratory features of, 200t

Progressive familial intrahepatic cholestasis, 25, *27*
bile duct paucity and, 20t, *21*
cirrhosis with, *92*
histologic and clinical/laboratory features of, 190t

Protoporphyria, erythropoietic, diagnostic features of, 30t
histology and clinical/laboratory findings in, *78,* 147t

Pseudomonas pseudomallei, infection with, histologic and clinical/laboratory features of, 178t

Pseudotumor, inflammatory, benign, *71*
histologic and clinical/laboratory features of, 170t

Pylephlebitis, characteristics of, 8
histologic and clinical/laboratory features of, 190t
portal veins in, 2

Pyogenic abscess, histologic and clinical/laboratory features of, 191t
in bacterial sepsis, 133t

Pyogenic cholangiohepatitis, recurrent. See *Cholangitis, recurrent pyogenic.*

Q fever, fatty change with, *42*
granulomas in, *46*
histologic and clinical/laboratory features of, 191t

Radiopaque pigments, drugs/toxins causing, 223t

Recurrent cholestasis with lymphedema, histologic and clinical/laboratory features of, 192t

Recurrent intrahepatic cholestasis of pregnancy, histologic and clinical/laboratory features of, 192t

Recurrent pyogenic cholangiohepatitis. See *Cholangiohepatitis, recurrent pyogenic.*

Red blood cells, extravasation of, adjacent to space-occupying lesions, 119t
in sinusoids, 4, 102, 102t, *102–103*
in veno-occlusive disease, 203t
trabecular lesions of, 102, 102t, *102–103*

Relapsing fever, histology and clinical/laboratory findings in, 134t

Reye's syndrome, histologic and clinical/laboratory features of, 193t

Rheumatoid arthritis, histologic and clinical/laboratory features of, 193t

Rickettsia conorii, infection with, histology and clinical/laboratory findings in, 135t

Ring granulomas, 191t

Rochalimaea infection, histology and clinical/laboratory findings in, 132t

Rubeanic acid stain, 73
bile duct paucity and, 19
copper on, in Wilson's disease, 77

Rubella virus infection, histologic and clinical/laboratory features of, 193t

Rubeola virus infection, histologic and clinical/laboratory features of, 194t

Salmonella typhi, infection with, histologic and clinical/laboratory features of, 194t

Salmonellosis, granulomas in, *47*
  histologic and clinical/laboratory features of, 194t
  necroinflammatory change with, *58*
  vasculitis in, *109*
Sandhoff's disease, histologic and clinical/laboratory findings in, 153t
Sanfilippo syndrome, histologic and clinical/laboratory features of, 180t
Sarcoidosis, granulomas in, *47*
  histologic and clinical/laboratory features of, 195t
  lymphocytic inflammation of bile ducts and, 13t
Satellitosis, 66, *66–67*
  in acute sclerosing hyaline necrosis, *94,* 117t
  in nonalcoholic steatohepatitis, 183t
Schaumann bodies, in sarcoidosis, 195t
Schistosomiasis, calcification and, 22t, *24*
  diagnostic features of, 30t
  granulomas in, *47*
  histologic and clinical/laboratory features of, *34,* 196t
Sclerosing cholangitis, primary, 4
  bile duct paucity and, 19, 20t, *21*
  cirrhosis with, *92*
  copper-binding protein in, *76*
  histologic and clinical/laboratory features of, 189t
  Mallory bodies and, *68*
  periductal fibrosis of bile ducts and, 18, 18t, *19*
Sclerosing hyaline necrosis, acute, 2, 5. See also *Hepatitis, alcoholic.*
  histology and clinical/laboratory findings in, 117t
  increased sinusoidal circulating neutrophils in, *104*
  lobular necrosis with inflammation in, *55*
  Mallory bodies and, 66, *66*
  portal neutrophils with, *83*
  sinusoidal collagen deposits in, *94*
  chronic, histologic and clinical/laboratory features of, 190t
Sepsis, bacterial. See *Bacterial sepsis.*
Shock, histologic and clinical/laboratory findings in, 155t
Sialidosis, histologic and clinical/laboratory features of, 180t
Sickle cell anemia, histologic and clinical/laboratory features of, 196t
  sinusoidal dilatation and congestion and, *99*
Sinusoids, assessment of, 4
  circulating cells in, 103, 103t, *104*
  collagen deposits in. See *Collagen deposits, sinusoidal.*
  dilatation and congestion of, 98, 98t, *98–99,* 136t
    adjacent to space-occupying lesions, 119t
    drugs/toxins causing, 221t
    in right-sided heart failure, 156t
  extramedullary hematopoiesis in, 105, 105t, *105–106*
  fibrosis of, *94, 94,* 95t, *95–97*
  hemorrhage of, 98, 98t, *99*
    drugs/toxins causing, 221t
  peliotic lesions of, 100, 100t, *100–101*
  red blood cell extravasation in, 102, 102t, *102–103*
Sly syndrome, histologic and clinical/laboratory features of, 180t
South American blastomycosis, histologic and clinical/laboratory features of, 184t
Space of Disse, red blood cell extravasation into, 102, 111, 136t
Space-occupying lesion(s), liver adjacent to, histology and clinical/laboratory findings in, 119t
  sinusoidal dilatation and congestion and, *98*
Sphingomyelin-cholesterol lipidosis, histologic and clinical/laboratory features of, 182t
Spontaneous [liver] rupture in pregnancy, histologic and clinical/laboratory features of, 197t
Stain(s), hematoxylin-eosin, extracellular (non-collagen) deposits on, 36, 36t, *36–37*
  immunocytochemical, for malignant mass lesions, 71
  immunoperoxidase, for HBsAg, in fibrosing cholestatic hepatitis of allograft, 124t
    for hepatoblastoma, 159t
    in alpha₁-antitrypsin deficiency, *29*
    in vasculitis, 108
  special, for copper visualization, 73
    for hepatocyte inclusions, 48

Stain(s) *(Continued)*
  granulomas and, 43
  in alpha₁-antitrypsin deficiency, *29*
  liver diseases diagnosed by, 29, *29,* 30t, *31–35*
  trichrome. See *Trichrome stain.*
Steatohepatitis, nonalcoholic, 2
  cirrhosis with, *92*
  fatty change with, *41*
  granulomas in, *46*
  histologic and clinical/laboratory features of, 183t
  inclusions on, *48*
  Mallory bodies and, *68*
  necroinflammatory change with, *58*
  sinusoidal collagen deposits in, *97*
Steatosis, 37. See also *Fatty change.*
Stigmata, of chronic liver disease, in acute sclerosing hyaline necrosis, 117t
Strongyloides stercoralis, infection with, histologic and clinical/laboratory features of, 198t
Strongyloidiasis, histologic and clinical/laboratory features of, 198t
Sulfatide lipidosis, histologic and clinical/laboratory features of, 179t
Sulfonamides, granulomas with, *45*
Sweat test, 143t
Syncytial giant cells, 106, 106t, *107–108*
  vs. multinucleated giant cells, 106
Syphilis, diagnostic features of, 30t
  histologic and clinical/laboratory features of, 199t
  vasculitis in, *110*
Systemic carnitine deficiency, histologic and clinical/laboratory features of, 199t
Systemic lupus erythematosus, histologic and clinical/laboratory features of, 200t

Tangier's disease, histologic and clinical/laboratory features of, 200t
Tay-Sachs disease, histologic and clinical/laboratory findings in, 153t
Tetracycline, fatty change with, *40*
Thorium dioxide pigment, in angiosarcoma, 77
Thrombosis, of hepatic arteries, allograft ischemia and, 125t
  of hepatic veins, in Budd-Chiari syndrome, 136t
  of nonsinusoidal vessels, 111, 111t, *111–113*
Tombstone lesions, in hepatitis A, 204t
Total parenteral nutrition, 166t
Toxemia of pregnancy, extracellular (non-collagen) deposits on, *37*
  histologic and clinical/laboratory features of, 200t
Toxic shock syndrome, histologic and clinical/laboratory features of, 201t
Toxocara canis infection, histologic and clinical/laboratory features of, 212t
Toxocariasis, histologic and clinical/laboratory features of, 212t
Toxoplasma gondii infection, histologic and clinical/laboratory features of, 201t
Toxoplasmosis, histologic and clinical/laboratory features of, 201t
Treponema pallidum infection (syphilis), diagnostic features of, 30t
  histologic and clinical/laboratory features of, 199t
  vasculitis in, *110*
Trichrome stain, alcoholic cirrhosis on, *89*
  cystic fibrosis on, *90*
  in amyloidosis, *31*
  in portal fibrosis leading to cirrhosis, *90–92*
  sinusoidal collagen deposits on, *95–97*
Tropical splenomegaly syndrome, 177t
Tuberculosis, granulomas in, *47*
  histologic and clinical/laboratory features of, 201t
Typhoid fever, histologic and clinical/laboratory features in, 194t
Typhoid nodule, 194t
Tyrosinemia, histologic and clinical/laboratory features in, 202t

Ulcerative colitis, 141t
  fatty change in, *40*
  histologic and clinical/laboratory features of, 202t
Uroporphyrinogen decarboxylase, defect of, 188t

Vanishing bile duct syndrome, 123t
Vascular channels, benign mass lesions of, conditions causing, 69t
   malignant mass lesions of, 71t
Vascular compromise, lobular necrosis with minimal to absent in-
      flammation, 61
   sinusoidal hemorrhage and, 98
Vasculitis, drugs/toxins causing, 221t
   lobular necrosis with minimal to absent inflammation with, 61
   nonsinusoidal, 108, 108t, *109–110*
Veins, endothelial inflammation of, in acute cellular allograft rejec-
      tion, 122t
   hepatic, occlusion of, in Budd-Chiari syndrome, 136t
      in veno-occlusive disease, 203t
   in vascular allograft rejection, 126t
   portal, assessment of, 2
      inflammation of, 4
      thrombophlebitis of, 190t
   thrombosis and occlusion of, hepatic injury with, 111, 111t, *111–
      113*
   vasculitis of, 108, 108t, *109–110*
Veno-occlusive disease, drugs/toxins causing, 221t
   histologic and clinical/laboratory features of, 203t
Venous outflow obstruction, adjacent to space-occupying lesions,
      119t
   chronic, 111
   drugs/toxins causing, 221t
   red blood cell extravasation and, 102, *102*
Venules, hepatic, veno-occlusive change of, 111, 111t
Vessels, nonsinusoidal, inflammation of, 108, 108t, *109–110*
   thrombosis and occlusion of, 111, 111t, *111–113*
   outflow, inflammation of, 4
Viral hepatitis, acute, classic, histologic and clinical/laboratory fea-
      tures of, 204t
      necroinflammatory change with, *59*
   hepatic cord structure in, 3
   type A, histologic and clinical/laboratory features of, 205t
      lobular confluent necrosis with, *65*
      plasma cells in, *86*
   type B, histologic and clinical/laboratory features of, 205t
      lobular confluent necrosis with, *65*
      necroinflammatory change with, *60*
   type B + delta, histologic and clinical/laboratory features of,
      206t
   type C, necroinflammatory change with, *60*
   type E, histologic and clinical/laboratory features of, 207t
   type G, histologic and clinical/laboratory features of, 207t
   type non A-G, histologic and clinical/laboratory features of, 207t
   with bridging necrosis, histologic and clinical/laboratory features
      of, 208t
   with impaired regeneration, histologic and clinical/laboratory
      features of, 208t
   with panacinar necrosis, bile duct proliferation and ectasia
      and, *17*
      histologic and clinical/laboratory features of, *65*, 208t

Viral hepatitis *(Continued)*
   chronic, classic, histologic and clinical/laboratory features of, 209t
      inclusions in, *51, 54*
      type B, histologic and clinical/laboratory features of, 210t
         histologic features of, *35*
         inclusions in, *51, 52*
         necroinflammatory change with, *60*
         periportal inflammation with piecemeal necrosis and, *82*
         plasma cells in, *86*
         regenerative nodules of cirrhosis in, *93*
      type B + delta, histologic and clinical/laboratory features of,
         210t
         necroinflammatory change with, *60*
      type C, fatty change with, *42*
         histologic and clinical/laboratory features of, 211t
         lymphocytic inflammation of bile ducts and, *15*
         portal lymphocytic infiltrates with, *80*
         sinusoidal collagen deposits in, *97*
      type G, histologic and clinical/laboratory features of, 211t
      type non A-G, histologic and clinical/laboratory features of, 212t
         multinucleated giant cells in, *108*
   diagnostic features of, 30t
Viruses, hepatotropic, viral hepatitis and, 3
Visceral larva migrans, histologic and clinical/laboratory features of,
      212t
   portal eosinophils with, *88*
Von Meyenberg complex, histology and clinical/laboratory findings
      in, 134t

Waldenström's macroglobulinemia, histologic and clinical/laboratory
      features of, 212t
Weber-Christian disease, histologic and clinical/laboratory features
      of, 212t
Weil's disease, histologic and clinical/laboratory features of, 173t
Whipple's disease, histologic and clinical/laboratory features of, 213t
Wilson's disease, copper in, 77
   fatty change with, *42*
   histologic and clinical/laboratory features of, 213t
   inclusions in, *50*
   Mallory bodies and, *68*
   regenerative nodules of cirrhosis in, *93*
   sinusoidal collagen deposits in, *97*
Wolman's disease, 139t
   histologic and clinical/laboratory features of, 214t

Yellow fever, histologic and clinical/laboratory features of, 214t

Zygomycosis, histologic and clinical/laboratory features of, 215t

ISBN 0-7216-7692-8